Light on the Yoga Sūtras of Patañjali

By the same author:

The Art of Yoga
The Concise Light on Yoga
Light on Prāṇāyāma
Light on Yoga
The Tree of Yoga

B.K.S. IYENGAR

Light on the Yoga Sūtras of Patañjali

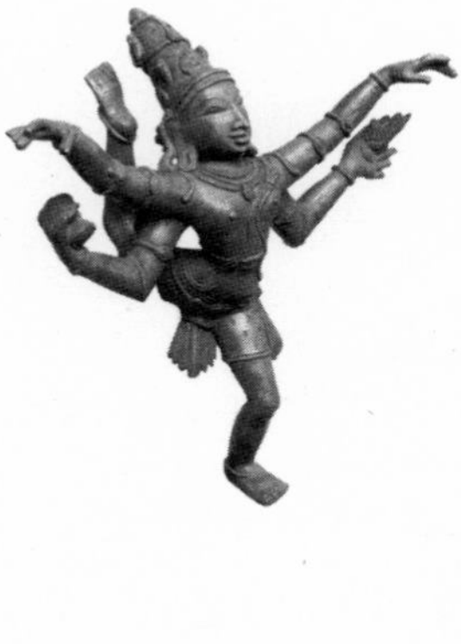

Thorsons

This work is my offering to
my Invisible, First and Foremost Guru
Lord Patañjali

Thorsons
An imprint of HarperCollins*Publishers*
1 London Bridge Street
London SE1 9GF

www.harpercollins.co.uk

First published in Great Britain by
George Allen & Unwin, 1966
Published by The Aquarian Press 1993
Published by Thorsons 1996
This edition published by Thorsons 2002

22

A catalogue record of this book is
available from the British Library

ISBN 978-0-00-714516-4

Printed and bound in Great Britain by
Clays Ltd, St Ives plc

Contents

A note from Sir Yehudi Menuhin vii
Foreword by Godfrey Devereux viii
Hints on Transliteration and Pronunciation ix
List of important terms in the text xi
Introduction to the New Edition by B.K.S. Iyengar xiii
On Yoga xvii
Acknowledgements xix

Patañjali 1
The Yoga Sūtras 3
Themes in the Four Pādas 11

Samādhi Pāda 11
Sādhana Pāda 22
Vibhūti Pāda 34
Kaivalya Pāda 39

Yoga Sūtras

Text, translation and commentary

Part I Samādhi Pāda 45
Part II Sādhana Pāda 105
Part III Vibhūti Pāda 173
Part IV Kaivalya Pāda 239

Epilogue 289
Appendices

Appendix I A thematic Key to the Yoga Sūtras 293
Appendix II Interconnection of Sūtras 298
Appendix III Alphabetical Index of Sūtras 302
Appendix IV Yoga in a Nutshell 309

List of Tables and Diagrams 318
Glossary 319
Index 351

Invocatory Prayers

yogena cittasya padena vācāṁ
malaṁ śarīrasya ca vaidyakena
yopākarottaṁ pravaraṁ munīnāṁ
patañjaliṁ prāñjalirānato'smi
ābāhu puruṣākāraṁ
śaṅkha cakrāsi dhāriṇam
sahasra śirasaṁ śvetaṁ
praṇamāmi patañjalim

Let us bow before the noblest of sages, Patañjali, who gave yoga for serenity and sanctity of mind, grammar for clarity and purity of speech, and medicine for perfection of health.

Let us prostrate before Patañjali, an incarnation of Ādiśeṣa, whose upper body has a human form, whose arms hold a conch and a disc, and who is crowned by a thousand-headed cobra.

Where there is yoga, there is prosperity and bliss with freedom.

yastyaktvā rūpamādyaṁ prabhavati jagato'nekadhānugrahāya
prakṣīṇakleśarāśirviṣamaviṣadharo'nekavaktraḥ subhogī
sarvajñānaprasūtirbhujagaparikaraḥ prītaye yasya nityaṁ
devohīṣaḥ sa vovyātsitavimalatanuryogado yogayuktaḥ

Let us prostrate before Lord Ādiśeṣa, who manifested himself on earth as Patañjali to grace the human race with health and harmony.

Let us salute Lord Ādiśeṣa of the myriad serpent heads and mouths carrying noxious poisons, discarding which he came to earth as single-headed Patañjali in order to eradicate ignorance and vanquish sorrow.

Let us pay our obeisance to Him, repository of all knowledge, amidst His attendant retinue.

Let us pray to the Lord whose primordial form shines with pure and white effulgence, pristine in body, a master of yoga who bestows on us his yogic light to enable mankind to rest in the house of the immortal soul.

A note from Sir Yehudi Menuhin

It is a remarkable accomplishment and a tribute to the continuity of human endeavour that today, some 2500 years after yoga was first described by the renowned Patañjali, his living heritage is being commented upon and introduced to the modern world by one of yoga's best exponents today, my own teacher B.K.S. Iyengar.

There are not many practical arts, sciences, and visions of human perfection of body, mind and soul which have been in practice over so long a period without attachment to a particular religious creed or catechism. *Anyone* can practise yoga, and this important contribution to the history of yoga and its validity today is for everyone.

YEHUDI MENUHIN

Foreword by Godfrey Devereux, author of *Dynamic Yoga*

Patañjali's *Yoga Sūtras* are the bible of yoga. However, their inaccessibility in the hands of scholars and academics has left yoga practitioners adrift with neither chart nor compass. B.K.S. Iyengar's translation, based on over fifty years of dedicated and accomplished practice and teaching, is unique in its relevance and utility to contemporary yoga practitioners. The depth of his practice and understanding shines through his elucidation of the often terse and obscure sūtras. Iyengar's ability to elucidate Patañjali in pragmatic terms is an extension of his clarification of the subtlety and integrity of yoga practice. This is most evident in the rigorous precision with which he understands and articulates the body in yoga postures. However, it goes further and much deeper than that. In his unique investigation of alignment, Iyengar not only reveals the therapeutic necessity of stuctural integrity in the body, but also its subtle and equally necessary impact on the flow of energy and consciousness in the mind.

What Iyengar has proved, for those willing to apply themselves to test it, is that the apparent divide between matter and spirit, body and soul, and physical and spiritual is only that: apparent. Through his insistence on structural integrity he has opened the spiritual doorway to millions of people for whom the mind would otherwise never give up its subtleties. Here, in his presentation of Patañjali, that door is flung wide open. This is especially clear, to even the least academically minded student, in his profound and practical interpretations of the sūtras relating to *āsana* and *prāṇāyāma*. Here, especially, Iyengar's genius comes as a great gift of clarity and insight that can only deepen the understanding and support the practice of any keen student.

Iyengar's incomparable experience as an Indian teacher of Westerners, combined with his experience as a Brahmin and participant in a genuine lineage of the yoga tradition, gives his perspective an authority and authenticity that is all too often lacking. It offers a lucid and pragmatic interpretation of the insights and subtleties of yoga's root guru. To practice yoga without the profound and panoramic inner cartography of the *Yoga Sūtras* is to be adrift in a difficult and potentially dangerous ocean. To use that map without the compass of Iyengar's deep and authoritative experience, is to handicap oneself unnecessarily. No yoga practitioner should be without this classic and invaluable work.

Hints on Transliteration* and Pronunciation

Sanskrit is an Indo-European language. It is ancient; the language of the Indian scriptures which claim to be eternal. They were recited or chanted in Sanskrit thousands of years ago, and still are today.

The word Sanskrit itself means 'perfect', 'perfected', 'literary', 'polished'. It is a highly organized language, with a complex grammar. However, some works are written in a simpler form which it is not so difficult for us to grasp. To these types of work belong the *Bhagavad Gītā*, the *Upaniṣads*, and also the *Yoga Sūtras of Patañjali*.

Sanskrit letters, both vowels and consonants, are arranged consecutively according to their organ of pronunciation, starting with throat (guttural), then palate (palatal), then a group of sounds called cerebral (modern 'retroflex', which may not originally belong to the Indo-European group), then dental and labial. After that come semi-vowels, sibilants, and a full aspirate. Philologists have given these sounds various names, but we are giving the approximate equivalent of their Sanskrit meanings.

These placings apply to vowels and to consonants.

The following is a list of vowels, which includes diphthongs, a nasal (half 'n' sound) and an aspirate ('h' sound). The vowels are short and long, the diphthongs long. The aspirate sound repeats its preceding vowel, (e.g. a: = aha, i: = ihi, etc.):

PRONUNCIATION		PRONUNCIATION	
a	as in **cut**	ā	as in **car**
i	as in **sit**	î	as in **seat**
u	as in **full**	ū	as in **pool**
ri/ru	as in **rich/rook**	rî/rū	as in **reach/root**
e	as in **air**, or French '**été**'	ai	as in **aisle**
o	as in **all**	au	as in **owl**
aṁ	as in **umbrella**, or French '**en**'	aḥ	as in **ahoy**, **aha**

The following are the consonants and semi-vowels. The first five groups consist of 1) a leading hard consonant, 2) its aspirated form, 3) a corresponding soft consonant, 4) its aspirated form, and 5) its nasal consonant.

* The transliteration marks used are internationally accepted.

GROUP	CONSONANTS					PRONUNCIATION	
I Guttural	k	kh	g	gh	ṅg	cake	bank-holiday
						gale	doghouse
						ink/anger	
II Palatal	ch	chh	j	jh	ñ	chain	church-hall
						join	hedgehog
						inch/angel	
III Cerebral/ retroflex	ṭ	ṭh	ḍ	ḍh	ṇ	talk	at home
						dawn	hardheaded
						under/unreal	
IV Dental	t	th	d	dh	n	take	fainthearted
						date	kindhearted
						ant/and	
V Labial	p	ph	b	bh	m	pain	uphill
						bill	abhor
						ample/amble	
VI Semi- vowels	y	r	l	v		year	rely
						love	vibration/way
VII Sibilants and	ś	ṣ	s			sheep	(palatal)
						shy (cerebral) salve	
aspirate	h					high	

The following should be noted:

1) The 'h' sound of the aspirated consonants should always be pronounced.
2) To pronounce the sounds in the 'cerebral' group, the tongue is curled back (retroflexed) and the roof of the palate is then hit with the back of the tip of the tongue.
3) The dental group is similar to English, only the tongue touches the back of the teeth in pronouncing them.
4) There are some local variants in pronunciation.
5) An oblique stroke under a consonant shows that it is pronounced without its intrinsic vowel.

The letters are put together to form a syllabary, and also to form 'conjunct' consonants in various combinations.

List of important terms in the text

Throughout the *Yoga Sūtras*, certain particularly important terms and concepts are repeatedly referred to and discussed. The reader who is not familiar with yoga philosophy or with Sanskrit may find the following short list of these vital terms helpful. A full list of Sanskrit words with their English equivalents is given in the Glossary.

yoga	Union of body, mind and soul, and with God
aṣṭāṅga yoga	Eight aspects of yoga described by Patañjali as follows:
yama	Restraints on behaviour
niyama	Spiritual observances
āsana	Seat, posture, practice of postures
prāṇāyāma	Expansion of vital energy through control of breath
pratyāhāra	Withdrawal of the senses
dhāraṇā	Concentration
dhyāna	Meditation
samādhi	Complete absorption
samyama	Integration (of *dhāraṇā, dhyāna* and *samādhi*)
citta	Consciousness, composed of three aspects, as follows:
manas	Mind
buddhi	Intelligence
ahaṁkāra	Ego
asmitā	Sense of self
vṛttis	Thought-waves
nirodha	Control, restraint, cessation
abhyāsa	Practice
vairāgya	Renunciation, detachment
sādhana	Practice; discipline in pursuit of a goal
sādhaka	Practitioner, aspirant
dharma	Science of duty, observance of duties
kośa	Sheath, layer
kleśa	Affliction
avidyā	Ignorance, lack of spiritual knowledge, the root cause of all afflictions
duḥkha	Sorrow, grief
karma	Action and its results; universal law of cause and effect

jñāna	Knowledge, wisdom
bhakti	Devotion
saṁskāra	Subliminal impressions
prāṇa	Life force, vital energy, breath
pāda	Part, quarter, chapter
puruṣa	The soul, the seer
prakṛti	Nature
mahat	The great principle of nature, cosmic intelligence
guṇas	The qualities of nature:
sattva	luminosity
rajas	vibrancy
tamas	dormancy, inertia
kaivalya	Liberation, emancipation
Īśvara	God
ātman	The individual spirit, seer, soul
Brahman	The Universal Spirit, Soul

Introduction to the New Edition by B.K.S. Iyengar

I express my sense of gratitude to Thorsons, who are bringing out my *Light on the Yoga Sūtras of Patañjali* in this new attractive design, as a feast not only for the physical eyes but also for the intellectual and spiritual eye.

As a mortal soul, it is a bit of an embarrassment for me with my limited intelligence to write on the immortal work of Patañjali on the subject of yoga.

If God is considered the seed of all knowledge *(sarvajña bijan)*, Patañjali is all knower, all wise *(sarvajñan)*, of all knowledge. The third part of his *Yoga Sūtras* (the *vibūti pāda)* makes it clear to us that we should respect him as a knower of all knowledge and a versatile personality.

It is impossible, even for sophisticated minds, to comprehend fully what knowledge he had. We find him speaking on an enormous range of subjects – art, dance, mathematics, astronomy, astrology, physics, chemistry, psychology, biology, neurology, telepathy, education, time and gravitational theory – with a divine spiritual knowledge.

He was a perfect master of cosmic energy; he knew the *prāṇic* energy centres in the body; his intelligence *(buddhi)* was as clean and clear as crystal and his words express him as a pure perfect being.

Patañjali's sūtras make use of his great versatility of language and mind. He clothes the righteous and virtuous aspects of religious matters with a secular fabric and in so doing is able to skilfully present the wisdom of both the material and the spiritual world, blending them as a universal culture.

Patañjali fills each sūtra with his experiential intelligence, stretching it like a thread *(sūtra)*, and weaving it into a garland of pearls of wisdom to flavour and savour by those who love and live in yoga, as wise-men in their lives.

Each *sūtra* conveys the practice as well as the philosophy behind the practice, as a practical philosophy for aspirants and seekers (*sādhakas*) to follow in life.

What is sādhanā?

Sādhanā is a methodical, sequential means to accomplish the *sādhaka*'s aims in life. The *sādhaka*'s aims are right duty (*dharma*), a rightful purpose and means (*artha*), right inclinations (*kāma*) and ultimate release or emancipation (*mokṣa*).

If *dharma* is the atonement of duty *(dharma śāstra)*, *artha* is the means to purification of action (*karma śāstra)*. Our inclinations (*kāma*) are made good through study of sacred texts and growth towards wisdom (*svādhyāya* and *jñāna śāstra*), and emancipation (*mokṣa*) is reached through devotion (*bhakti śāstra*) and meditation (*dhyāna śāstra*).

It is *dharma* that uplifts man who has fallen physically, mentally, morally, intellectually and spiritually, or who is about to fall. Therefore, *dharma* is that which upholds, sustains and supports man.

These aims are all stages on the road to perfect knowledge (*vedānta*). The term *vedānta* comes from *Veda,* meaning knowledge, and *anta* meaning the end of knowledge. The true end of knowledge is emancipation and liberation from all imperfections. Hence the journey, or *vedānta*, is an act of pursuit of the vision of wisdom to transform one's conduct and actions in order to experience the ultimate reality of life.

Due to lack of knowledge or misunderstanding, fear, love of the self, attachment and aversion with respect to the material world, one's actions and conduct become disturbed. This disturbance shows as lust *(kāma)*, wrath *(krodha)*, greed *(lobha)*, infatuation *(moha)*, intoxication *(mada)* and malice *(mātsarya)*. All of these emotional turbulences affect the psyche by veiling the intelligence.

The yoga *sādhanā* of Patañjali comes to us as a penance in order to minimise or eradicate these disturbed and destructive emotive thoughts and the actions that accrue from them.

The yoga *sādhanā* of Patañjali

The *Sādhanā* is a rhythmic, three-tiered practice (*sādhanā-traya*), covering the eight aspects or petals of yoga in a capsule as *kriyā yoga*, the yoga of action, whereby all actions are surrendered to the Divinity (see Sutra II.1 in the *sādhanā pāda*). These three tiers (*sādhanā-traya*) represent the body *(kāyā)*, the mind *(manasā)* and the speech *(vāk)*.

Hence:

- At the level of the body, *tapas*, or the drive towards purity, develops the student through practice on the path of right action *(karma mārga)*.
- At the level of the mind, through careful study of the self and the mind in it's consciousness, the student develops self-knowledge, *svādhyāya*, leading to the path of wisdom *(jñānamārga)*.
- Later, profound meditation using the voice to pronounce the universal aum (see Sūtras I.27 and 28) directs the self to abandon ego *(ahamkāra)*, and to feel virtuousness *(śīlatā)*, and so it becomes the path of devotion *(bhakti mārga)*.

Tapas is a burning desire for ascetic, devoted *sādhanā*, through *yama*, *niyama*, *āsana* and *prāṇāyāma*. This cleanses the body and senses *(karmendriya* and *jñānendriya)*, and frees one from afflictions *(kleśa nivṛtti)*.

Svādhyāya means the study of the *Vedas*, spiritual scriptures that define the real and the unreal, or the study of one's own self (from the body to the self). This study of spiritual science *(ātmā śāstra)* ignites and inspires the student for self-progression. Thus *svādhyāya* is for restraining the fluctuations *(mano vṛtti nirodha)* and in its wake comes tranquillity *(samādhāna citta)* in the consciousness. Here the petals of yoga are *pratyāhāra* and *dhāraṇā*, besides the former aspects of *tapas*.

Īśvara praṇidhāna is the surrender of oneself to God, and is the finest aspect of yoga *sādhanā*. Patañjali explains God as a Supreme Soul, who is eternally free from afflictions, unaffected by actions and their reactions or by their residue. He advises one to think of God through repeating His name *(japa)*, with profound thoughtfulness *(arthabhāvana)*, so that the seeker's speech can become sanctified and thus the seed of imperfection *(doṣa bija)* or defect be eradicated *(doṣa nivṛtti)* once and for all.

From here on, his *sādhanā* continues uninterruptedly with devotion *(anuṣṭhana)*. This practice, (*sādhanā-ana*) will go on generating knowledge until he touches the towering wisdom (see Sūtra II.28 in the *sādhanā pāda*).

Through the capsule of *kriyā* yoga, Patañjali explains the cosmogony of nature and how to ultimately co-ordinate nature, in body, mind and speech. Through discipline *tapas*, study – *svādhyāya*, and devotion – *Īśvara praṇidhāna*, the student can become free from nature's erratic play, remaining in the abode of the Self.

In Sūtra II.19 in the *sādhanā pāda*, Patañjali identifies the distinguishable, or physically manifest *(viśeṣa)* marks and the non-distinguishable, or subtle, *(aviśeṣa)* elements which comprise existence and which are transformed to take the individual to the noumenal *(liṅga)* state. Then through *aṣṭāṅga yoga*, coupled with *sādhanā-traya*, all nature, or *prakṛti (aliṅga)* becomes one, merged.

He defines the distinguishable marks of nature as the five elements: earth, water, fire, air and ether; *(pañca-bhuta)*; the five organs of action *(karmendriya)*; the five senses of perception *(jñānendriya)*, and the mind *(manas)*. The non-distinguishable marks are defined as the *tanmātra* (sound, touch, shape, taste and smell) and pride *(ahamkāra)*. These twenty-two principles have to merge in *mahat (liṅga)*, and then dissolve in nature *(prakṛti)*. The first sixteen distinguishable marks are brought under control by *tapas* – practice and discipline, the six undistinguishable ones by *svādhyāya* – study and *abhyāsa* – repetition. Nature, *prakṛti,* and *mahat*, the Universal Consciousness, become one through and in *Īśvara praṇidhāna*.

At this point all oscillations of the *guṇas* that shape existence terminate and *prakṛtijāya,* a mastery over nature, takes place. From this quiet silence of *prakṛti*, Self *(puruṣa)* shines forth like the never fading sun.

In the *Haṭhayoga Pradipika* Svātmārāmā explains something very similar. He says that the body, being inert, *tāmasic*, is uplifted to the level of the active, *rājasic*, mind through *āsana* and *prāṇāyāma* with *yama* and *niyama.* When the body is made as vibrant as the mind, through study, *svādhyāya* and through practice and repetitions, *abhyāsa*, both mind and body are lifted towards the noumenal state of *sattva guṇa.* From *sattva guṇa* the *sādhaka* follows *Īśvara praṇidhāna* to become a *guṇatītan* (free from *guṇas*).

Patañjali also addresses Svātmārāmā's explanation of the different capabilities and therefore expectations for weak (*mṛdu*), average (*madhyāma*) and outstanding (*adhimātra*) students (see I.22). He guides the most basic beginner *(*the *tāmasic sādhaka)* to follow *yama*, *niyama*, *āsana*, and *prāṇāyāma* as *tapas*, to become *madhyādhikārins* (vibrant and *rājasic)*, and to intensify this practice into *pratyāhāra* (withdrawal of the senses) and *dhāraṇā* (intense focus and concentration) as their path of study, *svādhyāya*, and then to proceed towards *sattva guṇa* through *dhyāna* (devotion), and to *guṇatītan* (the state uninfluenced by the guṇas) into *samādhi*, the most profound state of meditiation – through *Īśvara praṇidhāna.*

By this graded practice, according to the level of the *sādhaka*, all *sādhakas* have to touch the *puruṣa (hrdayasparṣi)*, sooner or later through *tīvra samvega sādhanā* (I.21).

Hence, *kriyā yoga sādhanā-traya* envelopes all the aspects of *aṣṭāṅga yoga*, each complimenting *(pūraka)* and supplementing *(poṣaka)* the others. When *sādhanā* becomes subtle and fine, then *tapas*, *svādhyāya* and *Īśvara praṇidhāna*, work in unison with the eight-petals of *aṣṭāṅga yoga*, and the *sādhaka's* mind *(manas)*, intelligence *(buddhi)* and 'I' ness or 'mineness' *(ahamkāra)* are sublimated. Only then does he become a yogi. In him friendliness, compassion, gladness and oneness *(samānata)* flows benevolently in body, consciousness and speech to live in beatitude *(divya ānanda).*

This is the way of the practice *(sādhanā)*, as explained by Patañjali that lifts even a raw *sādhaka* to reach ripeness in his *sādhanā* and experience emancipation.

I am indebted to Thorsons for this special edition of *Light on the Yoga Sūtras of Patañjali*, enabling readers to take a dip in *sādhanā* and savour the nectar of immortality.

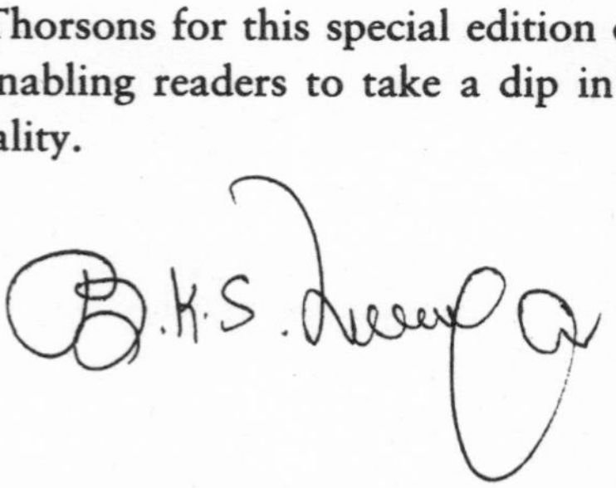

B.K.S. IYENGAR
14 December 2001

On Yoga

Yoga is an art, a science and a philosophy. It touches the life of man at every level, physical, mental, and spiritual. It is a practical method for making one's life purposeful, useful and noble.

As honey is sweet from any part of the honeycomb, so is yoga. It enables every part of the human system to become attuned to its essence, the conscious seer within. Yoga alone enables the practitioner to perceive and experience the world within and around himself, to touch the divine joy of all creation, and then to share that nectar of divine wealth and happiness with his fellow beings.

The *Yoga Sūtras* of Patañjali are concise and compact. No word is superfluous. They are compiled in such a way as to cover all the various facets of life, exploring each in depth. Patañjali shows the initiated as well as the uninitiated, the intelligent and the unintelligent, ways of adopting the principles of yoga and adapting its techniques, of plumbing each sūtra, so that one may grasp it with integrity, purity and divinity.

Yoga is a friend to those who embrace it sincerely and totally. It lifts its practitioners from the clutches of pain and sorrow, and enables them to live fully, taking a delight in life. The practice of yoga helps the lazy body to become active and vibrant. It transforms the mind, making it harmonious. Yoga helps to keep one's body and mind in tune with the essence, the soul, so that all three are blended into one.

For a number of years, my pupils and friends have been asking me to express the profound depths of each sūtra of Patañjali's yoga with a simple and lucid translation, together with my explanatory comments, to help people understand and follow the path of evolution. I have therefore, after some hesitation, undertaken this work for the benefit of my pupils and others interested in the subject.

In ancient times, knowledge in the form of traditional lore such as the Vedas and Upaniṣads was passed on orally. Now, most of this teaching is lost. We have to depend upon written sources in order to gain access to the past, to grasp this heritage which is concerned with the science of knowing and realizing the spiritual oasis which lies within us.

It is difficult to learn through books, but they are our only means of progress until we come across that rarity, a true teacher or master. Mindful of my limitations and my comparatively restricted ability to explore the fine nuances of each sūtra, I have nevertheless undertaken this task in an attempt to help my fellow practitioners, so that they may be aided by this practical guide in their search for their own inner identity.

There are a number of commentaries and works on Patañjali's *Yoga Sūtras*, but very few deal with the practical needs of genuine seekers. The translations are sometimes difficult to understand and the commentaries are heavy and obscure. All interpretations differ. Even intellectual giants like Vyāsa, Vācaspati Miśra and Vijñāna Bhikṣu, on whom all later commentators depend, are in disagreement with one another. Various differing translations are available, creating confusion in the mind of the seeker. Will my commentary suffer the same fate? I sincerely hope not, for in my heart of hearts I am satisfied that the task of helping my fellow travellers on the path of yoga, by providing a commentary such as this, is well worth undertaking, owing to the scarcity of practical guidance in this domain.

I am neither a learned pundit nor a scholarly academician. To help yoga practitioners with less knowledge than myself, I have introduced several dictionary definitions for each word contained in the sūtras. I have selected those which carry conviction for me, in the light of my own firm practice and experience.

Yoga is an ocean of lore, and this book is just a drop in that ocean. I ask forgiveness if I have erred or digressed from the subject. It is my duty to seek knowledge, and I shall be glad to receive constructive criticisms and suggestions, for incorporation in future editions.

May this manual act as fuel to the fire of practice, so that aspirants may gain some glimmer of light, until such time as they find teachers who can further enhance their knowledge and experience.

I hope that those who read this book in conjunction with my other works, *Light on Yoga*, *Light on Prāṇāyāma*, *The Art of Yoga* and *The Tree of Yoga* (HarperCollins*Publishers*), may derive even greater advantage by adapting the various interpretations of the meaning of the sūtras to the light of their own experience.

If this work helps those who practise yoga, I shall feel that I have contributed my humble share.

Acknowledgements

First of all, I should express my gratitude to my esteemed friend, the late Mr Gerald Yorke, reader for Allen & Unwin who originally published *Light on Yoga* and *Light on Prāṇāyāma*. He taught me a tremendous amount about the writing of books through his collaboration in these earlier works. In his admonitions about my style, Mr Yorke was as forceful as my guru, Sri T. Krishnamachārya, was about my yoga.

Though I was a teacher with thirty years of experience, I had never attempted to write even an article on yoga. Also, my English in those days was not good. The first writing I attempted was *Light on Yoga*, which was to become a standard textbook.

When he first saw my 600-odd photographs together with the text, he was impressed by the illustrations and their explanations. He acknowledged the quality and originality of the technical part, but thought the introductory section was too full of literary allusions and needed explanatory notes.

'You have to rewrite and bring the introduction up to the level of the practical side or else the book will never see publication,' he told me. 'No doubt with your direct techniques you are a first-class teacher, but as a writer, you have *everything* to learn.'

Gerald Yorke took immense trouble to give me guidelines for reworking the text so that rhythm and style should accord and bring homogeneity to the book. His encouragement was my touchstone, spurring me to express my thoughts in as exact and precise a form as possible. Since then I hold him to be my 'literary guru'.

When I was in England in the 1980s, I called on him with the manuscript of *The Art of Yoga*. He disclaimed any knowledge of art, and suggested instead that I write on the *Yoga Sūtras* of Patañjali, promising, as philosophy was his interest, to help me with it. Nevertheless, on our parting, he said, 'Leave the *Art of Yoga* with me and let me see.' Within a few days of my return home he sent the manuscript back, saying that he might not live to see it through. His premonition was sadly fulfilled, as I received the manuscript on the same day that he left the earth.

So this work is the fruit of his initiative combined with the subsequent insistence of my pupils. May it fulfil all these hopes.

My thanks are also due to Mrs Shirley D. French and to my daughter Geeta for going through the manuscript and for their valuable suggestions.

I am grateful to Sri C. V. Tendulkar for retyping the manuscript several times with much patience, and to my pupil Mr Patxi Lizardi of Spain, for elegantly typing the final copy with great devotion and style. My thanks are also due to Mrs Silva Mehta for reading the proofs.

Finally, I would like to thank my friends and pupils, Mrs Odette Plouvier and Mr John Evans for their help in completing this work. Mrs Plouvier generously made it possible for John to make lengthy stays in Pune, where he was able to correct my English and offer useful suggestions for the presentation of the work. Having him near me helped me to formulate my ideas and bring to life aspects of the sūtras which might otherwise have lain dormant. I am grateful to them for their help.

I express my gratitude to Julie Friedeberger for the care she took in editing the book, retaining my style and tone.

I am also indeed grateful to HarperCollins*Publishers* for publishing and presenting my work to a worldwide public.

In ending this preface, I pray Patañjali to bless the readers so that the illuminative rays of yoga may penetrate and reach them, and that poise and peace may flow in them as a perennial river flows into the sea of spiritual wisdom.

Patañjali

First I would like to tell you something about Patañjali, who he was and what was his lineage. Historically, Patañjali may have lived some time between 500 and 200 B.C., but much of what we know of the master of yoga is drawn from legends. He is referred to as a *svayaṁbhū*, an evolved soul incarnated of his own will to help humanity. He assumed human form, experienced our sorrows and joys, and learned to transcend them. In the *Yoga Sūtras* he described the ways of overcoming the afflictions of the body and the fluctuations of the mind: the obstacles to spiritual development.

Patañjali's words are direct, original and traditionally held to be of divine provenance. After more than twenty centuries they remain fresh, fascinating and all-absorbing, and will remain so for centuries to come.

Patañjali's 196 aphorisms or sūtras cover all aspects of life, beginning with a prescribed code of conduct and ending with man's vision of his true Self. Each word of the sūtras is concise and precise. As individual drops of rain contribute towards the formation of a lake, so each word contained in the sūtras conveys a wealth of thought and experience, and is indispensable to the whole.

Patañjali chose to write on three subjects, grammar, medicine and yoga. The *Yoga Sūtras*, his culminating work, is his distillation of human knowledge. Like pearls on a thread, the *Yoga Sūtras* form a precious necklace, a diadem of illuminative wisdom. To comprehend their message and put it into practice is to transform oneself into a highly cultured and civilized person, a rare and worthy human being.

Though I have practised and worked in the field of yoga for more than fifty years, I may have to practice for several more lifetimes to reach perfection in the subject. Therefore, the explanation of the most abstruse sūtras lies yet beyond my power.

It is said that once Lord Viṣṇu was seated on Ādiśeṣa, Lord of serpents, His couch, watching the enchanting dance of Lord Śiva. Lord Viṣṇu was so totally absorbed in the dance movements of Lord Śiva that His body began to vibrate to their rhythm. This vibration made Him heavier and heavier, causing Ādiśeṣa to feel so uncomfortable that he was gasping for breath and was on the point of collapse. The moment the dance came to an end, Lord Viṣṇu's body became light again. Ādiśeṣa was amazed and asked his master the cause of these stupendous changes. The Lord explained that the grace, beauty, majesty and grandeur of Lord Śiva's dance had created corresponding vibrations in His own body, making it heavy. Marvelling at this, Ādiśeṣa professed a desire to learn to dance so as to exalt his Lord. Viṣṇu became thoughtful, and predicted that soon Lord Śiva would grace Ādiśeṣa to write a commentary on grammar, and that he would then also be able to devote himself to perfection in the art of dance. Ādiśeṣa was over-joyed by these words and looked forward to the descent of Lord Śiva's grace.

Ādiśeṣa then began to meditate to ascertain who would be his mother on earth. In meditation, he had the vision of a *yoginī* by the name of Goṇikā who was praying for a worthy son to whom she could impart her knowledge and wisdom. He at once realized that she would be a worthy mother for him, and awaited an auspicious moment to become her son.

Goṇikā, thinking that her earthly life was approaching its end, had not found a worthy son for whom she had been searching. Now, as a last resort, she looked to the Sun God, the living witness of God on earth and prayed to Him to fulfil her desire. She took a handful of water as a final oblation to Him, closed her eyes and meditated on the Sun. As she was about to offer the water, she opened her eyes and looked at her palms. To her surprise, she saw a tiny snake moving in her palms who soon took on a human form. This tiny male human being prostrated to Goṇikā and asked her to accept him as her son. This she did and named him Patañjali.

Pata means falling or fallen and *añjali* is an oblation. *Añjali* also means 'hands folded in prayer'. Goṇikā's prayer with folded hands thus bears the name Patañjali. Patañjali, the incarnation of Ādiśeṣa, Lord Viṣṇu's bearer, became not only the celebrated author of the *Yoga Sūtras* but also of treatises on *āyurveda* and grammar.

He undertook the work at Lord Śiva's command. The *Mahābhāsya*, his great grammar, a classical work for the cultivation of correct language, was followed by his book on *āyurveda*, the science of life and health. His final work on yoga was directed towards man's mental and spiritual evolution. All classical dancers in India pay their homage to Patañjali as a great dancer.

Together, Patañjali's three works deal with man's development as a whole, in thought, speech and action. His treatise on yoga is called *yoga darśana*. *Darśana* means 'vision of the soul' and also 'mirror'. The effect of yoga is to reflect the thoughts and actions of the aspirant as in a mirror. The practitioner observes the reflections of his thoughts, mind, consciousness and actions, and corrects himself. This process guides him towards the observation of his inner self.

Patañjali's works are followed by yogis to this day in their effort to develop a refined language, a cultured body and a civilized mind.

The Yoga Sūtras

The book is divided into four chapters or *pādas* (parts or quarters), covering the art, science and philosophy of life. The 196 sūtras are succinct, precise, profound, and devout in approach. Each contains a wealth of ideas and wisdom to guide the aspirant (*sādhaka*) towards full knowledge of his own real nature. This knowledge leads to the experience of perfect freedom, beyond common understanding. Through ardent study of the sūtras, and through devotion, the *sādhaka* is finally illumined by the lamp of exalted knowledge. Through practice, he radiates goodwill, friendliness and compassion. This knowledge, gained through subjective experience gives him boundless joy, harmony and peace.

As with the *Bhagavad Gītā*, different schools of thought have interpreted the sūtras in various ways, placing the emphasis on their particular path towards Self-Realization, whether on *karma* (action), *jñāna* (wisdom) or *bhakti* (devotion). Each commentator bases his interpretations on certain key or focal themes and weaves around them his thoughts, feelings and experiences. My own interpretations are derived from a lifelong study of yoga, and from experiences gained from the practice of *āsana*, *prāṇāyāma* and *dhyāna*. These are the key aspects of yoga which I use to interpret the sūtras in the simplest and most direct way, without departing from traditional meanings given by successive teachers.

The four chapters or *pādas* of the book are:

1 *Samādhi pāda* (on contemplation)
2 *Sādhana pāda* (on practice)
3 *Vibhūti pāda* (on properties and powers)
4 *Kaivalya pāda* (on emancipation and freedom)

The four *pādas* correspond to the four *varṇas* or divisions of labour; the four *āśramas* or stages of life; the three *guṇas* or qualities of nature and the fourth state beyond them (*sattva*, *rajas*, *tamas* and *guṇātīta*) and the four *puruṣārthas* or aims of life. In the concluding sūtra of the fourth pāda, Patañjali speaks of the culmination of *puruṣārthas* and *guṇas* as the highest goal of yoga *sādhana*. These concepts must have been wholly understood in Patañjali's time, and therefore implicit in the earlier chapters, for him to speak of them explicitly only at the very end of the book.

The ultimate effect of following the path laid out by Patañjali is to experience the effortless, indivisible state of the seer.

The first *pāda* amounts to a treatise on *dharmaśāstra*, the science of religious duty. *Dharma* is that which upholds, sustains, and supports one who has fallen or is falling, or is about to fall in the sphere of ethics, physical or mental practices, or spiritual discipline. It appears to me that Patañjali's whole concept of yoga is based on *dharma*, the law handed down in perpetuity through Vedic tradition. The goal of the law of *dharma* is emancipation.

If *dharma* is the seed of yoga, *kaivalya* (emancipation) is its fruit. This explains the concluding sūtra, which describes *kaivalya* as the state which is motiveless and devoid of all worldly aims and qualities of nature. In *kaivalya*, the yogi shines in his own intelligence which sprouts from the seer, *ātman*, independent of the organs of action, senses of perception, mind, intelligence and consciousness. Yoga is, in fact, the path to *kaivalya*.

Dharma, the orderly science of duty is part of the eightfold path of yoga (*aṣṭāṅga yoga*), which Patañjali describes in detail. When the eight disciplines are followed with dedication and devotion, they help the *sādhaka* to become physically, mentally and emotionally stable so that he can maintain equanimity in all circumstances. He learns to know the Supreme Soul, *Brahman*, and to live in speech, thought and action in accordance with the highest truth.

Samādhi Pāda

The first chapter, *samādhi pāda*, defines yoga and the movement of the consciousness, *citta vṛtti*. It is directed towards those who are already highly evolved to enable them to maintain their advanced state of cultured, matured intelligence and wisdom. Rare indeed are such human souls who experience *samādhi* early in life, for *samādhi* is the last stage of the eightfold path of yoga. *Samādhi* is seeing the soul face to face, an absolute, indivisible state of existence, in which all differences between body, mind and soul are dissolved. Such sages as Hanumān, Śuka, Dhruva, Prahlāda, Śaṅkarācārya, Jñāneśvar, Kabīr, Svāmi Rāmdās of Mahārāṣṭra, Rāmakṛṣṇa Paramahaṁsa and Ramaṇa Maharṣi, evolved straight to *kaivalya* without experiencing the intermediate stages of life or the various stages of yoga. All the actions of these great seers arose from their souls, and they dwelled throughout their lives in a state of unalloyed bliss and purity.

The word *samādhi* is made up of two components. *Sama* means level, alike, straight, upright, impartial, just, good and virtuous; and *ādhi* means over and above, i.e. the indestructible seer. *Samādhi* is the tracing of the source of consciousness – the seer – and then diffusing its essence, impartially and evenly, throughout every particle of the intelligence, mind, senses and body.

We may suppose that Patañjali's intention, in beginning with an exegesis of *samādhi*, was to attract those rare souls who were already on the brink of Self-Realization, and to guide them into experiencing the state of non-duality itself. For the uninitiated majority, the enticing prospect of *samādhi*, revealed so early in his work, serves as a lamp to draw us into yogic discipline, which will refine us to the point where our own soul becomes manifest.

Patañjali describes the fluctuations, modifications and modulations of thought which disturb the consciousness, and then sets out the various disciplines by which they may be stilled. This has resulted in yoga being called a mental *sādhana* (practice). Such a *sādhana* is possible only if the accumulated fruits derived from the good actions of past lives (*saṁskāras*) are of a noble order. Our *saṁskāras* are the fund of our past perceptions, instincts and subliminal or hidden impressions. If they are good, they act as stimuli to maintain the high degree of sensitivity necessary to pursue the spiritual path.

Consciousness is imbued with the three qualities (*guṇas*) of luminosity (*sattva*), vibrancy (*rajas*) and inertia (*tamas*). The *guṇas* also colour our actions: white (*sattva*), grey (*rajas*) and black (*tamas*). Through the discipline of yoga, both actions and intelligence go beyond these qualities and the seer comes to experience his own soul with crystal clarity, free from the relative attributes of nature and actions. This state of purity is *samādhi*. Yoga is thus both the means and the goal. Yoga is *samādhi* and *samādhi* is yoga.

There are two main types of *samādhi*. *Sabīja* or *saṁprajñāta samādhi* is attained by deliberate effort, using for concentration an object or idea as a 'seed'. *Nirbīja samādhi* is without seed or support.

Patañjali explains that before *samādhi* is experienced the functioning of consciousness depends upon five factors: correct perception, misperception (where the senses mislead), misconception or ambiguousness (where the mind lets one down), sleep, and memory. The soul is pure, but through the sullying or misalignment of consciousness it gets caught up in the spokes of joys and sorrows and becomes part of suffering, like a spider ensnared in its own web. These joys and sorrows may be painful or painless, cognizable or incognizable.

Freedom, that is to say direct experience of *samādhi*, can be attained only by disciplined conduct and renunciation of sensual desires and appetites. This is brought about through adherence to the 'twin pillars' of yoga, *abhyāsa* and *vairāgya*.

Abhyāsa (practice) is the art of learning that which has to be learned through the cultivation of disciplined action. This involves long, zealous, calm, and persevering effort. *Vairāgya* (detachment or renunciation) is the art of avoiding that which should be avoided. Both require a positive and virtuous approach.

Practice is a generative force of transformation or progress in yoga, but if undertaken alone it produces an unbridled energy which is thrown outwards to the material world as if by centrifugal force. Renunciation acts to shear off this energetic outburst, protecting the practitioner from entanglement with sense objects and redirecting the energies centripetally towards the core of being.

Patañjali teaches the *sādhaka* to cultivate friendliness and compassion, to delight in the happiness of others and to remain indifferent to vice and virtue so that he may maintain his poise and tranquillity. He advises the *sādhaka* to follow the ethical disciplines of *yama* and *niyama*, the ten precepts similar to the Ten Commandments, which govern behaviour and practice and form the foundation of spiritual evolution. He then offers several methods through which consciousness detaches itself from intellectual and emotional upheavals and assumes the form of the soul – universal, devoid of all personal and material identity. The *sādhaka* is now filled with serenity, insight and truth. The soul, which until now remained unmanifest, becomes visible to the seeker. The seeker becomes the seer: he enters a state without seed or support, *nirbīja samādhi*.

Sādhana Pāda

In the second chapter, *sādhana pāda*, Patañjali comes down to the level of the spiritually unevolved to help them, too, to aspire to absolute freedom. Here he coins the word *kriyāyoga*. *Kriyā* means action, and *kriyāyoga* emphasizes the dynamic effort to be made by the *sādhaka*. It is composed of eight yogic disciplines, *yama* and *niyama*, *āsana* and *prāṇāyāma*, *pratyāhāra* and *dhāraṇā*, *dhyāna* and *samādhi*. These are compressed into three tiers. The tier formed by the first two pairs, *yama* and *niyama, āsana* and *prāṇāyāma*, comes under *tapas* (religious spirit in practice). The second tier, *pratyāhāra* and *dhāraṇā*, is self-study (*svādhyāya*). The third, *dhyāna* and *samādhi*, is *Īśvara praṇidhāna*, the surrender of the individual self to the Universal Spirit, or God (*Īśvara*).

In this way, Patañjali covers the three great paths of Indian philosophy in the *Yoga Sūtras*. *Karmamārga*, the path of action is contained in *tapas*; *jñānamārga*, the path of knowledge, in *svādhyāya*; and *bhaktimārga*, the path of surrender to God, in *Īśvara praṇidhāna*.

In this chapter, Patañjali identifies *avidyā*, spiritual ignorance, as the source of all sorrow and unhappiness. *Avidyā* is the first of the five *kleśas*, or afflictions, and is the root of all the others: egoism, attachment, aversion and clinging to life. From these arise desires, sowing the seeds of sorrow.

Afflictions are of three types. They may be self-inflicted, hereditary, or caused through imbalance of elements in the body. All are consequences of one's actions, in this or previous lifetimes, and are to be overcome through practice and renunciation in the eight yogic disciplines which cover purification of the body, senses and mind, an intense discipline whereby the seeds are incinerated, impurities vanish, and the seeker reaches a state of serenity in which he merges with the seer.

For one who lacks ethical discipline and perfect physical health, there can be no spiritual illumination. Body, mind and spirit are inseparable: if the body is asleep, the soul is asleep.

The seeker is taught to perform *āsanas* so that he becomes familiar with his body, senses and intelligence. He develops alertness, sensitivity, and the power of concentration. *Prāṇāyāma* gives control over the subtle qualities of the elements – sound, touch, shape, taste and smell. *Pratyāhāra* is the withdrawal into the mind of the organs of action and senses of perception.

Sādhana pāda ends here, but Patañjali extends *dhāraṇā*, *dhyāna* and *samādhi*, the subtle aspects of *sādhana*, into the next chapter, *vibhūti pāda*. These three withdraw the mind into the consciousness, and the consciousness into the soul.

The journey from *yama* to *pratyāhāra*, described in *sādhana pāda*, ends in the sea of tranquillity, which has no ripples. If *citta* is the sea, its movements (*vṛttis*) are the ripples. Body, mind and consciousness are in communion with the soul; they are now free from attachments and aversions, memories of place and time. The impurities of body and mind are cleansed, the dawning light of wisdom vanquishes ignorance, innocence replaces arrogance and pride, and the seeker becomes the seer.

Vibhūti Pāda

The third chapter speaks of the divine effects of yoga *sādhana*. It is said that the *sādhaka* who in this state has full knowledge of past, present and future, as well as of the solar system. He understands the minds of others. He acquires the eight supernatural powers or *siddhis*: the ability to become small and large, light and heavy, to acquire, to attain every wish, to gain supremacy and sovereignty over things.

These achievements are dangerous. The *sādhaka* is cautioned to ignore their temptations and pursue the spiritual path.

Sage Vyāsa's commentary on the sūtras gives examples of those who became ensnared by these powers and those who remained free. Nahūṣa, who belonged to the mortal world, became the Lord of heaven, but misused his power, fell from grace and was sent back to earth in the form of a snake. Ūrvaṣi, a famous mythical nymph, the daughter of Nara Nārāyaṇa (the son of Dharma and grandson of Brahma), became a creeping plant. Ahalyā, who succumbed to sensual temptation, was cursed by Gautama and became a stone. On the other hand, Nandi, the bull, reached Lord Śiva. Matsya, the fish, became Matsyendranāth, the greatest *haṭha yogi* on earth.

If the *sādhaka* succumbs to the lure of the *siddhis*, he will be like a person running away from a gale only to be caught in a whirlwind. If he resists, and perseveres on the spiritual path, he will experience *kaivalya*, the indivisible, unqualified, undifferentiated state of existence.

Kaivalya Pāda

In the fourth chapter, Patañjali distinguishes *kaivalya* from *samādhi*. In *samādhi*, the *sādhaka* experiences a passive state of oneness between seer and seen, observer and observed, subject and object. In *kaivalya*, he lives in a positive state of life, above the *tāmasic*, *rājasic* and *sāttvic* influences of the three *guṇas* of nature. He moves in the world and does day-to-day work dispassionately, without becoming involved in it.

Patañjali says it is possible to experience *kaivalya* by birth, through use of drugs, by repetition of *mantra*, or by *tapas* (intense, disciplined effort) and through *samādhi*. Of these, only the last two develop mature intelligence and lead to stable growth.

Man may make or mar his progress through good actions or bad. Yogic practices lead to a spiritual life; non-yogic actions bind one to the world. The ego, *ahaṁkāra*, is the root cause of good and bad actions. Yoga removes the weed of pride from the mind and helps the seeker to trace the source of all actions, the consciousness, wherein all past impressions (*saṁskāras*) are stored. When this ultimate source is traced through yogic practices, the *sādhaka* is at once freed from the reactions of his actions. Desires leave him. Desire, action and reaction are spokes in the wheel of thought, but when consciousness has become steady and pure, they are eliminated. Movements of mind come to an end. He becomes a perfect yogi with skilful actions. As wick, oil and flame combine to give light, so thought, speech and action unite, and the yogi's knowledge becomes total. For others, whose knowledge and understanding are limited, an object may be one thing, experience of the object another, and the word quite different from both. These vacillations of mind cripple one's capacity for thought and action.

The yogi differentiates between the wavering uncertainties of thought processes and the understanding of the Self, which is changeless. He does his work in the world as a witness, uninvolved and uninfluenced. His mind reflects its own form, undistorted, like a crystal. At this point, all speculation and deliberation come to an end and liberation is experienced. The yogi lives in the experience of wisdom, untinged by the emotions of desire, anger, greed, infatuation, pride, and malice. This seasoned wisdom is truth-bearing (*ṛtambharā prajñā*). It leads the *sādhaka* towards virtuous awareness, *dharma megha samādhi*, which brings him a cascade of knowledge and wisdom. He is immersed in *kaivalya*, the constant burning light of the soul, illuminating the divinity not only in himself, but also in those who come in contact with him.

I end this prologue with a quotation from the *Viṣṇu Purāṇa* given by Śri Vyāsa in his commentary on the *Yoga Sūtras*: 'Yoga is the teacher of yoga; yoga is to be understood through yoga. So live in yoga to realize yoga; comprehend yoga through yoga; he who is free from distractions enjoys yoga through yoga.'

Themes in the Four Pādas

I: Samādhi Pāda

Patañjali's opening words are on the need for a disciplined code of conduct to educate us towards spiritual poise and peace under all circumstances.

He defines yoga as the restraint of *citta*, which means consciousness. The term *citta* should not be understood to mean only the mind. *Citta* has three components: mind (*manas*), intelligence (*buddhi*) and ego (*ahaṁkāra*) which combine into one composite whole. The term 'self' represents a person as an individual entity. Its identity is separate from mind, intelligence and ego, depending upon the development of the individual.

Self also stands for the subject, as contrasted with the object, of experience. It is that out of which the primeval thought of 'I' arises, and into which it dissolves. Self has a shape or form as 'I', and is infused with the illuminative, or *sāttvic*, quality of nature (*prakṛti*). In the temples of India, we see a base idol, an idol of stone that is permanently fixed. This represents the soul (*ātman*). There is also a bronze idol, which is considered to be the icon of the base idol, and is taken out of the temple in procession as its representative, the individual self. The bronze idol represents the self or the individual entity, while the base idol represents the universality of the Soul.

Eastern thought takes one through the layers of being, outwards from the core, the soul, towards the periphery, the body; and inwards from the periphery towards the core. The purpose of this exploration is to discover, experience and taste the nectar of the soul. The process begins with external awareness: what we experience through the organs of action or *karmendriyas* (the arms, legs, mouth, and the organs of generation and excretion) and proceeds through the senses of perception or *jñānendriyas* (the ears, eyes, nose, tongue and skin). That awareness begins to penetrate the mind, the intelligence, the ego, the consciousness, and the individual self (*asmitā*), until it reaches the soul (*ātma*). These sheaths may also be penetrated in the reverse order.

Asmitā's existence at an empirical level has no absolute moral value, as it is in an unsullied state. It takes its colour from the level of development of the individual practitioner (*sādhaka*). Thus, 'I-consciousness' in its grossest form may manifest as pride or egoism, but in its subtlest form, it is the innermost layer of being, nearest to the *ātman*. *Ahaṁkāra*, or ego, likewise has changing qualities, depending on whether it is *rājasic*, *tāmasic* or *sāttvic*. *Sāttvic ahaṁkāra* usually indicates an evolved *asmitā*.

The chameleon nature of *asmitā* is apparent when we set ourselves a challenge. The source of the challenge lies in the positive side of *asmitā*, but the moment fear arises negatively, it inhibits our initiative. We must then issue a counter-challenge to disarm that fear. From this conflict springs creation.

Āsana, for example, offers a controlled battleground for the process of conflict and creation. The aim is to recreate the process of human evolution in our own internal environment. We thereby have the opportunity to observe and comprehend our own evolution to the point at which conflict is resolved and there is only oneness, as when the river meets the sea. This creative struggle is experienced in the headstand: as we challenge ourselves to improve the position, fear of falling acts to inhibit us. If we are rash, we fall, if timorous, we make no progress. But if the interplay of the two forces is observed, analysed and controlled, we can achieve perfection. At that moment, the *asmitā* which proposed and the *asmitā* which opposed become one in the *āsana* and assume a perfect form. *Asmitā* dissolves in bliss, or *satcitānanda* (purity-consciousness-bliss).

Ahaṁkāra, or ego, the sense of 'I', is the knot that binds the consciousness and the body through the inner sense, the mind. In this way, the levels of being are connected by the mind, from the soul, through the internal parts, to the external senses. The mind thus acts as a link between the objects seen, and the subject, the seer. It is the unifying factor between the soul and the body which helps us to uncover layer after layer of our being until the sheath of the self (*jīvātman*) is reached.

These layers, or sheaths, are the anatomical, skeletal, or structural sheath (*annamaya kośa*); the physiological or organic sheath (*prāṇamaya kośa*); the mental or emotional sheath (*manomaya kośa*); the intellectual or discriminative sheath (*vijñānamaya kośa*); and the pure blissful sheath (*ānandamaya kośa*). These *kośas* represent the five elements of nature, or *prakṛti*: earth, water, fire, air and ether. *Mahat*, cosmic consciousness, in its individual form as *citta*, is the sixth *kośa*, while the inner soul is the seventh *kośa*. In all, man has seven sheaths, or *kośas*, for the development of awareness.

The blissful spiritual sheath is called the causal body (*kāraṇa śarīra*), while the physiological, intellectual and mental sheaths form the subtle body (*ṣūkṣma śarīra*), and the anatomical sheath the gross body (*kārya śarīra*). The yoga aspirant tries to understand the functions of all these sheaths of the soul as well as the soul itself, and thereby begins his quest to experience the divine core of being: the *ātman*.

The mind permeates and engulfs the entire conscious and unconscious mental process, and the activities of the brain. All vital activities arise in the mind. According to Indian thought, though mind, intelligence and ego are parts of consciousness, mind acts as the outer cover of intelligence and ego and is considered to be the eleventh sense organ. Mind is as elusive as mercury. It senses, desires, wills, remembers, perceives, recollects and experiences emotional sensations such as pain and pleasure, heat and cold, honour and dishonour. Mind is inhibitive as well as exhibitive. When inhibitive, it draws nearer to the core of being. When exhibitive, it manifests itself as brain in order to see and perceive the external objects with which it then identifies.

It should be understood that the brain is a part of the mind. As such, it functions as the mind's instrument of action. The brain is part of the organic structure of the central nervous system that is enclosed in the cranium. It makes mental activity possible. It controls and co-ordinates mental and physical activities. When the brain is trained to be consciously quiet, the cognitive faculty comes into its own, making possible, through the intelligence, apprehension of the mind's various facets. Clarity of intelligence lifts the veil of obscurity and encourages quiet receptivity in the ego as well as in the consciousness, diffusing their energies evenly throughout the physical, physiological, mental, intellectual and spiritual sheaths of the soul.

What is soul?

God, *Paramātman* or *Puruṣa Viśeṣan*, is known as the Universal Soul, the seed of all (see I.24). The individual soul, *jīvātman* or *puruṣa*, is the seed of the individual self. The soul is therefore distinct from the self. Soul is formless, while self assumes a form. The soul is an entity, separate from the body and free from the self. Soul is the very essence of the core of one's being.

Like mind, the soul has no actual location in the body. It is latent, and exists everywhere. The moment the soul is brought to awareness of itself, it is felt anywhere and everywhere. Unlike the self, the soul is free from the influence of nature, and is thus universal. The self is the seed of all functions and actions, and the source of spiritual evolution through knowledge. It can also, through worldly desires, be the seed of spiritual destruction. The soul perceives spiritual reality, and is known as the seer (*dṛṣṭa*).

As a well-nurtured seed causes a tree to grow, and to blossom with flowers and fruits, so the soul is the seed of man's evolution. From this source, *asmitā* sprouts as the individual self. From this sprout springs consciousness, *citta*. From consciousness, spring ego, intelligence, mind, and the senses of perception and organs of action. Though the soul is free from influence, its sheaths come in contact with the objects of the world, which leave imprints on them through the intelligence of the brain and the mind. The discriminative faculty of brain and mind screens these imprints, discarding or retaining them. If discriminative power is lacking, then these imprints, like quivering leaves, create fluctuations in words, thoughts and deeds, and restlessness in the self.

These endless cycles of fluctuation are known as *vṛttis*: changes, movements, functions, operations, or conditions of action or conduct in the consciousness. *Vṛttis* are thought-waves, part of the brain, mind and consciousness as waves are part of the sea.

Thought is a mental vibration based on past experiences. It is a product of inner mental activity, a process of thinking. This process consciously applies the intellect to analyse thoughts arising from the seat of the mental body through the remembrance of past experiences. Thoughts create disturbances. By analysing them one develops discriminative power, and gains serenity.

When consciousness is in a serene state, its interior components, intelligence, ego, mind and the feeling of 'I', also experience tranquillity. At that point, there is no room for thought-waves to arise either in the mind or in the consciousness. Stillness and silence are experienced, poise and peace set in and one becomes cultured. One's thoughts, words and deeds develop purity, and begin to flow in a divine stream.

Study of consciousness

Before describing the principles of yoga, Patañjali speaks of consciousness and the restraint of its movements.

The verb *cit* means to perceive, to notice, to know, to understand, to long for, to desire and to remind. As a noun, *cit* means thought, emotion, intellect, feeling, disposition, vision, heart, soul, Brahman. *Cinta* means disturbed or anxious thoughts, and *cintana* means deliberate thinking. Both are facets of *citta*. As they must be restrained through the discipline of yoga, yoga is defined as *citta vṛtti nirodhaḥ*. A perfectly subdued and pure *citta* is divine and at one with the soul.

Citta is the individual counterpart of *mahat*, the universal consciousness. It is the seat of the intelligence that sprouts from conscience, *antaḥkaraṇa*, the organ of virtue and religious knowledge. If the soul is the seed of conscience, conscience is the source of consciousness, intelligence and mind. The thinking processes of consciousness embody mind, intelligence and ego. The mind has the power to imagine, think, attend to, aim, feel and will. The mind's continual swaying affects its inner sheaths, intelligence, ego, consciousness and the self.

Mind is mercurial by nature, elusive and hard to grasp. However, it is the one organ which reflects both the external and internal worlds. Though it has the faculty of seeing things within and without, its more natural tendency is to involve itself with objects of the visible, rather than the inner world.

In collaboration with the senses, mind perceives things for the individual to see, observe, feel and experience. These experiences may be painful, painless or pleasurable. Through their influence, impulsiveness and other tendencies or moods creep into the mind, making it a storehouse of imprints (*saṁskāras*) and desires (*vāsanas*), which create excitement and emotional impressions. If these are favourable they create good imprints; if unfavourable they cause repugnance. These imprints generate the fluctuations, modifications and modulations of consciousness. If the mind is not disciplined and purified, it becomes involved with the objects experienced, creating sorrow and unhappiness.

Patañjali begins the treatise on yoga by explaining the functioning of the mind, so that we may learn to discipline it, and intelligence, ego and consciousness may be restrained, subdued and diffused, then drawn towards the core of our being and absorbed in the soul. This is yoga.

Patañjali explains that painful and painless imprints are gathered by five means: *pramāṇa*, or direct perception, which is knowledge that arises from correct thought or right conception and is perpetual and true; *viparyaya*, or misperception and misconception, leading to contrary knowledge; *vikalpa*, or imagination or fancy; *nidrā* or sleep; and *smṛti* or memory. These are the fields in which the mind operates, and through which experience is gathered and stored.

Direct perception is derived from one's own experience, through inference, or from the perusal of sacred books or the words of authoritative masters. To be true and distinct, it should be real and self-evident. Its correctness should be verified by reasoned doubt, logic and reflection. Finally, it should be found to correspond to spiritual doctrines and precepts and sacred, revealed truth.

Contrary knowledge leads to false conceptions. Imagination remains at verbal or visual levels and may consist of ideas without a factual basis. When ideas are proved as facts, they become real perception.

Sleep is a state of inactivity in which the organs of action, senses of perception, mind and intelligence remain inactive. Memory is the faculty of retaining and reviving past impressions and experiences of correct perception, misperception, misconception and even of sleep.

These five means by which imprints are gathered shape moods and modes of behaviour, making or marring the individual's intellectual, cultural and spiritual evolution.

Culture of consciousness

The culture of consciousness entails cultivation, observation, and progressive refinement of consciousness by means of yogic disciplines. After explaining the causes of fluctuations in consciousness, Patañjali shows how to overcome them, by means of practice, *abhyāsa*, and detachment or renunciation, *vairāgya*.

If the student is perplexed to find detachment and renunciation linked to practice so early in the *Yoga Sūtras*, let him consider their symbolic relationship in this way. The text begins with *atha yogānuśāsanam. Anuśāsanam* stands for the practice of a disciplined code of yogic conduct, the observance of instructions for ethical action handed down by lineage and tradition. Ethical principles, translated from methodology into deeds, constitute practice. Now, read the word 'renunciation' in the context of sūtra I.4: 'At other times, the seer identifies with the fluctuating consciousness.' Clearly, the fluctuating mind lures the seer outwards towards pastures of pleasure and valleys of pain, where enticement inevitably gives rise to attachment. When mind starts to drag the seer, as if by a stout rope, from the seat of being towards the gratification of appetite, only renunciation can intervene and save the *sādhaka* by cutting the rope. So we see, from sūtras I.1 and I.4, the interdependence from the very beginning of practice and renunciation, without which practice will not bear fruit.

Abhyāsa is a dedicated, unswerving, constant, and vigilant search into a chosen subject, pursued against all odds in the face of repeated failures, for indefinitely long periods of time. *Vairāgya* is the cultivation of freedom from passion, abstention from worldly desires and appetites, and discrimination between the real and the unreal. It is the act of giving up all sensuous delights. *Abhyāsa* builds confidence and refinement in the process of culturing the consciousness, whereas *vairāgya* is the elimination of whatever hinders progress and refinement. Proficiency in *vairāgya* develops the ability to free oneself from the fruits of action.

Patañjali speaks of attachment, non-attachment, and detachment. Detachment may be likened to the attitude of a doctor towards his patient. He treats the patient with the greatest care, skill and sense of responsibility, but does not become emotionally involved with him so as not to lose his faculty of reasoning and professional judgement.

A bird cannot fly with one wing. In the same way, we need the two wings of practice and renunciation to soar up to the zenith of Soul realization.

Practice implies a certain methodology, involving effort. It has to be followed uninterruptedly for a long time, with firm resolve, application, attention and devotion, to create a stable foundation for training the mind, intelligence, ego and consciousness.

Renunciation is discriminative discernment. It is the art of learning to be free from craving, both for worldly pleasures and for heavenly eminence. It involves training the mind and consciousness to be unmoved by desire and passion. One must learn to renounce objects and ideas which disturb and hinder one's daily yogic practices. Then one has to cultivate non-attachment to the fruits of one's labours.

If *abhyāsa* and *vairāgya* are assiduously observed, restraint of the mind becomes possible much more quickly. Then, one may explore what is beyond the mind, and taste the nectar of immortality, or Soul-realization. Temptations neither daunt nor haunt one who has this intensity of heart in practice and renunciation. If practice is slowed down, then the search for Soul-realization becomes clogged and bound in the wheel of time.

Why practice and renunciation are essential

Avidyā (ignorance) is the mother of vacillation and affliction. Patañjali explains how one may gain knowledge by direct and correct perception, inference and testimony, and that correct understanding comes when trial and error ends. Here, both practice and renunciation play an important role in gaining spiritual knowledge.

Attachment is a relationship between man and matter, and may be inherited or acquired.

Non-attachment is the deliberate process of drawing away from attachment and personal affliction, in which, neither binding oneself to duty nor cutting oneself off from it, one gladly helps all, near or far, friend or foe. Non-attachment does not mean drawing inwards and shutting oneself off, but involves carrying out one's responsibilities without incurring obligation or inviting expectation. It is between attachment and detachment, a step towards detachment, and the *sādhaka* needs to cultivate it before thinking of renunciation.

Detachment brings discernment: seeing each and every thing or being as it is, in its purity, without bias or self-interest. It is a means to understand nature and its potencies. Once nature's purposes are grasped, one must learn to detach onself from them to achieve an absolute independent state of existence wherein the soul radiates its own light.

Mind, intelligence and ego, revolving in the wheel of desire (*kāma*), anger (*krodha*), greed (*lobha*), infatuation (*moha*), pride (*mada*) and malice (*mātsarya*), tie the *sādhaka* to their imprints; he finds it exceedingly difficult to come out of the turmoil and to differentiate between the mind and the soul. Practice of yoga and renunciation of sensual desires take one towards spiritual attainment.

Practice demands four qualities from the aspirant: dedication, zeal, uninterrupted awareness and long duration. Renunciation also demands four qualities: disengaging the senses from action, avoiding desire, stilling the mind and freeing oneself from cravings.

Practitioners are also of four levels, mild, medium, keen and intense. They are categorized into four stages: beginners; those who understand the inner functions of the body; those who can connect the intelligence to all parts of the body; and those whose body, mind and soul have become one. (See table 1.)

Effects of practice and renunciation

Intensity of practice and renunciation transforms the uncultured, scattered consciousness, *citta*, into a cultured consciousness, able to focus on the four states of awareness. The seeker develops philosophical curiosity, begins to analyse with sensitivity, and learns to grasp the ideas and purposes of material objects in the right perspective (*vitarka*). Then he meditates on them to know and understand fully the subtle aspects of matter (*vicāra*). Thereafter he moves on to experience spiritual elation or the pure bliss (*ānanda*) of meditation, and finally sights the Self. These four types of awareness are collectively termed *saṁprajñāta samādhi* or *saṁprajñāta samāpatti*. *Samāpatti* is thought transformation or contemplation, the act of coming face to face with oneself.

From these four states of awareness, the seeker moves to a new state, an alert but passive state of quietness known as *manolaya*. Patañjali cautions the *sādhaka* not to be caught in this state, which is a crossroads on the spiritual path, but to intensify his *sādhana* to experience a still higher state known as *nirbīja samādhi* or *dharma megha samādhi*. The *sādhaka* may not know which road to follow beyond *manolaya*, and could be stuck there forever, in a spiritual desert. In this quiet state of void, the hidden tendencies remain inactive but latent. They surface and become active the moment the alert passive state disappears. This state should therefore not be mistaken for the highest goal in yoga.

This resting state is a great achievement in the path of evolution, but it remains a state of suspension in the spiritual field. One loses body consciousness and is undisturbed by nature, which signifies conquest of matter. If the seeker is prudent, he realizes that this is not the aim and end, but only the beginning of success in yoga. Accordingly, he further intensifies his effort (*upāya pratyaya*) with faith and vigour, and uses his previous experience as

Table 1: *Levels of* sādhaka, *levels of* sādhana *and stages of evolution*

Levels of *sādhaka*	*Abhyāsa* (practice)	Body, mind, soul	*Vairāgya* (renunciation)	Four stages of evolution
a *Mṛdu* (mild)	Slow, indefinite, undecided practice	Physical (*annamaya*) (*indriyamaya*)	*Yatamāna* (disengaging the senses from action)	*Ārambhāvasthā* The state of commencement (surface and peripheral movement)
b *Madhya* (medium)	Methodical, disciplined practice	Physiological (*prāṇamaya,* cells, glands, circulatory, respiratory and other organs)	*Vyatireka* (keeping away from desire)	*Ghaṭavasthā* The state of fullness (using the physical and physiological sheaths to understand the inner functions of the body)
c *Adhimātra* (intense)	Scientific, meaningful, purposeful and decisive practice	Mental, intellectual (*manomaya*) (*vijñānamaya*)	*Ekendriya* (stilling the mind)	*Paricayāvasthā* (the state of intimate knowledge. Mind linking *annamaya* and *prāṇamaya* kośas to *vijñānamaya* kosa)
d *Tivra saṁvegiṅ adhimātrataman* (supremely intense)	Religiousness and purity in practice	Practice with attentive consciousness surrender to the Supreme Soul (*citta maya*) (*ātma maya*)	*Vaśīkāra* (freeing oneself from cravings)	*Niṣpattyāvasthā* (the state of perfection and ripeness) (consummation)

a guide to proceed from the state of void or loneliness, towards the non-void state of aloneness or fullness, where freedom is absolute.

If the *sādhaka*'s intensity of practice is great, the goal is closer. If he slackens his efforts, the goal recedes in proportion to his lack of willpower and intensity.

Universal Soul or God (*Īśvara, Puruṣa Viśeṣan* or *Paramātman*)

There are many ways to begin the practice of yoga. First and foremost, Patañjali outlines the method of surrender of oneself to God (*Īśvara*). This involves detachment from the world and attachment to God, and is possible only for those few who are born as adepts. Patañjali defines God as the Supreme Being, totally free from afflictions and the fruits of action. In Him abides the matchless seed of all knowledge. He is First and Foremost amongst all masters and teachers, unconditioned by time, place and circumstances.

His symbol is the syllable *ĀUṀ*. This sound is divine: it stands in praise of divine fulfilment. *ĀUṀ* is the universal sound (*śabda brahman*). Philosophically, it is regarded as the seed of all words. No word can be uttered without the symbolic sound of these three letters, *ā*, *u* and *ṁ*. The sound begins with the letter *ā*, causing the mouth to open. So the beginning is *ā*. To speak, it is necessary to roll the tongue and move the lips. This is symbolized by the letter *u*. The ending of the sound is the closing of the lips, symbolized by the letter *ṁ*. *ĀUṀ* represents communion with God, the Soul and with the Universe.

ĀUṀ is known as *praṇava*, or exalted praise of God. God is worshipped by repeating or chanting *ĀUṀ*, because sound vibration is the subtlest and highest expression of nature. *Mahat* belongs to this level. Even our innermost unspoken thoughts create waves of sound vibration, so *ĀUṀ* represents the elemental movement of sound, which is the foremost form of energy. *ĀUṀ* is therefore held to be the primordial way of worshipping God. At this exalted level of phenomenal evolution, fragmentation has not yet taken place. *ĀUṀ* offers complete praise, neither partial nor divided: none can be higher. Such prayer begets purity of mind in the *sādhaka*, and helps him to reach the goal of yoga. *ĀUṀ*, repeated with feeling and awareness of its meaning, overcomes obstacles to Self-Realization.

The obstacles

The obstacles to healthy life and Self-Realization are disease, indolence of body or mind, doubt or scepticism, carelessness, laziness, failing to avoid desires and their gratification, delusion and missing the point, not being able to concentrate on what is undertaken and to gain ground, and inability to maintain concentration and steadiness in practice once attained. They are further aggravated through sorrows, anxiety or frustration, unsteadiness of the body, and laboured or irregular breathing.

Ways of surmounting the obstacles and reaching the goal

The remedies which minimize or eradicate these obstacles are: adherence to single-minded effort in *sādhana*, friendliness and goodwill towards all creation, compassion, joy, indifference and non-attachment to both pleasure and pain, virtue and vice. These diffuse the mind evenly within and without and make it serene.

Patañjali also suggests the following methods to be adopted by various types of practitioners to diminish the fluctuations of the mind.

> Retaining the breath after each exhalation (the study of inhalation teaches how the self gradually becomes attached to the body; the study of exhalation teaches non-attachment as the self recedes from the contact of the body; retention after exhalation educates one towards detachment); involving oneself in an interesting topic or object contemplating a luminous, effulgent and sorrowless light; treading the path followed by noble personalities; studying the nature of wakefulness, dream and sleep states, and maintaining a single state of awareness in all three; meditating on an object which is all-absorbing and conducive to a serene state of mind.

Effects of practice

Any of these methods can be practised on its own. If all are practised together, the mind will diffuse evenly throughout the body, its abode, like the wind which moves and spreads in space. When they are judiciously, meticulously and religiously practised, passions are controlled and single-mindedness develops. The *sādhaka* becomes highly sensitive, as flawless and transparent as crystal. He realizes that the seer, the seeker and the instrument used to see or seek are nothing but himself, and he resolves all divisions within himself.

This clarity brings about harmony between his words and their meanings, and a new light of wisdom dawns. His memory of experiences steadies his mind, and this leads both memory and mind to dissolve in the cosmic intelligence.

This is one type of *samādhi*, known as *sabīja samādhi*, with seed, or support. From this state, the *sādhaka* intensifies his *sādhana* to gain unalloyed wisdom, bliss and poise. This unalloyed wisdom is independent of anything heard, read or learned. The *sādhaka* does not allow himself to be halted in his progress, but seeks to experience a further state of being: the *amanaskatva* state.

If *manolaya* is a passive, almost negative, quiet state, *amanaskatva* is a positive, active state directly concerned with the inner being, without the influence of the mind. In this state, the *sādhaka* is perfectly detached from external things. Complete renunciation has taken place, and he lives in harmony with his inner being, allowing the seer to shine brilliantly in his own pristine glory.

This is true *samādhi*: seedless or *nirbīja samādhi*.

II: Sādhana Pāda

Why did Patañjali begin the *Yoga Sūtras* with a discussion of so advanced a subject as the subtle aspect of consciousness? We may surmise that intellectual standards and spiritual knowledge were then of a higher and more refined level than they are now, and that the inner quest was more accessible to his contemporaries than it is to us.

Today, the inner quest and the spiritual heights are difficult to attain through following Patañjali's earlier expositions. We turn, therefore, to this chapter, in which he introduces *kriyāyoga*, the yoga of action. *Kriyāyoga* gives us the practical disciplines needed to scale the spiritual heights.

My own feeling is that the four *pādas* of the Yoga Sūtras describe different disciplines of practice, the qualities or aspects of which vary according to the development of intelligence and refinement of consciousness of each *sādhaka*.

Sādhana is a discipline undertaken in the pursuit of a goal. *Abhyāsa* is repeated practice performed with observation and reflection. *Kriyā*, or action, also implies perfect execution with study and investigation. Therefore, *sādhana, abhyāsa*, and *kriyā* all mean one and the same thing. A *sādhaka*, or practitioner, is one who skilfully applies his mind and intelligence in practice towards a spiritual goal.

Whether out of compassion for the more intellectually backward people of his time, or else foreseeing the spiritual limitations of our time, Patañjali offers in this chapter a method of practice which begins with the organs of action and the senses of perception. Here, he gives those of average intellect the practical means to strive for knowledge, and to gather hope and confidence to begin yoga: the quest for Self-Realization. This chapter involves the *sādhaka* in the art of refining the body and senses, the visible layers of the soul, working inwards from the gross towards the subtle level.

Although Patañjali is held to have been a self-incarnated, immortal being, he must have voluntarily descended to the human level, submitted himself to the joys and sufferings, attachments and aversions, emotional imbalances and intellectual weaknesses of average individuals, and studied human nature from its nadir to its zenith. He guides us from our shortcomings towards emancipation through the devoted practice of yoga. This chapter, which may be happily followed for spiritual benefit by anyone, is his gift to humanity.

Kriyāyoga, the yoga of action, has three tiers: *tapas, svādhyāya* and *Īśvara praṇidhāna. Tapas* means burning desire to practise yoga and intense effort applied to practice. *Svādhyāya* has two aspects: the study of scriptures to gain sacred wisdom and knowledge of moral and spiritual values; and the study of one's own self, from the body to the inner self. *Īśvara praṇidhāna* is faith in God and surrender to God. This act of surrender teaches humility. When these three aspects of *kriyāyoga* are followed with zeal and earnestness, life's sufferings are overcome, and *samādhi* is experienced.

Sufferings or afflictions (*Kleśas*)

Kleśas (sufferings or afflictions) have five causes: ignorance, or lack of wisdom and understanding (*avidyā*), pride or egoism (*asmitā*), attachment (*rāga*), aversion (*dveṣa*), and fear of death and clinging to life (*abhiniveśa*). The first two are intellectual defects, the next two emotional, and the last instinctual. They may be hidden, latent, attenuated or highly active.

Avidyā, ignorance, or lack of wisdom, is a fertile ground in which afflictions can grow, making one's life a hell. Mistaking the transient for the eternal, the impure for the pure, pain for pleasure, and the pleasures of the world for the bliss of the spirit constitutes *avidyā*.

Identifying the individual ego (the 'I') with the real soul is *asmitā*. It is the false identification of the ego with the seer.

Encouraging and gratifying desires is *rāga*. When desires are not gratified, frustration and sorrow give rise to alienation or hate. This is *dveṣa*, aversion.

The desire to live forever and to preserve one's individual self is *abhiniveśa*. Freedom from such attachment to life is very difficult for even a wise, erudite and scholarly person to achieve. If *avidyā* is the mother of afflictions, *abhiniveśa* is its offspring.

All our past actions exert their influence and mould our present and future lives: as you sow, so shall you reap. This is the law of *karma*, the universal law of cause and effect. If our actions are good and virtuous, afflictions will be minimized; wrong actions will bring sorrow and pain. Actions may bear fruit immediately, later in life or in lives to come. They determine one's birth, span of life and the types of experiences to be undergone. When spiritual wisdom dawns, one perceives the tinge of sorrow attached even to pleasure, and from then on shuns both pleasure and pain. However, the fruits of actions continue to entrap ordinary beings.

How to minimize afflictions

Patañjali counsels dispassion towards pleasures and pains and recommends the practice of meditation to attain freedom and beatitude. First he describes in detail the eightfold path of yoga. Following this path helps one to avoid the dormant, hidden sufferings which may surface when physical health, energy and mental poise are disturbed. This suggests that the eightfold path of yoga is suitable for the unhealthy as well as for the healthy, enabling all to develop the power to combat physical and mental diseases.

Cause of afflictions

The prime cause of afflictions is *avidyā*: the failure to understand the conjunction between the seer and the seen: *puruṣa* and *prakṛti*. The external world lures the seer towards its pleasures, creating desire. The inevitable non-fulfilment of desires in turn creates pain, which suffocates the inner being. Nature and her beauties are there for enjoyment and pleasure (*bhoga*) and also for freedom and emancipation (*yoga*). If we use them indiscriminately, we are bound by the chains of pleasure and pain. A judicious use of them leads to the bliss which is free from pleasure mixed with pain. The twin paths to this goal are practice (*abhyāsa*), the path of evolution, of going forward; and detachment or renunciation (*vairāgya*), the path of involution, abstaining from the fruits of action and from worldly concerns and engagements.

Cosmology of nature

In *sāṁkhya* philosophy, the process of evolution and the interaction of spirit and matter, essence and form, are carefully explained.

To follow nature's evolution from its subtlest concept to its grossest or most dense manifestation, we must start with root nature, *mūla-prakṛti*. At this phase of its development, nature is infinite, attributeless and undifferentiated. We may call this phase 'noumenal' or *aliṅga* (without mark): it can be apprehended only by intuition. It is postulated that the qualities of nature, or *guṇas*, exist in *mūla-prakṛti* in perfect equilibrium; one third *sattva*, one third *rajas* and one third *tamas*.

Root nature evolves into the phenomenal stage, called *liṅga* (with mark). At this point a disturbance or redistribution takes place in the *guṇas*, giving nature its turbulent characteristic, which is to say that one quality will always predominate over the other two (though never to their entire exclusion; for example, the proportion might be 7/10 *tamas*, 2/10 *rajas*, 1/10 *sattva*, or any other disproportionate rate). The first and most subtle stage of the phenomenal universe is *mahat*, cosmic intelligence. *Mahat* is the 'great principle', embodying a spontaneous motivating force in nature, without subject or object, acting in both creation and dissolution.

Nature further evolves into the stage called *aviśeṣa* (universal or non-specific) which can be understood by the intellect but not directly perceived by the senses. To this phase belong the subtle characteristics of the five elements, which may be equated with the infra-atomic structure of elements. These may be explained at a basic level as the inherent quality of smell in earth (*pṛthvi*), of taste in water (*āp*), of sight or shape in fire (*tej*), of touch in air (*vāyu*) and of sound in ether (*ākāśa*). The 'I' principle is also in this group.

The final stage, *viśeṣa*, in which nature is specific and obviously manifest, includes the five elements, the five senses of perception (ears, eyes, nose, tongue and skin), the five organs of action (arms, legs, mouth, generative and excretory organs), and lastly the mind, or the eleventh sense. So in all, there are twenty-four principles (*tattvas*) of nature, and a twenty-fifth: *puruṣa*, *ātman*, or soul. *Puruṣa* permeates and transcends nature, without belonging to it.

(When *puruṣa* stirs the other principles into activity, it is the path of evolution. Its withdrawal from nature is the path of involution. If *puruṣa* interacts virtuously with the properties of nature, bliss is experienced; for such a *puruṣa*, *prakṛti* becomes a heaven. If wrongly experienced, it becomes a hell.

Sometimes, *puruṣa* may remain indifferent, yet we know that nature stirs on its own through the mutation of the *guṇas*, but takes a long time to surface. If *puruṣa*, gives a helping hand, nature is disciplined to move in the right way, whether on the path of evolution or involution.)

The sixteen principles of the *viśeṣa* stage are the five elements, the five senses of perception and five organs of action, and the mind. They are definable and distinguishable. At the *aviśeṣa* stage, all five *tanmātras* – smell, taste, sight or shape, touch and sound – and *ahaṁkāra*, ego, are undistinguishable and indefinable, yet nevertheless entities in themselves. At the material level of creation, *tamas* is greater than *rajas* and *sattva*, whereas at the psycho-sensory level, *rajas* and *sattva* together predominate.

The interaction of the *guṇas* with these sixteen principles shapes our destiny according to our actions. Effectively, our experiences in life derive from the gross manifestations of nature, whether painful or pleasurable; that is, whether manifesting as physical affliction or as art. The delusion that this is the only 'real' level can lead to bondage, but fortunately the evolutionary or unfolding structure of nature has provided the possibility of involution, which is the return journey to the source. This is achieved by re-absorbing the specific principles into the non-specific, then back into the *aliṅga* state, and finally by withdrawing and merging all phenomenal nature back into its noumenal root, the unmanifested *mūla-prakṛti*, rather as one might fold up a telescope.

At the moment when the seer confronts his own self, the principles of nature have been drawn up into their own primordial root and remain quietly there without ruffling the serenity of the *puruṣa*. It is sufficient to say here that the involutionary process is achieved by the intervention of discriminating intelligence, and by taming and re-balancing the *guṇas* to their noumenal perfect proportions, so that each stage of re-absorption can take place. Yoga shows us how to do this, starting from the most basic manifest level, our own body.

Once the principles have been withdrawn into their root, their potential remains dormant, which is why a person in the state of *samādhi is* but can not *do*; the outward form of nature has folded up like a bird's wings. If the *sādhaka* does not pursue his *sādhana* with sufficient zeal, but rests on his laurels, the principles of nature will be re-activated to ill effect. Nature's turbulence will again obscure the light of the *puruṣa* as the *sādhaka* is again caught up in the wheel of joy and sorrow. But he who has reached the divine union of *puruṣa* and *prakṛti*, and then redoubles his efforts, has only *kaivalya* before him.

Characteristics of *Puruṣa*

Puruṣa, the seer or the soul, is absolute pure knowledge. Unlike nature (*prakṛti*), which is subject to change, *puruṣa* is eternal and unchanging. Free from the qualities of nature, it is an absolute knower of everything. The seer is beyond words, and indescribable. It is the intelligence, one of nature's sheaths, which enmeshes the seer in the playground of nature and influences and contaminates its purity. As a mirror, when covered with dust, cannot reflect clearly, so the seer, though pure, cannot reflect clearly if the intelligence is clouded. The aspirant who follows the eightfold path of yoga develops discriminative understanding, *viveka*, and learns to use the playground of nature to clear the intelligence and experience the seer.

Fulfilment

Everyone has an inborn desire to develop sensitivity and maturity in intelligence. That is why God has provided the principles of nature – so that the seer can commune with them and make the fullest use of them for his intellectual and spiritual growth. Nature is there to serve its master, the seer, *puruṣa* or *ātman*, the inner being of man. It becomes an obstacle to spiritual enlightenment when used for sensual pleasure, but on the other hand it can help its master to realize his potential and true stature. It is not the fault of nature if human beings abuse it or fall prey to its temptations. Nature is always ready to oblige, or to remain ineffectual, according to our deeds. When we have overcome our intellectual and emotional defects, nature's gifts readily serve us for realization of the soul. Having fulfilled their functions, they withdraw.

This true Self-Realization is the peak of development of intelligence. It must be sustained, with uninterrupted awareness, in thought, word and deed: then the purpose of nature's contact with and withdrawal from the seer are fully understood. All sorrows and hatred are washed away, and everlasting unalloyed peace come to the seeker. Nature continues to taunt throughout life, with afflictions and uncertainties, those who have no discriminative power and awareness.

Seven states of wisdom

After explaining the functions of nature and of the seer, Patañjali speaks of the seven states of understanding or wisdom (*prajñā*) that emerge from the release of nature's contact with the seer. First let us identify the seven corresponding states of ignorance, or *avidyā*:

1. smallness, feebleness, insignificance, inferiority, meanness
2. unsteadiness, fickleness, mutability
3. living with pains, afflictions, misery, agony
4. living with the association of pain
5. mistaking the perishable body for the Self
6. creating conditions for undergoing sorrow
7. believing that union with the soul (yoga) is impossible, and acting as though that were so

The seven states of wisdom are:

1. knowing that which has to be known
2. discarding that which is to be discarded
3. attaining that which has to be attained
4. doing that which has to be done
5. winning the goal that is to be won
6. freeing the intelligence from the pull of the three *guṇas* of nature
7. achieving emancipation of the soul so that it shines in its own light

These seven states of wisdom are interpreted as right desire, right reflection, disappearance of memory and mind, experiencing pure *sattva* or the truth (reality), indifference to praise and blame, reabsorption of phenomenal creation, and living in the vision of the soul. They may be further simplified as:

1. understanding the body within and without
2. understanding energy and its uses
3. understanding mind
4. consistency of will
5. awareness of experience
6. awareness of pure quintessence, sentiment and beauty
7. understanding that the individual soul, *jīvātman*, is a particle of the Universal Spirit, *Paramātman*

The *Yoga Vasiṣṭa* correlates this sūtra (II.27) with the seven stages of individual development:

1 study and cultivation of the company of wise men
2 capacity to solve problems
3 development of non-attachment
4 dissolution of inherent faults
5 working towards the bliss in which a half-sleeping and half-wakeful state is experienced
6 experience of a deep sleep state
7 attaining a state in which purity, tranquillity and compassion flow out towards others.

The seven frontiers of awareness also correlate with the five sheaths or *kośas* of the body. Consciousness is the sixth, and the inner self, the seventh.

Patañjali describes the seven states of awareness as:

1 emerging consciousness (*vyutthāna citta*)
2 refraining consciousness (*nirodha citta*)
3 tranquil consciousness (*śānta citta*)
4 one-pointed consciousness (*ekāgra citta*)
5 sprouted consciousness (*nirmāṇa citta*)
6 rent consciousness (*chidra citta*)
7 pure consciousness (*divya citta*)
(See III.9, 10, 11; IV.27 and 29.)

It is also possible to consider the ethical, physical, physiological, neurological, emotional, intellectual and spiritual domains as the seven states of awareness. When one rests on the vision of the soul, divinity is felt in this empirical state.

The Yogic disciplines

The yogic disciplines are *yama* (restraint) and *niyama* (practice or observance). These disciplines channel the energies of the organs of action and the senses of perception in the right direction. *Āsana* (posture) results in balance, stillness of mind, and power to penetrate the intelligence. Through *āsana* we learn to know the body well and to distinguish between motion and action: motion excites the mind while action absorbs it. *Prāṇāyāma* (control of energy through restraint of breath) and *pratyāhāra* (withdrawal of the senses) help the *sādhaka* to explore his hidden facets, and enable him to penetrate the core of his being. *Dhāraṇā* (concentration), *dhyāna* (meditation) and *samādhi* (total absorption) are the fulfilment of yogic discipline, the essence or natural constituents of yoga. They develop when the other five disciplines have been mastered. Actually, all eight intermingle and interweave to form the whole seamless body of yoga.

Yama

There are five *yamas*: *ahiṁsā* (non-violence or non-injury), *satya* (truthfulness), *asteya* (non-stealing), *brahmacarya* (continence) and *aparigraha* (freedom from avarice or non-covetousness).

Intending no harm in word, thought or deed; being sincere, honest and faithful; being careful not to misappropriate another's wealth; being chaste and not coveting the possessions of others or accepting gifts, are the practices of *yama*. It is essential they be observed and followed. They are to be practised individually and collectively irrespective of lineage, place, time, condition or career. The *yamas* are mighty universal vows, says Patañjali.

Effects of *Yama*

If the *sādhaka* adheres to the principles of *ahiṁsā*, all beings around him abandon their hostile behaviour. By observance of *satya*, spoken words fructify into action. All kinds of treasures are bestowed on him who observes *asteya*. For a *brahmacārī* (a chaste or celibate person), vigour, vitality, energy and spiritual knowledge flow like a river. One who observes *aparigraha* will come to know of his past and future lives.

Niyama

The five *niyamas* are to be followed not merely as individual, but also as spiritual, disciplines. They are: *śauca* (cleanliness or purity), *santoṣa* (contentment), *tapas* (religious fervour), *svādhyāya* (study of the sacred scriptures and of one's own self) and *Īśvara praṇidhāna* (surrender of the self to God).

Śauca is of two types, external and internal. One's daily bath is external; *āsana* and *prāṇāyāma* cleanse one internally. They help to cleanse one's thoughts, words and actions, and make the body fit for its Lord to dwell in. *Saṇtoṣa* brings about a state of cheerfulness and benevolence. *Tapas* is a burning effort involving purification, self-discipline and austere practice. It is religiousness or devoutness in the practice of yoga. *Tapaṣ* purges and purifies the body, senses and mind. *Svādhyāya* enlightens the practitioner with the knowledge of his inner immortal being. *Īśvara praṇidhāna* brings the inner being to his creator, the Supreme God.

Actually, the observance of *yama* brings about niyama, and the practice of *niyama* disciplines one to follow the principles of *yama*. For example, non-violence brings purity of thought and deed, truthfulness leads to contentment, non-covetousness leads to *tapas*. Chastity leads to the study of the self, and non-possessiveness to surrender to God. Similarly, cleanliness leads towards non-violence, and contentment towards truthfulness. *Tapas* guides one not to misappropriate another's wealth. Study of the self leads towards chastity, and surrender to God frees one from possessiveness.

By now, the reader is acquainted with the causes of afflictions. Not only do *yama* and *niyama* help to minimize and uproot them; they are also the firm foundation of spiritual experience. They are the ethical disciplines which show us what must be done and what must be discarded. They are the golden keys to unlock the spiritual gates.

Sooner or later, improper use of words, impure thoughts and wrong actions result in pain. Pain may be self-inflicted (*ādhyātmika*), due to fate or heredity (*ādhidaivika*), or to imbalance of elements in the body (*ādhibhautika*). It may be caused by lust, anger or greed, indulged in directly, by provocation or by compliancy. The resulting sorrows may be mild, moderate or intense.

The causes of lust, anger and greed can be countered directly by self-analysis, or subdued by invoking their opposites: balance, poise, peace and harmony. Because the latter dualistic approach may cause one to hide from the facts, the former is the better approach. The use of analysis, study and investigation requires courage, strength and discretion. The evocation of opposite tendencies is not a cure, but a help. The first is a direct method of purification; the second an indirect method of appeasement. Patañjali suggests that both should be followed to speed progress.

Āsana and its effects

Āsana means posture, the positioning of the body as a whole with the involvement of the mind and soul. *Āsana* has two facets, pose and repose. Pose is the artistic assumption of a position. 'Reposing in the pose' means finding the perfection of a pose and maintaining it, reflecting in it with penetration of the intelligence and with dedication. When the seeker is closer to the soul, the *āsanas* come with instantaneous extension, repose and poise.

In the beginning, effort is required to master the *āsanas*. Effort involves hours, days, months, years and even several lifetimes of work. When effortful effort in an *āsana* becomes effortless effort, one has mastered that *āsana*. In this way, each *āsana* has to become effortless. While performing the *āsanas*, one has to relax the cells of the brain, and activate the cells of the vital organs and of the structural and skeletal body. Then intelligence and consciousness may spread to each and every cell.

The conjunction of effort, concentration and balance in *āsana* forces us to live intensely in the present moment, a rare experience in modern life. This actuality, or being in the present, has both a strengthening and a cleansing effect: physically in the rejection of disease, mentally by ridding our mind of stagnated thoughts or prejudices; and, on a very high level where perception and action become one, by teaching us instantaneous correct action; that is to say, action which does not produce reaction. On that level we may also expunge the residual effects of past actions.

The three origins of pain are eradicated by *āsana* as we progress from clear vision through right thinking to correct action.

To the new student or non-practitioner of yoga a relentless pursuit of perfection in *āsana* may seem pointless. To advanced students, a teacher teaches a whole *āsana* in relationship to what is happening in a single action. At this subtlest level, when we are able to observe the workings of *rajas*, *tamas* and *sattva* in one toe, and to adjust the flow of energy in *iḍā*, *piṅgalā* and *suṣumnā* (the three principal *nāḍīs*, or energy channels), the macrocosmic order of nature is perceived in even the smallest aspects. And when the student then learns how the minutest modifications of a toe can modify the whole *āsana*, he is observing how the microcosm relates to the whole, and the organic completeness of universal structure is grasped.

The body is the temple of the soul. It can truly become so if it is kept healthy, clean and pure through the practice of *āsana*.

Āsanas act as bridges to unite the body with the mind, and the mind with the soul. They lift the *sādhaka* from the clutches of afflictions and lead him towards disciplined freedom. They help to transform him by guiding his consciousness away from the body towards awareness of the soul.

Through *āsana*, the *sādhaka* comes to know and fully realize the finite body, and merge it with the infinite – the soul. Then there is neither the known nor the unknown and only then does the *āsana* exist wholly. This is the essence of a perfect *āsana*.

Prāṇāyāma and its effects

Patañjali states that there must be a progression from *āsana* to *prāṇāyāma*, but does not mention such a progression in the other branches of yoga. He states that *prāṇāyāma* should be attempted only after perfection is attained in *āsana*. This does not mean one *āsana* alone, as is sometimes suggested.

It should be understood why one *āsana* is not a sufficient basis for the study of *prāṇāyāma*. In *prāṇāyāma*, the spine and the spinal muscles are the sources of action and the lungs are the receiving instruments. They must be trained to open and to extend backwards, forwards, upwards and outwards, and the spinal muscles straightened, cultured and toned to create space and stimulate the spinal nerves to draw energy from the breath. Inverted postures, forward bends, backbends – the whole range of postures – are therefore essential if we are to derive from *prāṇāyāma* the maximum benefit with the minimum strain.

Normal breath flows irregularly, depending on one's environment and emotional state. In the beginning, this irregular flow of breath is controlled by a deliberate process. This control creates ease in the inflow and outflow of the breath. When this ease is attained, the breath must be regulated with attention. This is *prāṇāyāma*.

Prāṇa means life force and *āyāma* means ascension, expansion and extension. *Prāṇāyāma* is the expansion of the life force through control of the breath. In modern terms, *prāṇa* is equated to bio-energy and works as follows. According to *sāṁkhya* and yoga philosophies, man is composed of the five elements: earth, water, fire, air and ether. The spine is an element of earth and acts as the field for respiration. Distribution and creation of space in the torso is the function of ether. Respiration represents the element of air. The remaining elements, water and fire, are by nature opposed to one another. The practice of *prāṇāyāma* fuses them to produce energy. This energy is called *prāṇa*: life force or bio-energy.

Āyāma means extension, vertical ascension, as well as horizontal expansion and circumferential expansion of the breath, lungs and ribcage.

Prāṇāyāma by nature has three components: inhalation, exhalation and retention. They are carefully learned by elongating the breath and prolonging the time of retention according to the elasticity of the torso, the length and depth of breath and the precision of movements. This *prāṇāyāma* is known as deliberate or *sahita prāṇāyāma* as one must practise it consciously and continuously in order to learn its rhythm.

To inhalation, exhalation and retention, Patañjali adds one more type of *prāṇāyāma* that is free from deliberate action. This *prāṇāyāma*, being natural and non-deliberate, transcends the sphere of breath which is modulated by mental volition. It is called *kevala kuṁbhaka* or *kevala prāṇāyāma*.

The practice of *prāṇāyāma* removes the veil of ignorance covering the light of intelligence and makes the mind a fit instrument to embark on meditation for the vision of the soul. This is the spiritual quest.

(For further details see *Light on Yoga, The Art of Yoga* and *Light on*

Prāṇāyāma (HarperCollins*Publishers*) and *The Tree of Yoga* (Fine Line Books).

Pratyāhāra

Through the practices of *yama*, *niyama*, *āsana* and *prāṇāyāma*, the body and its energy are mastered. The next stage, *pratyāhāra*, achieves the conquest of the senses and mind.

When the mind becomes ripe for meditation, the senses rest quietly and stop importuning the mind for their gratification. Then the mind, which hitherto acted as a bridge between the senses and the soul, frees itself from the senses and turns towards the soul to enjoy its spiritual heights. This is the effect of disciplines laid out in *sādhana pāda*. *Pratyāhāra*, the result of the practice of *yama*, *niyama*, *āsana* and *prāṇāyāma*, forms the foundation for *dhāraṇā*, *dhyāna* and *samādhi*. Through practice of these five stages of yoga, all the layers or sheaths of the self from the skin to the consciousness are penetrated, subjugated and sublimated to enable the soul to diffuse evenly throughout. This is true *sādhana*.

III. Vibhūti Pāda

In *samādhi pāda*, Patañjali explains why the intelligence is hazy, sluggish and dull, and gives practical disciplines to minimize and finally eliminate the dross which clouds it. Through these, the *sādhaka* develops a clear head and an untainted mind, and his senses of perception are then naturally tamed and subdued. The *sādhaka*'s intelligence and consciousness can now become fit instruments for meditation on the soul.

In *vibhūti pāda*, Patañjali first shows the *sādhaka* the need to integrate the intelligence, ego and 'I' principle. He then guides him in the subtle disciplines: concentration (*dhāraṇā*), meditation (*dhyāna*) and total absorption (*samādhi*). With their help, the intelligence, ego and 'I' principle are sublimated. This may lead either to the release of various supernatural powers or to Self-Realization.

Saṁyama

Patañjali begins this *pāda* with *dhāraṇā*, concentration, and points out some places within and outside the body to be used by the seeker for concentration and contemplation. If *dhāraṇā* is maintained steadily, it flows into *dhyāna* (meditation). When the meditator and the object meditated upon become one, *dhyāna* flows into *samādhi*. Thus, *dhāraṇā*, *dhyāna* and *samādhi* are interconnected. This integration is called by Patañjali *saṁyama*. Through *saṁyama* the intelligence, ego and sense of individuality withdraw into their seed. Then the *sādhaka*'s intelligence shines brilliantly with the lustre of wisdom, and his understanding is enlightened. He turns his attention to a progressive exploration of the core of his being, the soul.

Intelligence

Having defined the subtle facets of man's nature as intelligence, ego, the 'I' principle and the inner self, Patañjali analyses them one by one to reveal their hidden content. He begins with the intellectual brain, which oscillates between one-pointed and scattered attention. If the *sādhaka* does not recollect how, where and when his attention became disconnected from the object contemplated, he becomes a wanderer: his intelligence remains untrained. By careful observation, and reflection on the qualities of the intelligence, the *sādhaka* distinguishes between its multi-faceted and its one-pointed manifestation, and between the restless and silent states. To help him, Patañjali explains how the discriminative faculty can be used to control emerging thought, to suppress the emergence of thought waves and to observe the appearance of moments of silence. If the *sādhaka* observes and holds these intermittent periods of silence, he experiences a state of restfulness. If this is deliberately prolonged, the stream of tranquillity will flow without disturbance.

Holding this tranquil flow of calmness without allowing the intelligence to forget itself, the seeker moves towards the seer. This movement leads to inner attention and awareness, which is in turn the basis for drawing the consciousness towards integration with the inner self. When this integration is established, the seeker realizes that the contemplator, the instrument used for contemplation, and the object of contemplation are one and the same, the seer or the soul: in other words, subject, object and instrument become one.

Bringing the intelligence, *buddhi*, to a refined, tranquil steadiness is *dhāraṇā*. When this is achieved, *buddhi* is re-absorbed by a process of involution into the consciousness, *citta*, whose inherent expression is a sharp awareness but without focus. This is *dhyāna*. The discrimination and unwinking observation which are properties of *buddhi* must constantly be ready to prevent consciousness from clouding and *dhyāna* from slipping away. *Buddhi* is the activator of pure *citta*.

When the *sādhaka* has disciplined and understood the intelligence, the stream of tranquillity flows smoothly, uninfluenced by pleasure or pain. Then he learns to exercise his awareness, to make it flow with peace and poise. This blending of awareness and tranquillity brings about a state of virtue, which is the powerful ethic, or *śakti*, of the soul, the culmination of intelligence and consciousness. This culturing of intelligence is an evolution, and virtue is its special quality. Maintenance of this civilized, cultured, virtuous state leads to a perfect propriety, wherein the intelligence continues to be refined, and the *sādhaka* moves ever closer to the spiritual zenith of yoga.

Properties of yoga

Patañjali guides the refined *sādhaka* in tracing the movements, order and sequence of each action and thought that arises. By retracing his steps through yogic discipline, the *sādhaka* coordinates his thoughts and actions so that there is no time gap between them. When there is absolute synchronicity of thought and action, the yogi is freed from the material limitations of time and space and this generates extraordinary powers. Patañjali describes these powers as *vibhūtis*, or properties, of yoga.

The properties of yoga are many. Experiencing even one of their extraordinary effects is an indication that the *sādhaka* is on the right path in his practice of yoga. However, see the next section, 'Caution', on page 37.

1 He begins to know the past and future
2 He understands the language of all people, birds and animals
3 He knows his past and future lives
4 He reads the minds of others
5 If necessary, he can define even the precise details of what is in the minds of others
6 He becomes invisible at will
7 He can arrest the senses: hearing, touch, sight, taste and smell
8 He knows the exact time of his death by intuition or through omens
9 He is friendly and compassionate to all
10 He becomes strong as an elephant and his movements are as graceful as a peacock
11 He clearly sees objects near and far, gross and fine, and concealed
12 He knows the working of the solar system
13 He knows the functions of the lunar system and through that, the position of the galaxies
14 He reads the movements of stars from the pole star and predicts world events

15 He knows his body and its orderly functions
16 He conquers hunger and thirst
17 He makes his body and mind immobile like a tortoise
18 He has visions of perfected beings, teachers and masters
19 He has the power to perceive anything and everything
20 He becomes aware of the properties of consciousness
21 By knowing the properties of consciousness he uses consciousness to light the lamp of the soul
22 Divine faculties which are beyond the range of ordinary senses come to him because of his enlightened soul
23 He leaves his body consciously and enters others' bodies at will
24 He walks over water, swamp and thorns
25 He creates fire at will
26 He hears distant sounds
27 He levitates
28 He frees himself from afflictions at will and often lives without a body
29 He controls nature's constituents, qualities and purposes
30 He becomes lord of the elements and their counterparts
31 He possesses an excellent body with grace, strength, perfect complexion and lustre
32 He has perfect control over his senses and mind, and their contact with the lower self or the 'I' consciousness
33 He transforms body, senses, mind, intelligence and consciousness to utmost sharpness and speed in tune with his very soul
34 He gains dominion over all creation and all knowledge

Caution

These powers are extraordinary. The appearance of any one of them indicates that the *sādhaka* has followed methods appropriate to his evolution. But he should not mistake these powers for the goal of his search. For onlookers they may seem to be great accomplishments, but for the *sādhaka* they are hindrances to *samādhi*. Even celestial beings try to seduce the *sādhaka*. If he succumbs to these temptations, misfortunes overwhelm him.

If a yogi gets carried away by supernatural powers and uses them for fame, he fails in his *sādhanā*. He is like a man who tries to save himself from the wind only to get caught up in a whirlwind. A yogi who attains certain powers and misconstrues them for his goal is caught in their effects and exposes himself to their afflictions. Therefore, Patañjali warns the *sādhaka* to renounce these accomplishments, so that the gates of everlasting bliss may open for him. He is counselled to develop non-attachment which destroys pride, a cardinal pitfall for those who acquire powers.

Adherence to the practice of *yama* and *niyama*, as described in *sādhana pāda*, will ensure that the *sādhaka* does not get caught up in these powers, or misuse them.

Moment and movement

Moment is subjective and movement is objective. Patañjali explains that the moment is the present and the present is the eternal now: it is timeless, and real. When it slips from attention, it becomes movement, and movement is time. As moment rolls into movement, the past and the future appear and the moment disappears. Going with the movements of moments is the future; retraction of this is the past. The moment alone is the present.

Past and future create changes; the present is changeless. The fluctuations of consciousness into the past and future create time. If the mind, intelligence and consciousness are kept steady, and aware of moments without being caught in movements, the state of no-mind and no-time is experienced. This state is *amanaskatva*. The seer sees directly, independent of the workings of the mind. The yogi becomes the mind's master, not its slave. He lives in a mind-free, time-free state. This is known as *vivekaja jñānam*: vivid, true knowledge.

Pure intelligence

Exalted intelligence is pure and true, untainted and uncontaminated. It distinguishes, clearly and instantly, the difference between similar entities, without analysing them according to rank, creed, quality and place.

This intelligence is true, pure and clean, as is the very soul. The yogi who possesses it is free from pride and prejudice. His intelligence and consciousness now rise to the level of the soul. As honey tastes the same from whichever side of the honeycomb it is taken, so, in the yogi, the body cells, senses, mind, intelligence, consciousness and conscience equally reflect the light of the soul. All parts of the seer appear as the soul. This is *kaivalya*. It comes when the powers which attract the misguided, but distract the yogi's consciousness, are renounced.

IV: Kaivalya Pāda

Kaivalya means exclusiveness, or eternal emancipation. It is release from *karma*: the consequences and obligations of our actions. *Kaivalya* is an absolute, indivisible state of existence. In it, the yogi is stripped of thoughts, mind, intellect and ego, and freed from the play of the *guṇas* of nature, *sattva*, *rajas* and *tamas*. He becomes a *guṇātītan*, a pure, flawless person.

In *vibhūti pāda*, Patañjali describes the supernatural powers that attend such exalted yogis and how the renunciation of these powers results in *kaivalya*: the crowning end of the yogic *sādhana*, a state of fullness of the soul and of unique aloneness.

This chapter, *Kaivalya pāda*, is impressive and exhaustive. One of its main themes is that the content of consciousness is pure, absolute and divine, provided it is unsullied by action, be it white (*sāttvic*), grey (*rājasic*) or black (*tāmasic*). The absolute nature of consciousness is to be realized by propitious birth, spiritual fervour and meditation. The cleansing transformation of consciousness liberates life-energy which accelerates the process of self-evolution. Progressively, one disentangles oneself from life's preoccupations with *dharma*, duty; *artha*, means of livelihood; and *kāma*, worldly enjoyment. This transcendence leads to freedom, or *mokṣa*. Consciousness, released from the attributes of nature, dissolves in the soul, *puruṣa*.

This chapter deals with the necessary rejection by yogis of the supernatural powers which attend their spiritual ascent, and indicates how such men and women, who have in a sense left the world behind, may then serve the world.

Five types of Yogis

Kaivalya pāda opens with the contention that prodigious yogic powers may be inborn, acquired by merit accumulated through practice in former lives. They may also be attained through use of herbs (*auṣadhi*), incantation (*mantra*), devoted discipline (*tapas*), meditation (*dhyāna*) and total absorption (*samādhi*).

In these five types of yogis, nature's energy, which later becomes known as *kuṇḍalini*, flows with ever-increasing abundance, preparing them to receive the infinite light of the soul. If misused, this energetic current will vanish, after destroying its user. This is why *tapas* and *samādhi* are held to be the best of the five: they provide a firm foundation for stable growth, which prevents the yogi from misusing the energy built up through his practices.

The yogi's judicious use of natural forces can be compared to the farmer who floods his fields one by one within their earthen banks, letting the water thoroughly drench the soil before breaking open a new channel into another. For safety's sake, the yogi employs method and restraint so as to use nature's energy (*śakti*) intelligently to gain wisdom.

Talent

It takes talent to grasp nature's potential and measure its use. The danger is that power leads to pride and builds ego, eclipsing one's essential divinity. The root of the ego is the same pure consciousness; it is its contact with external phenomena that generates desire, the seed of impurity. Purity is humility. When sullied by cleverness it becomes pride, which causes consciousness to dissipate itself in the fluctuations of thought. *Tapas* and *samādhi* are the most reliable means to acquire yogic talent.

Actions

Actions are of four types. They are black, white, grey, or without these attributes. The last is beyond the *guṇas* of *rajas*, *tamas* and *sattva*, free from intention, motivation and desire, pure and sourceless, and outside the law of cause and effect that governs all other actions. Motivated action leads eventually to pride, affliction and unhappiness; the genuine yogi performs only actions which are motiveless: free of desire, pride and effect.

The chain of cause and effect is like a ball endlessly rebounding from the walls and floor of a squash court. Memory, conscious or sublimated, links this chain, even across many lives. This is because every action of the first three types leaves behind a residual impression, encoded in our deepest memory, which thereafter continues to turn the karmic wheel, provoking reaction and further action. The consequences of action may take effect instantaneously, or lie in abeyance for years, even through several lives. *Tāmasic* action is considered to give rise to pain and sorrow, *rājasic* to mixed results, and *sāttvic* to more agreeable ones. Depending on their provenance, the fruits of action may either tie us to lust, anger and greed, or turn us towards the spiritual quest. These residual impressions are called *saṃskāras*: they build the cycles of our existence and decide the station, time and place of our birth. The yogi's actions, being pure, leave no impressions and excite no reactions, and are therefore free from residual impressions.

Desires and impressions

Desires, and knowledge derived from memory or residual impressions, exist eternally. They are as much a part of our being as is the will to cling to life. In a perfect yogi's life, desires and impressions have an end; when the mechanism of cause and effect is disconnected by pure, motiveless action, the yogi transcends the world of duality and desires and attachment wither and fall away.

Time

Yogic discipline eradicates ignorance, *avidyā*. When illusion is banished, time becomes timeless. Though time is a continuum, it has three movements: past, present and future. Past and future are woven into the present and the present is timeless and eternal. Like the potter's wheel, the present – the moment – rolls into movement as day and night, creating the impression that time is moving. The mind, observing the movement of time, differentiates it as past, present and future. Because of this, the perception of objects varies at different times.

Though the permanent characters of time, the object and the subject remain in their own entities, the mind sees them differently according to the development of its intelligence, and creates disparity between observation and reflection. Hence, actions and fulfilments differ. An illustration of this would be that we recognize the difference between what is involved when a murderer kills for money, a soldier kills for his country and a man kills defending his family against bandits. It is all killing, but the implications are radically different in each case, according to the development of the individual.

The yogi is alert to, and aware of, the present, and lives in the present, using past experience only as a platform for the present. This brings changelessness in the attitude of the mind towards the object seen.

Subject and object

Earlier chapters point out that whereas nature is eternal, its qualities or *guṇas*, are ever-changing. This blending of the *guṇas* creates diversity in the mind so that it sees objects in different ways. The object is the same and the mind, too, is the same. But the same mind has many qualities of mood and behaviour. This fragmentation is the cause of *avidyā*. The mind divided by the *guṇas* moulds and remoulds man. As the *guṇas* move in rhythmic unity, intellectual development differs qualitatively in each person and each one sees objects differently, though their essence does not change.

The yogi studies the uniqueness of that rhythmic mutation, keeps aloof from it, and rests in his own essence, his soul. This essence, and the essence of the perceived object, are the same for him. Through self-examination, he realizes that objects do not change, but that he himself fabricates their apparent changes. He learns to perceive without prejudice, aware that objects exist independently, irrespective of his cognition of them. His clear, unpolluted mind sees objects as they are, separate from him and therefore unable to leave an impression on him. Being free from bias, he is free from *karma*.

Cit and *citta* (universal and individual consciousness)

The unalterable seer (*cit*) is the Lord of the consciousness. He is ever-present, changeless, constant, ever-luminous. The seer can be both subject and object at the same time. He is aware of all mutations taking place in his mind, intelligence and consciousness. He knows that they are his products and that they may taint him as long as *avidyā* and *asmitā* survive.

The seer is the seed, and consciousness the seedling. Mind is the stem, and *vṛittis*, the fluctuations or thought-waves, are the leaves, relayed via mind through the single consciousness, the stem, back to the seed.

Consciousness and its branches, intelligence, mind and thought, become objects of the seer. The branches have no existence of their own without consciousness, and consciousness has none without the seer. It borrows light from the seer and extends towards intelligence, mind and thought. As it is not self-illumined it cannot be at once subject and object. It is a knowable object to the seer just as the objects of the world are knowable to it.

The *cit* (seer, soul, cosmic consciousness) is a passive, omniscient witness, whereas the *citta* (created or 'sprouted' consciousness) is active, impressionable and engaged, because it is involved in a direct relationship with the outside world. But when that involvement is analysed, controlled and brought to stillness, the *citta* gravitates towards its source, the *cit*, and takes on its characteristics, so that for the realized being *cit* and *citta* become one. The problem is that for the average person, the sprouted consciousness appears to be the seer, while in reality it merely masks the seer. Studying *citta*, we come to understand that it has no light of its own, but is dependent on its progenitor, the seer. Until this realization dawns, consciousness acts as a prism, distorting vision. Once it merges with the seer it becomes a perfect reflector, as well as a reflection, mirroring its own pure image, the soul reflecting on the soul.

So we see that *citta* can be pulled in two directions: outwards towards its mother, nature, *prakṛti*, or inwards towards its father, spirit, *puruṣa*. The role of yoga is to show us that the ultimate goal of *citta* is to take the second path, away from the world to the bliss of the soul. Yoga both offers the goal and supplies the means to reach it. He who finds his soul is *Yogeśvara*, Lord or God of yoga, or *Yogirāja*, a King among yogis.

Now, nothing is left to be known or acquired by him.

Caution

Patañjali warns that even such exalted yogis are not beyond all danger of relapse. Even when oneness between *cit* and *citta* is achieved, inattention, carelessness, or pride in one's achievement await opportunity to return, and fissure the consciousness. In this loss of concentration, old thoughts and habits may re-emerge to disturb the harmony of *kaivalya*.

If this takes place, the yogi has no alternative but to resume his purificatory struggle in the same way as less evolved people combat their own grosser afflictions.

The dawn of spiritual and sorrowless light

If the *Yogeśvara*'s indivisible state is unwaveringly sustained, a stream of virtue pours from his heart like torrential rain: *dharma megha samādhi*, or rain-cloud of virtue or justice. The expression has two complementary overtones. *Dharma* means duty; *megha* means cloud. Clouds may either obscure the sun's light or clear the sky by sending down rain to reveal it. If *citta*'s union with the seer is fissured it drags its master towards worldly pleasures (*bhoga*). If union is maintained it leads the aspirant towards *kaivalya*. Through yogic discipline, consciousness is made virtuous so that its possessor can become, and be, a yogi, a *jñānin*, a *bhaktan* and a *paravairāgin*.

All actions and reactions cease in that person who is now a *Yogeśvara*. He is free from the clutches of nature and *karma*. From now on, there is no room in his *citta* for the production of effects; he never speaks or acts in a way that binds him to nature. When the supply of oil to a lamp is stopped, the lamp is extinguished. In this yogi, when the fuel of desires dries out, the lamp of the mind cannot burn, and begins to fade on its own. Then infinite wisdom issues forth spontaneously.

The knowledge that is acquired through senses, mind and intellect is insignificant beside that emanating from the vision of the seer. This is the real intuitive knowledge.

When the clouds disappear, the sky clears and the sun shines brilliantly. When the sun shines, does one need artificial light to see? When the light of the soul blazes, the light of consciousness is needed no longer.

Nature and its qualities cease to affect the fulfilled yogi. From now on they serve him devotedly, without interfering with or influencing his true glory. He understands the sequence of time and its relationship with nature. He is crowned with the wisdom of living in the eternal Now. The eternal Now is Divine and he too is Divine. All his aims of life are fulfilled. He is a *kṛthārthan*, a fulfilled soul, one without equal, living in benevolent freedom and beatitude. He is alone and complete. This is *kaivalya*.

Patañjali begins the *Yoga Sūtras* with *atha*, meaning 'now', and ends with *iti*, 'that is all'. Besides this search for the soul, there is nothing.

part one

समाधिपादः ।

Samādhi Pāda

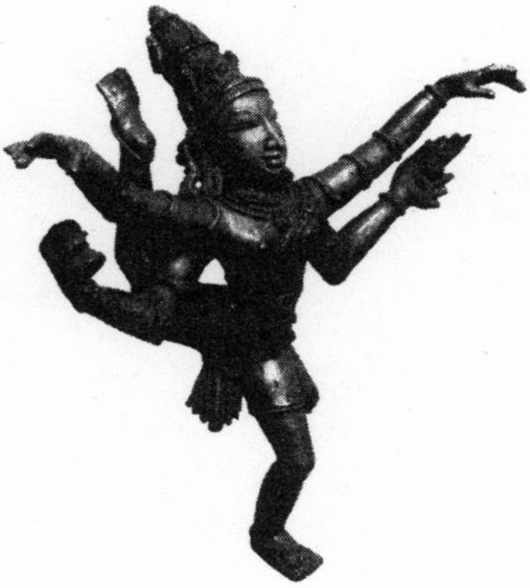

Samādhi means yoga and yoga means *samādhi*. This *pāda* therefore explains the significance of yoga as well as of *samādhi*: both mean profound meditation and supreme devotion.

For aspirants endowed with perfect physical health, mental poise, discriminative intelligence and a spiritual bent, Patañjali provides guidance in the disciplines of practice and detachment to help them attain the spiritual zenith, the vision of the soul (*ātma-darśana*).

The word *citta* has often been translated as 'mind'. In the West, it is considered that mind not only has the power of conation or volition, cognition and motion, but also that of discrimination.

But *citta* really means 'consciousness'. Indian philosophers analysed *citta* and divided it into three facets: mind (*manas*), intelligence (*buddhi*) and ego, or the sense of self (*ahaṁkāra*). They divided the mental body into two parts: the mental sheath and the intellectual sheath. People have thus come to think of consciousness and mind as the same. In this work, consciousness refers both to the mental sheath (*manomaya kośa*) as mind, and to the intellectual sheath (*vijñānamaya kośa*) as wisdom. Mind acquires knowledge objectively, whereas intelligence learns through subjective experience, which becomes wisdom. As cosmic intelligence is the first principle of nature, so consciousness is the first principle of man.

अथ योगानुशासनम् ।१।

I.1 atha yogānuśāsanam

atha now, auspiciousness, a prayer, a blessing, benediction, authority, a good omen

yoga joining, union, junction, combination, application, use, means, result, deep meditation, concentration, contemplation of the Supreme Spirit

anuśāsanam advice, direction, order, command, instructions, laying down rules and precepts, a revised text, introduction, or guide given in procedural form. Thus, it means guidance in the codes of conduct which are to be observed, and which form the base from which to cultivate one's ethical and spiritual life.

With prayers for divine blessings, now begins an exposition of the sacred art of yoga.

Now follows a detailed exposition of the discipline of yoga, given step by step in the right order, and with proper direction for self-alignment.

Patañjali is the first to offer us a codification of yoga, its practice and precepts, and the immediacy of the new light he is shedding on a known and ancient subject is emphasized by his use of the word 'now'. His reappraisal, based on his own experience, explores fresh ground, and bequeathes us a lasting, monumental work. In the cultural context of his time his words must have been crystal clear, and even to the spiritually impoverished modern mind they are never confused, although they are often almost impenetrably condensed.

The word 'now' can also be seen in the context of a progression from Patañjali's previous works, his treatises on grammar and on *āyurveda*. Logically we must consider these to predate the *Yoga Sūtras*, as grammar is a prerequisite of lucid speech and clear comprehension, and āyurvedic medicine of bodily cleanliness and inner equilibrium. Together, these works served as preparation for Patañjali's crowning exposition of yoga: the cultivation and eventual transcendence of consciousness, culminating in liberation from the cycles of rebirth.

These works are collectively known as *mokṣa śāstras* (spiritual sciences), treatises which trace man's evolution from physical and mental bondage towards ultimate freedom. The treatise on yoga flows naturally from the *āyurvedic* work, and guides the aspirant (*sādhaka*) to a trained and balanced state of consciousness.

In this first chapter Patañjali analyses the components of consciousness and its behavioural patterns, and explains how its fluctuations can be stilled in order to achieve inner absorption and integration. In the second, he reveals the whole linking mechanism of yoga, by means of which ethical conduct, bodily vigour and health and physiological vitality are built into the structure of the human evolutionary progress towards freedom. In the third chapter, Patañjali prepares the mind to reach the soul. In the fourth, he shows how the mind dissolves into the consciousness and consciousness into the soul, and how the *sādhaka* drinks the nectar of immortality.

The *Brahma Sūtra*, a treatise dealing with Vedanta philosophy (the knowledge of Brahman), also begins with the word *atha* or 'now': *athāto Brahma jijñāsā*. There, 'now' stands for the desire to know Brahman. Brahman is dealt with as the object of study and is discussed and explored throughout as the object. In the *Yoga Sūtras*, it is the seer or the true Self who is to be discovered and known. Yoga is therefore considered to be a subjective art, science and philosophy. 'Yoga' has various connotations as mentioned at the outset, but here it stands for *samādhi*, the indivisible state of existence.

So, this sūtra may be taken to mean: 'the disciplines of integration are here expounded through experience, and are given to humanity for the exploration and recognition of that hidden part of man which is beyond the awareness of the senses'.

योगश्चित्तवृत्तिनिरोधः ।२।

I.2 yogaḥ cittavṛtti nirodhaḥ

yogaḥ — union or integration from the outermost layer to the innermost self, that is, from the skin to the muscles, bones, nerves, mind, intellect, will, consciousness and self

citta — consciousness, which is made up of three factors: mind (*manas*), intellect (*buddhi*) and ego (*ahaṁkāra*). *Citta* is the vehicle of observation, attention; aims and reason; it has three functions, cognition, conation or volition, and motion

vṛtti — state of mind, fluctuations in mind, course of conduct, behaviour, a state of being, mode of action, movement, function, operation

nirodhaḥ — obstruction, stoppage, opposition, annihilation, restraint, control, cessation

Yoga is the cessation of movements in the consciousness.

Yoga is defined as restraint of fluctuations in the consciousness. It is the art of studying the behaviour of consciousness, which has three functions: cognition, conation or volition, and motion. Yoga shows ways of understanding the functionings of the mind, and helps to quieten their movements, leading one towards the undisturbed state of silence which dwells in the very seat of consciousness. Yoga is thus the art and science of mental discipline through which the mind becomes cultured and matured.

This vital sūtra contains the definition of yoga: the control or restraint of the movement of consciousness, leading to their complete cessation.

Citta is the vehicle which takes the mind (*manas*) towards the soul (*ātmā*). Yoga is the cessation of all vibration in the seat of consciousness. It is extremely difficult to convey the meaning of the word *citta* because it is the subtlest form of cosmic intelligence (*mahat*). *Mahat* is the great principle, the source of the material world of nature (*prakṛti*), as opposed to the soul, which is an offshoot of nature. According to *sāṁkhya* philosophy, creation is effected by the mingling of *prakṛti* with *Puruṣa*, the cosmic Soul. This view of cosmology is also accepted by the yoga philosophy. The principles of *Puruṣa* and *prakṛti* are the source of all action, volition and silence.

Words such as *citta*, *buddhi* and *mahat* are so often used interchangeably that the student can easily become confused. One way to structure one's understanding is to remember that every phenomenon which has reached its full evolution or individuation has a subtle or cosmic counterpart. Thus, we translate *buddhi* as the individual discriminating intelligence, and consider *mahat* to be its cosmic counterpart. Similarly, the individuated consciousness, *citta*, is matched by its subtle form *cit*. For the purpose of Self-Realization, the highest awareness of consciousness and the most refined faculty of intelligence have to work so much in partnership that it is not always useful to split hairs by separating them. (See Introduction, part I – Cosmology of Nature.)

The thinking principle, or conscience (*antaḥkaraṇa*) links the motivating principle of nature (*mahat*) to individual consciousness which can be thought of as a fluid enveloping ego (*ahaṁkāra*), intelligence (*buddhi*) and mind (*manas*). This 'fluid' tends to become cloudy and opaque due to its contact with the external world via its three components. The *sādhaka*'s aim is to bring the consciousness to a state of purity and translucence. It is important to note that consciousness not only links evolved or manifest nature to non-evolved or subtle nature; it is also closest to the soul itself, which does not belong to nature, being merely immanent in it.

Buddhi possesses the decisive knowledge which is determined by perfect action and experience. *Manas* gathers and collects information through the five senses of perception, *jñānendriyas*, and the five organs of action, *karmendriyas*. Cosmic intelligence, ego, individual intelligence, mind, the five senses of perception and the five organs of action are the products of the five elements of nature – earth, water, fire, air and ether (*pṛthvi, āp, tejas, vāyu* and *ākāśa*) – with their infra-atomic qualities of smell, taste, form or sight, touch and sound (*gandha, rasa, rūpa, sparṣa* and *śabda*).

In order to help man to understand himself, the sages analysed humans as being composed of five sheaths, or *kośas*:

Sheath	Corresponding element
Anatomical (*annamaya*)	Earth
Physiological (*prāṇamaya*)	Water
Mental (*manomaya*)	Fire
Intellectual (*vijñānamaya*)	Air
Blissful (*ānandamaya*)	Ether

The first three sheaths are within the field of the elements of nature. The intellectual sheath is said to be the layer of the individual soul (*jīvātman*), and the blissful sheath the layer of the universal Soul (*paramātman*). In effect, all five sheaths have to be penetrated to reach emancipation. The innermost content of the sheaths, beyond even the blissful body, is *puruṣa*, the indivisible, non-manifest One, the 'void which is full'. This is experienced in *nirbīja samādhi*, whereas *sabīja samādhi* is experienced at the level of the blissful body.

If *ahaṁkāra* (ego) is considered to be one end of a thread, then *antarātma* (Universal Self) is the other end. *Antaḥkaraṇa* (conscience) is the unifier of the two.

The practice of yoga integrates a person through the journey of intelligence and consciousness from the external to the internal. It unifies him from the intelligence of the skin to the intelligence of the self, so that his self merges with the cosmic Self. This is the merging of one half of one's being (*prakṛti*) with the other (*puruṣa*). Through yoga, the practitioner learns to observe and to think, and to intensify his effort until eternal joy is attained. This is possible only when all vibrations of the individual *citta* are arrested before they emerge.

Yoga, the restraint of fluctuating thought, leads to a *sāttvic* state. But in order to restrain the fluctuations, force of will is necessary: hence a degree of *rajas* is involved. Restraint of the movements of thought brings about stillness, which leads to deep silence, with awareness. This is the *sāttvic* nature of the *citta*.

Stillness is concentration (*dhāraṇā*) and silence is meditation (*dhyāna*).

Concentration needs a focus or a form, and this focus is *ahaṁkāra*, one's own small, individual self. When concentration flows into meditation, that self loses its identity and becomes one with the great Self. Like two sides of a coin, *ahaṁkāra* and *ātma* are the two opposite poles in man.

The *sādhaka* is influenced by the self on the one hand and by objects perceived on the other. When he is engrossed in the object, his mind fluctuates. This is *vṛtti*. His aim should be to distinguish the self from the objects seen, so that it does not become enmeshed by them. Through yoga, he should try to free his consciousness from the temptations of such objects, and bring it closer to the seer. Restraining the fluctuations of the mind is a process which leads to an end: *samādhi*. Initially, yoga acts as the means of restraint. When the *sādhaka* has attained a total state of restraint, yogic discipline is accomplished and the end is reached: the consciousness remains pure. Thus, yoga is both the means and the end.

(See I.18; II.28.)

तदा द्रष्टुः स्वरूपेऽवस्थानम् ।३।

I.3 tadā draṣṭuḥ svarūpe avasthānam

tadā	then, at that time
draṣṭuḥ	the soul, the seer
svarūpe	in his own, in his state
avasthānam	rests, abides, dwells, resides, radiates

Then, the seer dwells in his own true splendour.

When the waves of consciousness are stilled and silenced, they can no longer distort the true expression of the soul. Revealed in his own nature, the radiant seer abides in his own grandeur.

Volition being the mode of behaviour of the mind, it is liable to change our perception of the state and condition of the seer from moment to moment. When it is restrained and regulated, a reflective state of being is experienced. In this state, knowledge dawns so clearly that the true grandeur of the seer is seen and felt. This vision of the soul radiates without any activity on the part of *citta*. Once it is realized, the soul abides in its own seat.

(See I.16, 29, 47, 51; II.21, 23, 25; III.49, 56; IV.22, 25, 34.)

वृत्तिसारूप्यमितरत्र ॥४॥

I.4 vṛtti sārūpyam itaratra

vṛtti	behaviour, fluctuation, modification, function, state of mind
sārūpyam	identification, likeness, closeness, nearness
itaratra	at other times, elsewhere

At other times, the seer identifies with the fluctuating consciousness.

When the seer identifies with consciousness or with the objects seen, he unites with them and forgets his grandeur.

The natural tendency of consciousness is to become involved with the object seen, draw the seer towards it, and move the seer to identify with it. Then the seer becomes engrossed in the object. This becomes the seed for diversification of the intelligence, and makes the seer forget his own radiant awareness.

When the soul does not radiate its own glory, it is a sign that the thinking faculty has manifested itself in place of the soul.

The imprint of objects is transmitted to *citta* through the senses of perception. *Citta* absorbs these sensory impressions and becomes coloured and modified by them. Objects act as provender for the grazing *citta*, which is attracted to them by its appetite. *Citta* projects itself, taking on the form of the objects in order to possess them. Thus it becomes enveloped by thoughts of the object, with the result that the soul is obscured. In this way, *citta* becomes murky and causes changes in behaviour and mood as it identifies itself with things seen. (See III.36.)

Although in reality *citta* is a formless entity, it can be helpful to visualize it in order to grasp its functions and limitations. Let us imagine it to be like an optical lens, containing no light of its own, but placed directly above a source of pure light, the soul. One face of the lens, facing inwards towards the light, remains clean. We are normally aware of this internal facet of *citta* only when it speaks to us with the voice of conscience.

In daily life, however, we are very much aware of the upper surface of the lens, facing outwards to the world and linked to it by the senses and mind. This surface serves both as a sense, and as a content of consciousness, along with ego and intelligence. Worked upon by the desires and fears of turbulent worldly life, it becomes cloudy, opaque, even dirty and scarred, and prevents the soul's light from shining through it. Lacking inner illumination, it seeks all the more avidly the artificial lights of conditioned existence.

The whole technique of yoga, its practice and restraint, is aimed at dissociating consciousness from its identification with the phenomenal world, at restraining the senses by which it is ensnared, and at cleansing and purifying the lens of *citta*, until it transmits wholly and only the light of the soul.

(See II.20; IV.22.)

वृत्तयः पञ्चतय्यः क्लिष्टाक्लिष्टाः ।५।

I.5 vṛttayaḥ pañcatayyaḥ kliṣṭā akliṣṭāḥ

vṛttayaḥ	movements, modification
pañcatayyaḥ	fivefold
kliṣṭā	afflicting, tormenting, distressing, painful
akliṣṭāḥ	untroubling, undisturbing, unafflicting, undistressing, pleasing

The movements of consciousness are fivefold. They may be cognizable or non-cognizable, painful or non-painful.

Fluctuations or modifications of the mind may be painful or non-painful, cognizable or non-cognizable. Pain may be hidden in the non-painful state, and the non-painful may be hidden in the painful state. Either may be cognizable or non-cognizable.

When consciousness takes the lead, naturally the seer takes a back seat. The seed of change is in the consciousness and not in the seer. Consciousness sees objects in relation to its own idiosyncrasies, creating fluctuations and modifications in one's thoughts. These modifications, of which there are five, are explained in the next sūtra. They may be visible or hidden, painful or not, distressing or pleasing, cognizable or non-cognizable.

The previous sūtra explains that the consciousness involves the seer with the objects seen by it, and invites five types of fluctuations which can be divided and subdivided almost infinitely.

Thoughts, when associated with anguish, are known as painful (*kliṣṭā*) conditions of the mind and consciousness. For example, a live coal covered with ash appears to be ash. If one touches it, it burns the skin at once. The live coal was in an incognizable, or *akliṣṭā* state. The moment the skin was burned, it became cognizable, or *kliṣṭā*. As anguish predominates in pain, the pleasing state cannot be identified with it, though it exists side by side.

The pleasure of sex ends in the agony of labour pain at the time of delivery, to be followed by all the cycles of joy, worry and sadness associated with parenthood.

Even highly evolved souls, who have reached a certain spiritual height, as in I.18 which describes a non-painful, blissful state, are cautioned by Patañjali in I.19. He warns that, though the yogi remains free while the virtuous potencies continue to be powerful, the moment they fade away he has to strive again, a painful end to the attainment of the spiritual pinnacle. Alternatively, the pains may be hidden, and may appear as non-painful for a long time, until they surface. For example, cancer can remain undetected for a long time until it reaches a painful and tormenting state.

Cognizable pains and anguishes are controlled or annihilated by the practice of yoga, and by willpower. Incognizable pains are prevented from rising to the state of cognition by freedom from desires (*vāsanas*) and by non-attachment (*vairāgya*), in addition to yogic *sādhana*.

In II.12, Patañjali uses the words *dṛṣṭa* (visible) and *adṛṣṭa* (unperceived, invisible). These may be compared to *kliṣṭā* and *akliṣṭā*. Nature causes the five fluctuations to appear in their affictive *kliṣṭā* forms, whereas *puruṣa* tends to bring them to the *akliṣṭā* state. For example, the *kliṣṭā* form of memory is bondage in psychological time, the *akliṣṭā* form is the function of discrimination. Both the painful and non-painful states can be visible or hidden. The known, visible pains and pleasures can be reduced or eradicated. In painful states the 'non-pains' may be hidden, and consequently the virtues are difficult to recognize or perceive. Both these states must be stopped by yogic practice and renunciation. In sūtras I.23, 27, 28, 33–39, and in II.29, Patañjali underlines the means of reaching the zenith of virtue, which is freedom and beatitude.

The *citta* acts as the wheel, while *kliṣṭā* and *akliṣṭā* states are like the two spokes of the wheel which cause fluctuations and modulations in one's self. The *vṛttis* in their *kliṣṭā* and *akliṣṭā* manifestations are not separate parallel entities, but feed and support each other. For example, the dullness which is the negative aspect of sleep supports the wrong perception of the other modulations of consciousness, whereas the positive experience of sleep (the passive, virtuous state experienced immediately on waking, when the 'I' is silent) gives a glimmer of a higher state, encouraging the efforts of right knowledge and discrimination. If the wheel is at rest, the spokes remain steady, and the *citta* becomes free from *vṛttis*.

(For afflictions, see I.30, 31; II.3, 12, 16, 17.)

प्रमाणविपर्ययविकल्पनिद्रास्मृतयः ।६।

I.6 pramāṇa viparyaya vikalpa nidrā smṛtayaḥ

pramāṇa	valid knowledge, experienced knowledge, correct knowledge which is studied and verified, proof, or evidence
viparyaya	inverted, perverse, contrary
vikalpa	doubt, indecision, hesitation, fancy, imagination, or day-dreaming
nidrā	sleep, a state of emptiness
smṛtayaḥ	memory

They are caused by correct knowledge, illusion, delusion, sleep and memory.

These five-fold fluctuations or modifications of consciousness are based on real perception, or correct knowledge based on fact and proof; unreal or perverse perception, or illusion; fanciful or imaginary knowledge; knowledge based on sleep; and memory.

Consciousness has five qualitative types of intelligence: *mūḍha* (silly, stupid, or ignorant), *kṣipta* (neglected or distracted), *vikṣipta* (agitated or scattered), *ekāgra* (one-pointed or closely attentive) and *niruddha* (restrained or controlled). Since conscious intelligence is of five types, fluctuations are also classified into five kinds: correct knowledge, perverse perception, imagination, knowledge based on sleep, and memory. These five conscious states of intelligence and five classes of fluctuations may disturb the *sādhaka*, or help him to develop maturity of intelligence and attain emancipation.

Wrong perceptions (*viparyaya*) are gathered by the senses of perception and influence the mind to accept what is felt by them (as in the story of the six blind men and the elephant). Fanciful knowledge (*vikalpa*) causes the mind to live in an imaginary state without consideration of the facts. Memory (*smṛti*) helps one to recollect experiences for right understanding. Sleep (*nidrā*) has its own peculiarity. As a jar when empty is filled with air, so consciousness is empty in sleep. It exists in space, without a place, and is filled with dormancy. In sleep, one has a glimpse of a quiet state of mind, *manolaya*. This dormant state of mind is felt only on waking. Just as a flower when at rest is in its bud, so the consciousness rests in its bud, the conscience. Correct knowledge (*pramāṇa*) is direct knowledge from the core of the being. It is intuitive, therefore pure, and beyond the field of intellect.

Direct knowledge leads man beyond the conscious state. This state of consciousness is called *amanaskatva*.

प्रत्यक्षानुमानागमाः प्रमाणानि ॥७॥

I.7 pratyakṣa anumāna āgamāḥ pramāṇāni

pratyakṣa	direct perception
anumāna	inference
āgamāḥ	traditional sacred texts or scriptural references, a person who is a scriptural authority and whose word can be relied on
pramāṇāni	kinds of proof

Correct knowledge is direct, inferred or proven as factual.

Correct knowledge is based on three kinds of proof: direct perception, correct inference or deduction, and testimony from authoritative sacred scriptures or experienced persons.

Initially, individual perception should be checked by reasoned logic, and then seen to correspond to traditional or scriptural wisdom. This process involves the enlightened intelligence, or *buddhi*.

In modern intellectual terms, we take *buddhi* to be a monolithic entity. This is unhelpful when trying to understand its true role in our lives and in our yogic practice. Let us first separate it from mind, in which brain, whose function is to receive sensory information, to think and to act, has its source. Thinking expresses itself in the form of electro-magnetic waves.

Intellect is more subtle than mind. It is concerned with the knowledge of facts and the reasoning faculty, and becomes discernible only through its inherent quality, intelligence, which is closer to consciousness than to the mind/thought process. Intelligence is inherent in every aspect of our being, from the physical to the blissful. It is non-manifest only in the *ātman/puruṣa*, the core of being.

The quality of intelligence is inherent but dormant, so our first step must be to awaken it. The practice of *āsana* brings intelligence to the surface of the cellular body through stretching and to the physiological body by maintaining the pose. Once awakened, intelligence can reveal its dynamic aspect, its ability to discriminate. Then we strive for equal extensions to achieve a balanced, stable pose, measuring upper arm stretch against lower, right leg against left, inner against outer, etc. This precise, thorough process of measuring and discriminating is the apprenticeship, or culturing, of intelligence; it is pursued in the internal sheaths by *prāṇāyāma*, *pratyāhāra* and the further stages of yoga.

We can thus see that discrimination is a weighing process, belonging to the world of duality. When what is wrong is discarded, what is left must be correct.

When discrimination has been cultivated and intelligence is full and bright, ego and mind retreat, and *citta* becomes sharp and clear. But spiritual intelligence, which is true wisdom, dawns only when discrimination ends. Wisdom does not function in duality. It perceives only oneness. It does not discard the wrong, it sees only the right. (Patañjali calls this exalted intelligence, or *vivekaja jñānam*, III.55.) Wisdom is not mingled with nature, and is indeed unsuitable for the problems of life in a dualistic world. It would be of no use to a politician, for example, however high his motives, for he must choose and decide in the relative and temporal world. Spiritual wisdom does not decide, it *knows*. It is beyond time.

However, the progressive refinement of intelligence is essential in the search for freedom. The discriminating intellect should be used to 'defuse' the negative impact of memory, which links us in psychological time to the world of sensory pleasure and pain.

All matter, from rocks to human cells, contains its own inherent intelligence, but only man has the capacity to awaken, culture and finally transcend intelligence. Just as the totally pure *citta*, free from sensory entanglements, gravitates towards the *ātman*, so, once intelligence has achieved the highest knowledge of nature, it is drawn inwards towards the soul (IV.26). *Buddhi* has the capacity to perceive itself: its innate virtue is honesty (I.49).

विपर्ययो मिथ्याज्ञानमतद्रूपप्रतिष्ठम् ।८।

I.8 viparyayaḥ mithyājñānam atadrūpa pratiṣṭham

viparyayaḥ perverse, unreal
mithyājñānam illusory knowledge
atadrūpa not in its own form
pratiṣṭham occupying, standing, seeing, beholding

Illusory or erroneous knowledge is based on non-fact or the non-real.

Perverse, illusory or wrong knowledge is caused by error or misconception, or by mistaking one thing for another. It is based on the distortion of reality.

Wrong understanding and false conceptions generate wrong feelings and taint the consciousness. This hinders the *sādhaka* in his efforts to experience the seer, and may create a dual or split personality.

(See II.5.)

शब्दज्ञानानुपाती वस्तुशून्यो विकल्पः ।९।

I.9 śabdajñāna anupātī vastuśūnyaḥ vikalpaḥ

śabdajñāna verbal knowledge
anupātī followed in sequence, pursued, phased in regular succession
vastuśūnyaḥ devoid of things, devoid of substance or meaning
vikalpaḥ imagination, fancy

Verbal knowledge devoid of substance is fancy or imagination.

Playing with fanciful thoughts or words, and living in one's own world of thoughts and impressions which have no substantial basis, is *vikalpa*, a vague and uncertain knowledge which does not correspond to reality. In such a state of delusion, one is like the hare in the fable who imagined it had horns.

If *vikalpa* is brought to the level of factual knowledge by analysis, trial, error, and discrimination, it can awaken a thirst for correct or true knowledge, and delusion can be transformed into vision and discovery. Unless and until such a transformation takes place, knowledge based on imagination remains without substance.

अभावप्रत्ययालम्बना वृत्तिर्निद्रा ।१०।

I.10 abhāva pratyaya ālambanā vṛttiḥ nidrā

abhāva non-existence, a feeling of non-being, absence of awareness
pratyaya going towards conviction, trust, confidence, reliance, usage, knowledge, understanding, instrument, means, intellect

ālambanā support, abode, dependence on a prop, mental exercise to bring before one's thoughts the gross form of the eternal
vṛttiḥ function, condition, thought-wave
nidrā sleep without dreams

Sleep is the non-deliberate absence of thought-waves or knowledge.

Dreamless sleep is an inert state of consciousness in which the sense of existence is not felt.

Sleep is a state in which all activities of thought and feeling come to an end. In sleep, the senses of perception rest in the mind, the mind in the consciousness and the consciousness in the being. Sleep is of three types. If one feels heavy and dull after sleep, that sleep has been *tāmasic*. Disturbed sleep is *rājasic*. Sleep that brings lightness, brightness and freshness is *sāttvic*.

In the states of correct knowledge, perverse knowledge, fanciful knowledge, and knowledge born of memory, one is awake. Mind and consciousness are drawn by the senses into contact with external objects: thus, one gains knowledge. In deep sleep, these four types of knowledge are absent: the senses of perception cease to function because their king, the mind, is at rest. This is *abhāva*, a state of void, a feeling of emptiness.

The *sādhaka*, having experienced this negative state of void in sleep, tries to transform it into a positive state of mind while awake. Then he experiences that pure state in which the self is free from the knowledge of things seen, heard, acquired or felt through the senses and the mind. When he has learned to silence all the modulations of mind and consciousness, then he has reached *kaivalya*. He has sublimated the *vṛttis* and become a master: his *citta* is submerged in the soul.

Sleep gives one a glimpse of the seer, but only indistinctly because the light of discrimination, *viveka*, is clouded. Simulation of this state of sleep when one is awake and aware is *samādhi*, wherein the seer witnesses his own form.

अनुभूतविषयासंप्रमोषः स्मृतिः ।११।

I.11 anubhūta viṣaya asaṁpramoṣaḥ smṛtiḥ

anubhūta	perceived, apprehended, experienced, knowledge derived from direct perception, inference and comparison, verbal knowledge
viṣaya	an object, a sense of object, an affair, a transaction
asaṁpramoṣaḥ	not allowing to slip away, without stealing from anything else
smṛtiḥ	memory of a thing experienced, recollection of words or experiences

Memory is the unmodified recollection of words and experiences.

Memory is a modification of consciousness allowing us to recapture past experiences.

Memory is the collection of the modulations and impressions of correct knowledge, perverse knowledge, illusory knowledge and sleep. As perception changes, memory too may alter, but correctly used, it enables us to recall experiences in their true, pristine state. This ability is the foundation of the practice of discrimination.

The five properties of consciousness can be equated with the five fluctuations of consciousness: dullness with *nidrā*, negligence with *viparyaya*, agitation with *vikalpa*, one-pointedness with *smṛti* and restraint or control with *pramāṇa*.

(See II.5 for wrong impressions and wrong recollections.)

अभ्यासवैराग्याभ्यां तन्निरोधः ।१२।

I.12 abhyāsa vairāgyābhyāṁ tannirodhaḥ

abhyāsa	repeated practice
vairāgyābhyāṁ	freedom from desires, detachment, renunciation
tannirodhaḥ	their restraint

Practice and detachment are the means to still the movements of consciousness.

The fluctuations of consciousness, painful or non-painful, described in I.5 and I.6, are to be controlled through repeated yogic practice. Mental strength must also be developed, to attain detachment and freedom from desires.

Study of the consciousness and stilling it is practice (*abhyāsa*). Elsewhere (II.28) Patañjali has used another word: *anuṣṭhāna*. *Abhyāsa* conveys the sense of mechanical repetition, whereas *anuṣṭhāna* implies devotion, dedication, a religious attitude. Repeated effort made with a thorough understanding of the art and philosophy of yoga and with perfect communion of body, mind and soul is not a mechanical practice but a religious and spiritual one.

Practice is the positive aspect of yoga; detachment or renunciation (*vairāgya*) the negative. The two balance each other like day and night, inhalation and exhalation. Practice is the path of evolution; detachment and renunciation the path of involution. Practice is involved in all the eight limbs of yoga. Evolutionary practice is the onward march towards discovery of the Self, involving *yama*, *niyama*, *āsana* and *prāṇāyāma*. The involutionary path of renunciation involves *pratyāhāra*, *dhāraṇā*, *dhyāna* and *samādhi*. This inward journey detaches the consciousness from external objects.

Patañjali's practice represents the *ha* or 'sun' aspect, and renunciation the *ṭha* or 'moon' aspect of haṭha yoga. In *haṭha yoga*, *ha* represents the life-force and *ṭha*, the consciousness. *Ha* also represents the very being – the seer, while *ṭha* is the reflected light of the seer, representing *citta*. Through *Haṭhayoga* these two forces are blended, and then merged in the seer.

To be adept in yoga, *yama* and *niyama* must be observed carefully throughout the yogic *sādhana*. This is *abhyāsa*. The discarding of ideas and actions which obstruct progress in *sādhana* is *vairāgya*.

As we know, consciousness becomes involved with the objects seen, and identifies with them, drawing the seer with it. Then the seer becomes subordinate to the oscillating mind. The eight aspects of yoga, described in II.29, are given to us as a means to stop the wavering of the intelligence and to learn correct understanding. Although the first four relate to practice and the others to renunciation, practice and renunciation are interdependent and equally important. Without restraint, the forces generated by practice would spin out of control and could destroy the *sādhaka*. At the higher levels, *vairāgya* without *abhyāsa* could lead to stagnation and inner decay. The first four aspects are considered a building up process, and the last four one of inner consolidation. Once our initial *tāmasic* nature moves towards a dynamic state, restraint becomes necessary for our own inner security.

Vairāgya is a practice through which the *sādhaka* learns to be free from desires and passions and to cultivate non-attachment to things which hinder his pursuit of union with the soul.

The disciplines which are to be followed are explained in the succeeding sūtras.

(For yogic disciplines see II.29–32, II.35–53.)

तत्र स्थितौ यत्नोऽभ्यासः ।१३।

I.13 tatra sthitau yatnaḥ abhyāsaḥ

tatra	of these, under these circumstances, in that case
sthitau	as regards steadiness, as regards perfect restraint
yatnaḥ	continuous effort
abhyāsaḥ	practice

Practice is the steadfast effort to still these fluctuations.

Practice is the effort to still the fluctuations in the consciousness and then to move towards silencing it: to attain a constant, steady, tranquil state of mind.

In order to free the mind from fluctuations and oscillations and to reach a state of steadiness, the practitioner is advised to practise intensely all the yogic principles, from *yama* to *dhyāna*. These embrace all disciplines: moral, ethical, physical, mental, intellectual and spiritual. (For the application of the mind to the practice, see I.20.)

स तु दीर्घकालनैरन्तर्यसत्कारासेवितो दृढभूमिः ।१४।

I.14 sa tu dīrghakāla nairantarya satkāra
āsevitaḥ dṛḍhabhūmiḥ

sa	this
tu	and
dīrghakāla	for a long time
nairantarya	without interruption, continuous

satkāra dedication, devotion
āsevitaḥ zealously practised, performed assiduously
dṛḍhabhūmiḥ of firm ground, firmly rooted, well fixed

Long, uninterrupted, alert practice is the firm foundation for restraining the fluctuations.

When the effort is continued in accordance with yogic principles consistently and for a long time, with earnestness, attention, application and devotion, the yogic foundation is firmly established.

Profound wisdom is gained through steady, dedicated, attentive practice, and non-attachment through applied restraint. However, success may inflate the *sādhaka*'s ego, and he should be careful not to become a victim of intellectual pride which may drag him away from enlightenment. If this happens, he should re-establish his practice by taking guidance from a competent master, or through his own discrimination, so that humility replaces pride and spiritual wisdom dawns. This is correct practice.

दृष्टानुश्रविकविषयवितृष्णस्य वशीकारसंज्ञा वैराग्यम् ।१५।

I.15 dṛṣṭa ānuśravika viṣaya vitṛṣṇasya vaśīkārasaṁjñā vairāgyam

dṛṣṭa perceptible, visible
ānuśravika heard or listening, resting on the *Vedas* or on tradition according to oral testimony
viṣaya a thing, an object of enjoyment, matter
vitṛṣṇasya freedom from desire, contentment
vaśīkāra subjugation, supremacy, bringing under control
saṁjñā consciousness, intellect, understanding
vairāgyam absence of worldly desires and passions, dispassion, detachment, indifference to the world, renunciation

Renunciation is the practice of detachment from desires.

When non-attachment and detachment are learned there is no craving for objects seen or unseen, words heard or unheard. Then the seer remains unmoved by temptations. This is the sign of mastery in the art of renunciation.

Non-attachment and detachment must be learned through willpower. They consist of learning to be free from cravings, not only for worldly, but also heavenly pleasures. *Citta* is taught to be unmoved by thoughts of desire and passion, and to remain in a state of pure consciousness, devoid of all objects and free even from the qualities of *sattva*, *rajas* and *tamas*.

The mind is considered by the sages to be the eleventh sense. The eyes, ears, nose, tongue and skin are the five senses of perception. The arms, legs, mouth, generative and excretory organs are the five organs of action. These are the external senses: the mind is an internal sense organ.

There are five states in *vairāgya*.

1 Disengaging the senses from enjoyment of their objects, and controlling them, is *yatamāna*. As it is not possible to control all the senses at once, one should attempt to control them one by one to achieve mastery over them all.
2 By thoughtful control, one burns away the desires which obstruct *citta*'s movement towards the soul. This is *vyatireka*.
3 When the five senses of perception and five organs of action have been weaned away from contact with objects, the feeblest desires remain in a causal state and are felt only in the mind: this is *ekendriya*. The mind wants to play a dual role: to fulfil the desires of the senses, and also to experience Self-Realization. Once the senses have been silenced, the mind moves with one-pointed effort towards Soul Realization.
4 *Vaśīkāra* is attained when one has overcome all longings, and developed indifference to all types of attachment, non-attachment and detachment (see I.40). All eleven senses have been subjugated.
5 From these develops *paravairāgya*, the highest form of renunciation: it is free from the qualities of *sattva*, *rajas* and *tamas*. On attaining this state, the *sādhaka* ceases to be concerned with himself, or with others who remain caught in the web of pleasure (see Table 2 and II.19).

Often we come across renounced persons who get caught in the pleasures and comforts of life and neglect their *sādhana*. We should learn from such examples and guard ourselves so that we develop firmness in our *sādhana*.

A bird cannot fly with one wing. It needs two wings to fly. To reach the highest spiritual goal, the two wings of yoga, *abhyāsa* and *vairāgya* are essential.

तत्परं पुरुषख्यातेर्गुणवैतृष्ण्यम् ।१६।

I.16 tatparaṁ puruṣakhyāteḥ guṇavaitṛṣṇyam

tatparaṁ	that highest, that most excellent, the ultimate, the best, the purest, the supreme
puruṣakhyāteḥ	the highest knowledge of the soul, perception of the soul
guṇavaitṛṣṇyam	indifference to the qualities of nature, inertia or dormancy (*tamas*), passion or vibrance (*rajas*) and luminosity or serenity (*sattva*)

The ultimate renunciation is when one transcends the qualities of nature and perceives the soul.

Table 2: *Stages of* vairāgya *(detachment) and the involution of* prakṛti

Stage of *vairāgya*	Stage of involution of *prakṛti*	
1 *Yatamāna* (disengaging the senses from action)	*Viśeṣa* (specific)	11 *indriyas*
2 *Vyatireka* (keeping away from desire)		
3 *Ekendriya* (stilling the mind)		
4 *Vaśīkāra* (mastery of desire)	*Aviśeṣa* (non-specific)	5 *tanmātras* + *asmitā*
	Liṅga mātra (marked)	
5 *Paravairāgya* (supreme detachment)	*Aliṅga* (unmarked)	

The purest form of renunciation is when one is free from the qualities of nature. One realizes the soul at once. Clear intelligence of head and heart leads to this.

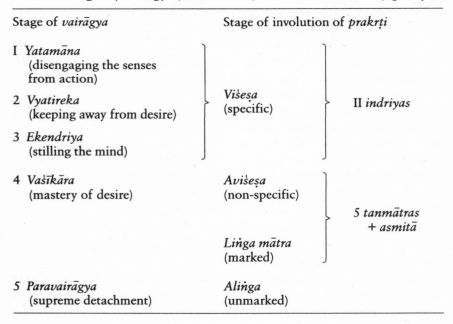

If through *abhyāsa* we activate and purify our energy, through *vairāgya* we

disentangle ourselves from involvement in even the subtlest manifestations of the phenomenal world. The creation of energy alone, without control or restraint, cannot lead to freedom. To understand the five levels of *vairāgya*, one should refer to the model of nature's evolution described in the introduction, in the section on *samādhi pāda*. Here, we see the unfolding of nature from its noumenal (*aliṅga*) state into the *liṅga* state, through *mahat*; then from the non-specific (*aviśeṣa*) phenomena including *ahaṁkāra*, ego or 'I-consciousness' to the manifest (*viśeṣa*) expressions of nature which form the basis of our experience of everyday reality (see II.19). The reverse or involutionary process, which is the path of yoga, can be seen as the ascension of a ladder. *Abhyāsa* gives us the necessary impetus for the ascent; by *vairāgya* we draw up the ladder behind us.

The lower rungs of renunciation are attempted by anyone who tries to disentangle himself from such a habit as smoking or drinking coffee. We cut down, then we stop, but the desire persists in the mind. When that mental desire has faded away, years later, our body cells may spontaneously rekindle attachment. Later still, we may find we become attached to the idea of ourselves as non-drinkers of coffee, so the ego is still attached to the idea of coffee even though it is now 'non-coffee'. This is self-conscious virtue. Gradually we may become totally indifferent to coffee, but coffee nevertheless still exists in our mind.

This sutra relates to the ultimate freedom achieved through *paravairāgya*: here phenomenal nature ceases to exist for us, as the *guṇas* are transcended, drawn back into their noumenal root. By transcending the *guṇas*, we unlock that which binds us to nature. When this is achieved in all our involvements, the soul is fully perceived.

The consciousness has now, by the power of wisdom, acquired everything that had to be acquired, and discarded everything that had to be discarded. The *sādhaka* is free from all bondage; there is no feeling of birth and death. *Kaivalya* is attained. This is the effect of the twin disciplines of *abhyāsa* and *vairāgya*, through which the *sādhaka* becomes wise and free, untainted by the influence of *citta*.

In IV.29 the word *prasaṅkhyāna*, meaning 'highest knowledge', has been used. Again in sūtra IV.31, there is the expression *sarvāvaraṇa malāpetasya* which means 'when all obscuring impurities are destroyed totally'. Then follows *puruṣakhyāti* signifying 'perception of the soul'.

(In sūtras I.17–51 Patañjali speaks of *samādhi*.) (See III.51 and IV.34.)

वितर्कविचारानन्दास्मितारूपानुगमात् संप्रज्ञातः ।१७।

I.17 vitarka vicāra ānanda asmitārūpa anugamāt saṁprajñātaḥ

vitarka	analytical thinking or analytical study, argument, inference, conjecture
vicāra	reason, meditation, insight, perfect intelligence where all logic comes to an end
ānanda	elation, bliss, felicity
asmitārūpa	consciousness of being one with oneself
anugamāt	by accompanying, by following, comprehending, grasping
saṁprajñātaḥ	distinguish, know actually, know accurately

Practice and detachment develop four types of samādhi: *self-analysis, synthesis, bliss, and the experience of pure being.*

Through practice and detachment, four types of awareness develop. Absorption of the consciousness, achieved through engrossment in conjecture, inference and analytical study; synthesis, consideration and discrimination; bliss or elation; and a state of pure being, constitute *saṁprajñāta samādhi.*

Here a distinction is recognized between the seer and the seen. *Saṁprajñāta samādhi* consists of *vitarka*, engrossment in analysis, *vicāra*, engrossment in reasoning, *ānanda*, experiencing a state of bliss, and *asmitā*, experiencing the state of 'I'.

Vitarka is an act of involvement by deliberate thinking and study, which leads to the final point or root cause. It is an attempt to distinguish the cause from the effect, a process of judicious experimental research from the gross to the subtle. Intellectual analysis, *vitarka saṁprajñāta*, being a function of the brain, produces relative and conditioned knowledge. It is gross and lacks refinement. It is further divided into deliberation, *savitarka* and non-deliberation, *nirvitarka.*

Vicāra means differentiating knowledge. It is a process of investigation, reflection and consideration through which the wandering conjectural brain is stilled and the *sādhaka* develops mental depth, acuteness, refinement and subtlety. *Vicāra* too is divided into reasoning, *savicāra* and non-reasoning, *nirvicāra.*

As the growing body of experience brings maturity, fulfilment is reached and a state of bliss, *ānanda*, ensues, freeing the *sādhaka* from the mechanism of study, investigation and fulfilment and leading him to dwell in the self alone. This state is called *asmitā rūpa saṁprajñāta samādhi*. Thus, all six gradations of *sabīja samādhi* (*samādhi* with support or seed) – *savitarka*, *nirvitarka*, *savicāra*, *nirvicāra*, *ānanda* and *asmitā* – are explained.

There is a seventh stage of *samādhi*, *virāma pratyaya*, so called *asaṁprajñāta samādhi*, and an eighth, called *dharma megha* or *nirbīja samādhi*.

As external objects are susceptible to change, deliberation may not be pure. One must go from the periphery to the source. *Vicāra* is beyond *vitarka*, *ānanda* is beyond *vitarka* and *vicāra*, and *asmitā* is beyond *vitarka*, *vicāra* and *ānanda*. This is the gradual progress from the gross body towards the subtle mind, and from the subtle mind towards the source, the core of being.

Savitarka and *nirvitarka samādhi* belong to the function of the brain, and are attained by contemplation on gross elements and objects knowable through the senses. *Savicāra* and *nirvicāra samādhi* belong to the realm of the mind and are attained by contemplation of subtle elements, and *ānanda* belongs to the realm of mature intelligence. *Ānanda* must be attributed not to the senses but to pure wisdom. Contemplation by the self of the self brings one close to *puruṣa*. Here, the self is devoid of ego.

It is said that the front of the brain is the analytical part (*savitarka*), while the back of the brain is the old, reasoning area (*savicāra*). The base of the brain is the seat of *ānanda*, and the crown of the head of the individual self, *asmitā*. *Sabīja samādhi* is achieved by drawing these four facets of the brain towards its stem.

When this synchronization has been achieved, a transitory state of quietness, *manolaya*, is experienced. Then, from the stem of the brain, consciousness is made to descend towards the source mind, the seat of the heart. Here it merges into a mindless, beginningless, endless state of being: *amanaskatva*, or *nirbīja samādhi* (*samādhi* without seed or support). It is the conquest of the spirit.

In between *sabīja* and *nirbīja samādhis*, Patañjali describes an intervening state, *virāma pratyaya*, which others call *asaṁprajñāta samādhi*. It is a spiritual plateau (*manolaya*), a transitory state or a resting place before one plunges into *nirbīja samādhi*.

(See II.18, 19, 21; III.45 and 48.)

Through practice and renunciation each and every part of man – the skin, the cells, the breath, the movements of thought, intelligence and reason become acquainted with the self. This is *saṁprajñāta samādhi*. The *sādhaka*'s intelligence spreads evenly within and around his body, like the surface of a lake without ripples. Then he sees things clearly. In this *saṁprajñāta samādhi* or contemplation, the disparity between the seer and the seen remains.

Take, for example, the performance of an *āsana*, or movements of breath in *prāṇāyāma*. In the beginning, these are done at a physical level. As understanding deepens, the body is penetrated internally, its movements are connected with the intelligence, and the *āsana* is grasped as a single unit in all directions: front to back, top to bottom, side to side. It is absorbed and held by the body's intelligence for the soul to perceive. One learns that one's body is the bow, the *āsana* is the arrow, and the target is the soul. When the *āsana* is perfected, the target is struck: the field and the knower of the field are united. The logic and reasoning of the *āsana* are fulfilled. The *sādhaka*, having lost the consciousness of the *āsana* and of his body, is one with himself. His *āsana*, his breath, his effort and his very being are one with the millions of cells in his body. He has reached *sāsmitā*, the auspicious state of *asmitā*.

Patañjali generally addresses us at several levels at once, so it is not unreasonable to explain *vitarka*, *vicāra*, *ānanda* and *asmitā* in relation to *āsana*.

When we begin to practise *āsana*, our method is largely hit or miss, 'let me try this; let me try that'. It is a process of trial and error based on conjecture. That is the nature of *vitarka*. It is adventurous rather than calculating but it does not forget its errors; we then evolve to the stage we may call *vicāra*, in which a body of experience has been built up from investigation, mature consideration and dawning discrimination. As our *āsanas* ripen, we reach a stage when skin-consciousness moves towards the centre of being, and the centre radiates towards the periphery. Movement is at once centripetal and centrifugal. This integrity brings bliss: *ānanda*. Finally, when the conscious mechanism by which we consider and perform *āsana* comes to an end, the process reaches a resting point. The *āsana* then rests only on the inner self which is in poise: the only support is *asmitā*.

विरामप्रत्ययाभ्यासपूर्वः संस्कारशेषोऽन्यः ।१८।

I.18 virāmapratyaya abhyāsapūrvaḥ saṁskāraśeṣaḥ anyaḥ

virāma	rest, repose, pause
pratyaya	going towards, firm conviction, reliance, confidence, usage, practice, a cause, instrument, means, device
abhyāsa	practice
pūrvaḥ	before, old, previous, foregoing

saṁskāraśeṣaḥ	balance of subliminal impressions
anyaḥ	other, another, different

The void arising in these experiences is another samādhi. *Hidden impressions lie dormant, but spring up during moments of awareness, creating fluctuations and disturbing the purity of the consciousness.*

As mentioned earlier, Patañjali indicates another state of *samādhi* in between *sabīja samādhi* and *nirbīja samādhi*, but does not name it. It is experienced with the cessation of all functions of the brain, leaving behind only the residual merits, or *saṁskāras*, of good practices. In this state one is free from passions, desires and appetites.

The word used for this state is *virāma pratyaya*. In it the *sādhaka* rests in a highly evolved state in which the intelligence is still. The nearest we come to *virāma pratyaya* in ordinary experience are those few moments before falling asleep, when the intellect relaxes its hold on thoughts and objects and the mind becomes silent, a state reminiscent of *manolaya*. Like a river joining the sea, the mind is dissolving into the self. We are given a momentary glimpse of the seer, abiding in the self. The moment one loses the feeling of 'I', one is in this state of *virāma pratyaya*, which is neither negative nor positive. It is a state of suspended animation in the consciousness. Patañjali calls this state a different type of *samādhi* (*anyaḥ*). It is not deliberate but natural.

In deliberate or *saṁprajñāta samādhi*, the intelligence dissolves but the sense of self remains. The *saṁskāras* of good practices remain and all other fluctuations cease. This state becomes a plateau, from which the aspirant may climb further up the spiritual ladder. As it is only a transitional state, one must take care that stagnation does not set in: it should not be taken as the goal. One should then, in fact, intensify one's *sādhana* to reach the state of the absolute, *nirbīja samādhi*. (For *nirbīja samādhi*, see I.50–51.)

In the next sūtra, it is said that those who remain in *virāma pratyaya* not only conquer the elements of nature but merge in them, while others live without a physical body as angels or *devatās*. We have the examples of Rāmakṛṣṇa Paramahaṁsa, Rāmaṇa Māharṣi and Śrī Aurobindo, who remained in that state for a long period without the awareness of their bodies, but emerged later to reach *nirbīja samādhi*. Such *sādhakas* are called *prakṛtilayas* (*laya* = merged in nature) or *videhins* (existing without a body). Other yogis who have reached a certain level of evolution in their search are caught at a crossroads, feeling that this is the end of their journey. If they stay there and do not attempt to go further in the practice of yoga, they fall from the grace of yoga. Lord Kṛṣṇa calls such aspirants *yoga bhraṣṭas*. In the *Bhagavad Gītā* (VI.41–43), he says that 'those yogis who have fallen deliberately from the grace of yoga are reborn in the houses of the pure and prosperous, where they live a contented life in a righteous way for many years; while the others, who have undeliberately fallen, are reborn into the families of poor yogis who are endowed with wisdom. Then they strive again for perfection, beginning from the state which they had reached in the previous life'. (See also IV.1–2.)

Virāma pratyaya is a precarious state. It may bind the *sādhaka* forever, or it may uplift him. Patañjali advises in I.20 that those who have reached *virāma pratyaya* should not stop there but should redouble their efforts with faith and courage, memory and contemplative awareness.

Śrī Vyāsa, the first commentator on Patañjali, calls this redoubled effort *upāya pratyaya* (*upāya* is the means by which one reaches one's aim, a stratagem). Through *upāya pratyaya* the evolved souls mentioned above reached *nirbīja samādhi.*

Patañjali clearly uses the word *saṁprajñāta* for the state of *samādhi* which is reached through *vitarka*, *vicāra*, *ānanda*, and *asmitā*. In this sūtra, he explains the deliberate maintenance of a thought-free state of consciousness. Hence, here he has not given a precise term, but uses the expression *anyaḥ*, meaning 'another', or a different type of *samādhi* and not *asaṁprajñāta samādhi*, as conveyed by many commentators.

भवप्रत्ययो विदेहप्रकृतिलयानाम् ।१९।

I.19 bhavapratyayaḥ videha prakṛtilayānām

bhava	arising or produced from, originating in, state of being, existence, origin, true condition, real disposition
pratyayaḥ	going towards, firm conviction, usage, means, device
videha	incorporeal, without material existence but an existence in contemplation of a law (the law of nature and of the spirit)
prakṛtilayānām	merged in nature

In this state, one may experience bodilessness, or become merged in nature. This may lead to isolation or to a state of loneliness.

In this *samādhi*, which is poised between *sabīja* and *nirbīja samādhi*, the *sādhaka* is freed from all fluctuations, but subliminal impressions, *saṁskāras*, spring to life the moment he comes out of that state. Some evolved entities move without a body, as spirits and angels, while others become absorbed in the elements of nature, *prakṛti*. Caught in the web of bodiless feeling, or merging in nature, they forget to climb to the topmost rung of the spiritual ladder, and fail to reach *nirbīja samādhi*. The *sādhaka*, having reached a state of isolation but not emancipation, must come out of it if he is not to lose the path of *kaivalya*.

A man who performs trance underground without ventilation becomes one with the earth. A person submerged in water becomes one with water. He is a *prakṛtilayan*: one with the elements. One whose spirit moves without a body is a *videhin*. When the *prakṛtilayan* is separated from earth or water, or the *videhin* comes in contact with his own body, subliminal impressions surface and create fluctuations in the mind (see III.44). This experience is the conquest of the principles or *tattvas* of nature: *prakṛtijaya*.

In I.10, Patañjali defines sleep as a state in which all thoughts and feelings are temporarily suspended, and the senses, mind, intellect and consciousness rest in the being. In dreamless sleep, there is absence of everything. If an average person, when awake, recollects the state of dreamless sleep, he glimpses a non-physical state of existence (*videha*) and also the state of merging in nature (*prakṛtilaya*). In sleep, these two phases remain unconscious until one wakes, whereas evolved souls in *samādhi* (as described in I.18) experience them consciously. Sleep is a natural condition of consciousness; *samādhi* is a superconscious state.

In sleep, everything is inert, *tāmasic*; in *samādhi* everything is luminous, untinged by the *guṇas*.

श्रध्दावीर्यस्मृतिसमाधिप्रज्ञापूर्वक इतरेषाम् ।२०।

I.20 śraddhā vīrya smṛti samādhiprajñā pūrvakaḥ itareṣām

śraddhā	trust which comes from revelation, faith, confidence, reverence
vīrya	vigour, physical and moral strength, mental power, energy, valour
smṛti	memory, recollection
samādhi	profound meditation, supreme devotion, identification of the contemplator with the subject of contemplation, perfect absorption of thoughts

prajñā	awareness of real knowledge acquired through intense contemplation
pūrvakaḥ	previous, prior, first
itareṣām	another, rest, different from, whereas

Practice must be pursued with trust, confidence, vigour, keen memory and power of absorption to break this spiritual complacency.

This sūtra guides those advanced souls who have attained a certain level in *samādhi*, to intensify their *sādhana*, with redoubled confidence, power, awareness and devotion.

Sage Vyāsa calls this state *upāya pratyaya.*

Highly evolved souls have the power to discriminate between isolation and emancipation. They are neither elated by their conquest of the elements nor delighted at their ability to move freely without their bodies. They adopt new means to intensify their practice with faith and vigour, and use memory as a guide to leap forward with wisdom, total absorption, awareness and attention.

It is said in the *purāṇas* that one Jaḍa Bhārata, having reached a state of *samādhi* became cold and unemotional. This is exactly what Patañjali means when he speaks of that intermediate state of *samādhi*, as *anyaḥ* or 'different'. Jaḍa Bhārata took three lives to come out of that state and then to proceed towards *nirbīja samādhi.*

Jaḍa Bhārata's father was a *rājarṣi* by the name of Ṛṣabha, who was a king of Bhārata; his mother, Jayavantyāmbikā was a pious lady. Being the son of such noble hearts, he was more inclined towards spiritual knowledge than to ruling the country.

He therefore made up his mind to renounce the kingdom and retired to the forest. One day, while he was bathing in a river, a pregnant doe came to drink. Frightened by a thunderous sound, it gave birth to a fawn and died. Jaḍa Bhārata took pity on the fawn, carried it to the hermitage and began tending it. He was so attached to it, that even at his last breath, he had only that deer in this thoughts. Hence, he was reborn as a deer but his previous *sādhana* remained as subliminal impressions. Later, he was reborn as a human being in the house of a realized soul, Āngirasa by name. He developed indifference to life and lived like a madman.

One day the king of the country wanted to perform a human sacrifice for Goddess Kālimātā. He commanded his attendants to bring a human being for the sacrifice. With great difficulty, they found a person who, however, escaped at the appointed time. The king, in rage, sent his attendants to find another person. This time they chanced upon Jaḍa Bhārata, who was moving about in the forest, unconcerned with life. He was brought for the sacrifice. As the king was about to kill him, Goddess Kālimātā appeared in her real form, destroyed the king and his attendants and set Jaḍa Bhārata free.

As a wandering sage, he moved to Sind. The king of the country wanted to sit at the feet of sage Kapilā to learn spiritual knowledge. One day, while he was travelling in a palanquin, his carriers spotted Jaḍa Bhārata and called him for help. He unhesitatingly consented to oblige, but moved in such a way as to disturb the rhythm of the others. They began scolding him, to which he replied that their abuses could not touch his Self as they were meant for his body. Hearing this, the king was wonderstruck; he climbed down and humbly prostrated before the sage asking his forgiveness. With a serene state of mind, Jaḍa Bhārata accepted the king's humble request and moved on to continue his *sādhana*. He had taken three lives to resume his *sādhana* from where he had left it.

This story aptly illustrates how the five dynamic qualities of faith, tenacity, perfect memory, absorption and awareness are necessary to hold on to what one has attained and to break out of that spiritual isolation which is not freedom.

Buddha says, in the *Dhammapada*, that all sorrows can be conquered through good conduct, reverential faith, enthusiasm, remembrance, concentration and right knowledge.

Śraddhā should not be understood simply as faith. It also conveys mental and intellectual firmness. (The next word, *vīrya*, stands for valour and power in the sense of physical and nervine strength.) Interestingly, Patañjali's first use of the word *śraddhā* is explicitly to encourage the *sādhaka* to intensify his *sādhana* in order to reach the highest goal.

The natural trust of the aspirant is confirmed by revelation, and transformed into the faith which permeates the consciousness of practitioners in any field of art, science and philosophy. If trust is instinctive, faith is intuitional.

After describing the experience of unbiased bliss and spiritual aura in I.17–19, Patañjali here expresses this felt trust as *śraddhā*.

तीव्रसंवेगानामासन्नः ।२१।

I.21 tīvrasaṁvegānām āsannaḥ

tīvra	vehement, intense, severe, sharp, acute, supreme, poignant
saṁvegānām	those who are quick, cheerful (*saṁvega* is a technical word like *saṁyama*, see III.4)
āsannaḥ	drawn near, approached, near in time, place or number

The goal is near for those who are supremely vigorous and intense in practice.

Samādhi is within reach for him who is honest and pure at heart, enthusiastic, intense and supremely energetic. He quickly reaches the highest goal of yoga, aided also by his residual accumulated virtues. However, sometimes even an intense aspirant may become mild or average, slow or moderate, in his practice.

In the *Śiva Saṁhitā*, chapter v.16, aspirants are categorized as feeble (*mṛdu*), moderate (*madhyama*), sharp in understanding and vigorous (*adhimātra*), and having colossal energy and supreme enthusiasm (*adhimātratama*).

मृदुमध्याधिमात्रत्वात् ततोऽपि विशेषः ।२२।

I.22 mṛdu madhya adhimātratvāt tataḥ api viśeṣaḥ

mṛdu	soft, feeble, mild, fickle
madhya	middle, intermediate, moderate, average
adhimātratvāt	ardent, steady minded, keen
tataḥ	thence, further
api	also
viśeṣaḥ	differentiation

There are differences between those who are mild, average and keen in their practices.

Table 3: *Levels of* sādhakas *and types of awareness*

Sādhaka	Awareness	
Mṛdu (mild)	1 *Vitarka prajñā*	intellectual analysis at the external level
	2 *Vicāra prajñā*	subtle differentiating knowledge and mental alertness
Madhya (medium)	3 *Ānanda prajñā*	knowledge of bliss
	4 *Asmitā prajñā*	knowledge of the self
Adhimātra (intense)	5 *Vaśīkāra prajñā*	subjugation of desire
	6 *Virāma pratyaya*	cessation of brain functions
	7 *Bhava pratyaya*	mental quietness
	8 *Upāya pratyaya*	skilful means
Tīvra saṁvegin or *adhimātratamān* (supremely intense)	9 *Paravairāgya*	supreme detachment

Sādhakas are of different levels of eagerness and intensity. For them, the goal is time-bound, depending on their level.

This sūtra further amplifies the distinction between yogis whose practices are feeble, average or keen, and who progress according to the level of their practice.

These types can be further subdivided. For example, a keen *sādhaka* may be feebly, moderately or intensely keen. Similar subdivisions can be made of the average and feeble types. The goal of yoga is near or far according to one's eagerness and one's efforts.

This sūtra refers to the different aptitudes of yogic practitioners. But if sūtras I.14–22 are examined as a group, it is clear that they refer to nine types of yogis who are highly evolved and whose standards of intelligence are far above ordinary human standards. They are of an ascending order of intensity. (See Table 3.)

Paravairāgya (supreme detachment) is for those who are clear of head and pure of heart, heroic and supremely energetic (*adhimātratamān* or *tīvra saṁvegin*). For these, the goal is at hand; for others, it is time-bound.

ईश्वरप्रणिधानाद्वा ।२३।

I.23 Īśvara praṇidhānāt vā

Īśvara	the Lord, God, and Universal Soul
praṇidhānāt	by profound religious meditation, contemplation, prayer, renunciation of the fruits of actions
vā	or

Or, the citta *may be restrained by profound meditation upon God and total surrender to Him.*

To contemplate on God, to surrender one's self to Him, is to bring everything face to face with God. *Praṇidhāna* is the surrender of everything: one's ego, all good and virtuous actions, pains and pleasures, joys and sorrows, elations and miseries to the Universal Soul. Through surrender the aspirant's ego is effaced, and the grace of the Lord pours down upon him like torrential rain.

क्लेशकर्मविपाकाशयैरपरामृष्टः पुरुषविशेष ईश्वरः ।२४।

I.24 kleśa karma vipāka āśayaiḥ aparāmṛṣṭaḥ puruṣaviśeṣaḥ Īśvaraḥ

kleśa	affliction, pain, distress, pain from disease
karma	act, action, performance
vipāka	ripe, mature, result
āśayaiḥ	seat, abode, reservoir
aparāmṛṣṭaḥ	untouched, unaffected, in no way connected
puruṣaviśeṣaḥ	a special person, a distinct *puruṣa*, or being
Īśvaraḥ	God

God is the Supreme Being, totally free from conflicts, unaffected by actions and untouched by cause and effect.

God is a special, unique Entity (*puruṣa*), who is eternally free from afflictions and unaffected by actions and their reactions, or by their residue.

Īśvara is the Supreme Soul, the Lord of all and master of everything. He is untouched by *kleśas* (afflictions), unaffected by the fruits of actions, abiding undisturbed in His own Being. He is eternally free and always sovereign (see II.3 for *kleśas*).

Human beings experience pain before reaching emancipation, but God is always detached from pain and pleasure, sorrow and joy, dejection and elation. God is ever free, but man has to wash away all his subliminal impressions before realizing freedom (see III.36).

There is a difference between *puruṣa* (individual soul) and *puruṣa viśeṣa* (Universal Soul). As God is distinct from the individual soul, He is called Īśvara.

तत्र निरतिशयं सर्वज्ञबीजम् ।२५।

I.25 tatra niratiśayaṁ sarvajñabījam

tatra	therein, in Him
niratiśayaṁ	matchless, unsurpassed, unrivalled
sarvajña	all knowing, omniscient, all wise
bījam	a seed, source, cause, origin, beginning

God is the unexcelled seed of all knowledge.

In Him abides the unrivalled, matchless source of all knowledge. He is the seed of omniscience, omnipresence and omnipotence.

In God rests all creation. He is eternal and one. He is Himself the seed of all knowledge, the seed of omniscience, whereas the yogi attains infinite knowledge but not the seed of that knowledge (see III.50 and IV.31).

स एष पूर्वेषामपि गुरुः कालेनानवच्छेदात् ।२६।

I.26 sa eṣaḥ pūrveṣām api guruḥ kālena anavacchedāt

sa	that
eṣaḥ	*Puruṣa* or God
pūrveṣām	first, foremost
api	also, too, besides, in addition to
guruḥ	master, preceptor
kālena	time
anavacchedāt	unbounded, unlimited, uninterrupted, undefined, continuous

God is the first, foremost and absolute guru, unconditioned by time.

This spiritual *Puruṣa*, the Supreme Spirit, is the first and foremost teacher, neither bound nor conditioned by place, space or time. He is all and all is He.

तस्य वाचकः प्रणवः ।२७।

I.27 tasya vācakaḥ praṇavaḥ

tasya	Him
vācakaḥ	connoting, denoting, signifying, sign, indicating
praṇavaḥ	the sacred syllable *Āuṁ*

He is represented by the sacred syllable āuṁ, *called* praṇava.

He is identified with the sacred syllable *āuṁ*. He is represented in *āuṁ*.

Āuṁ is considered to be the symbol of divinity. It is a sacred mantra, and is to be repeated constantly. *Āuṁ* is called *praṇava*, which stands for praise of the divine and fulfilment of divinity.

Sound is vibration, which, as modern science tells us, is at the source of all creation. God is beyond vibration, but vibration, being the subtlest form of His creation, is the nearest we can get to Him in the physical world. So we take it as His symbol.

The impersonal essence and source of all being is known as *hiranya garbha* (golden womb). It is also known as *Brahman*, who is within each heart. *Āuṁ* is the bow and the self is the arrow. With deep concentration, the aspirant has to hit the target, *Brahman*, so that the individual self and the Universal Soul become one.

Āuṁ is composed of three syllables, *ā*, *u*, *ṁ*. The word is written thus: ॐ. Without these three sounds, no words can begin, resound or end in any language. These three sounds are universal: they are the seed (*bīja*) of all words.

The letters *ā*, *u*, *ṁ* symbolize speech (*vāk*), mind (*manas*), and breath of life (*prāṇa*). As leaves are held together by a twig, all speech is held together by *āuṁ*. *Āuṁ* is the everlasting spirit, a symbol of serenity, divinity, majestic power, omnipotence and universality.

The three letters of *āuṁ* represent the three genders, the three *guṇas*, the three aspects of time: past, present and future, and the three *gurus*: the mother, the father and the preceptor.

They also represent the triad of divinity: *Brahma* the creator, *Viṣṇu* the sustainer, and *Śiva* the destroyer, of the Universe.

Āuṁ as a whole stands for the realization that liberates the human spirit from the confines of body, mind, intellect and ego. By meditating upon *Āuṁ*, the *sādhaka* remains steady, pure and faithful. He becomes a great soul (*mahātmā*). He finds the presence of the Supreme Spirit within, and earns the peace which is free from fear, dissolution and death.

(For further details on *āuṁ* see *Light on Yoga* and *Light on Prāṇāyāma* (HarperCollins*Publishers*).)

तज्जपस्तदर्थभावनम् ।२८।

I.28 tajjapaḥ tadarthabhāvanam

tat	that (*āuṁ*)
japaḥ	muttering in an undertone, whispering, repeating
tadarthabhāvanam	its aim, its purpose, its meaning with feeling, its identification

The mantra āuṁ *is to be repeated constantly, with feeling, realizing its full significance.*

Constant, reverential repetition of the *praṇava āuṁ*, with contemplation on its meaning and the feeling it evokes, helps the seer to reach the highest state in yoga.

Words, meaning and feeling are interwoven. As words are eternal, so are meaning and feeling. Meaning and feeling change according to one's intellectual calibre and understanding. This sūtra conveys the devotional aspects of the seed *mantra āuṁ*.

Japa is repetition of the *mantra*, with reverence and realization of its meaning. Practice of *japa* unites the perceiver, the instruments of perception, and the perceived: God. The *mantra āuṁ* is considered to be *Śabda Brahman* (Word of God, or Universal Sound) to be known with the organs of perception and action, mind, intelligence and consciousness (see I.23, 41 and II.1).

ततः प्रत्यक्चेतनाधिगमोऽप्यन्तरायाभावश्च ।२९।

I.29 tataḥ pratyakcetana adhigamaḥ api antarāya abhāvaḥ ca

tataḥ	then
pratyakcetana	individual soul, introspective mind
adhigamaḥ	to find, discover, accomplish, acquire mastery
api	also, too
antarāya	intervention, interference, impediment, hindrance, obstacle
abhāvaḥ	absence
ca	and

Meditation on God with the repetition of āuṁ *removes obstacles to the mastery of the inner self.*

The repetition of the *praṇava mantra* with feeling and understanding of its meaning leads to the discovery of the Self, and helps to remove impediments to Self-Realization (for impediments, see I.30 and 31).

When experience, the instruments of experience and the object experienced are interwoven, the soul manifests itself without the intervention of any impediments.

व्याधिस्त्यानसंशयप्रमादालस्याविरतिभ्रान्तिदर्शनालब्ध-
भूमिकत्वानवस्थितत्वानि चित्तविक्षेपास्तेऽन्तरायाः ।३०।

I.30 vyādhi styāna saṁśaya pramāda ālasya avirati bhrāntidarśana alabdhabhūmikatva anavasthitatvāni cittavikṣepaḥ te antarāyāḥ

vyādhi	disease
styāna	lack of perseverance, lack of interest, sluggishness, mental laziness
saṁśaya	doubt, indecision
pramāda	intoxication, carelessness, negligence, inattentiveness, inadvertence
ālasya	idleness, physical laziness
avirati	incontinence, lacking in moderation or control, sensual gratification
bhrāntidarśana	living under illusion, mistaken notion
alabdhabhūmikatva	missing the point, inability to hold on to what is achieved, disappointment in one's desired object
anavasthitatvāni	an unsettled state, inability to maintain the achieved progress
cittavikṣepaḥ	a scattered or oscillating mind causing distraction in the consciousness
te	these
antarāyāḥ	obstacles, impediments

These obstacles are disease, inertia, doubt, heedlessness, laziness, indiscipline of the senses, erroneous views, lack of perseverance, and backsliding.

This sūtra describes the nine obstacles or impediments which obstruct progress and distract the aspirant's consciousness.

These obstacles can be divided into physical, mental, intellectual and spiritual:

a	disease	physical
b	lack of interest or sluggishness	
c	lingering doubt	mental
d	pride or carelessness	
e	idleness	
f	sense gratification	

g	living in a world of delusion	intellectual
h	lack of perseverance or not being able to hold on to what has been undertaken	spiritual
i	inability to maintain the progress attained due to pride or stagnation in practices	

In I.29, Patañjali indicates that Self-Realization is possible only when consciousness is free from impediments.

दुःखदौर्मनस्याङ्गमेजयत्वश्वासप्रश्वासा विक्षेपसहभुवः ।३१।

I.31 duḥkha daurmanasya aṅgamejayatva śvāsapraśvāsāḥ vikṣepa sahabhuvaḥ

duḥkha	sorrow, pain, grief, distress, unhappiness
daurmanasya	mental pain, affliction, dejection, despair
aṅgamejayatva	unsteadiness of the body
śvāsapraśvāsāḥ	inspiration and expiration
vikṣepa	scattered, causing distraction
sahabhuvaḥ	existing at the same time, side by side, accompanying, concurrent

Sorrow, despair, unsteadiness of the body and irregular breathing further distract the citta.

Besides the obstacles mentioned in I.30, there are four more causes of distraction: sorrow, despair or evil disposition, tremor of the body and irregular or laboured breathing. (Possibly, laboured breathing shakes the body, creating instability, which in turn brings mental distress.) These cause further distractions which agitate the mind and consciousness.

These impediments are of three types: self-inflicted (*ādhyātmika*), imbalances of elements in the body (*ādhibhautika*) and problems brought about by fate, e.g. genetic defects (*ādhidaivika*). They need to be fought and conquered through yogic disciplines (see I.6; II.3, 17, 34).

तत्प्रतिषेधार्थमेकतत्त्वाभ्यासः ।३२।

I.32 tatpratiṣedhārtham ekatattva abhyāsaḥ

tatpratiṣedhārtham	for their prevention
eka	one, single
tattva	a real state, reality, truth, essential nature, the very essence, a principle, a doctrine
abhyāsaḥ	practice

Adherence to single-minded effort prevents these impediments.

To remove the thirteen impediments and prevent their recurrence, several specific methods have been described.

Though most commentators have concluded that *ekatattva* is devotion and surrender to God, it is beyond the average person's comprehension that surrender to God is the cure for all maladies. If surrender to God were possible for everyone, and could by itself eradicate all impediments, Patañjali need not have elaborated on all the other means of reaching the divine state. Only a few outstanding personalities like Rāmaṇa Māharṣi, Śrī Rāmakṛṣṇa Paramahaṁsa, Mahātmā Gāndhi, Jaḍa Bhārata and the great *ācāryas* of the past could surrender wholeheartedly to God, as they were angels in human form, highly evolved souls whose subliminal impressions from previous lives enabled them to assume their final human form in order to clear up the residues.

But total surrender to God is beyond the abilities of most ordinary men and women, who are still caught up in pleasure and pain, joy and sorrow, success and failure. Meditation undoubtedly helps to minimize the mental agitations of such persons, but to conquer all the obstacles to Self-Realization, all the eight stages of yoga must be followed.

Only when body, mind and intelligence are fully purified is it possible to surrender totally to God, without expecting any return. This is a surrender of the highest order, beyond the capacity of the average individual.

मैत्रीकरुणामुदितोपेक्षाणां सुखदुःखपुण्यापुण्यविषयाणां भावनातश्चित्तप्रसादनम् ।३३।

I.33 maitrī karuṇā muditā upekṣaṇaṁ sukha duḥkha puṇya apuṇya viṣayāṇāṁ bhāvanātaḥ cittaprasādanam

maitrī	friendliness
karuṇā	compassion, mercy
muditā	gladness, joy
upekṣaṇaṁ	to be indifferent and apathetic, to look at things without interest
sukha	happiness
duḥkha	sorrow
puṇya	virtue
apuṇya	vice
viṣayāṇāṁ	regarding an object, concerning a thing
bhāvanātaḥ	conception, remembrance, infusion, recollection, thoughtfulness
cittaprasādanam	graceful diffusion of the consciousness, favourable disposition

Through cultivation of friendliness, compassion, joy, and indifference to pleasure and pain, virtue and vice respectively, the consciousness becomes favourably disposed, serene and benevolent.

These qualities keep the mind in a state of well-being. Patañjali here lays the groundwork for our journey towards Self-Realization. *Citta vikṣepa* is a current of disturbed thoughts running like a river. In *citta prasādana*, graceful diffusion, the turbulent flow is dammed up and consciousness diffuses calmly like a lake.

If the *citta* is caught in the web of the senses, and the *sādhaka* fails to cultivate friendliness, compassion, delight and equanimity, sorrow and unhappiness arise in his heart. This sūtra asks us to rejoice with the happy, to be compassionate to the sorrowful, friendly to the virtuous, and indifferent to those who continue to live in vice despite attempts to change them. This mental adjustment builds social as well as individual health. Besides cultivating these qualities, one should follow the social virtues of *yama* (II.30) for the well-being of society as a whole. This approach to life keeps the mind of the *sādhaka* serene and pure.

प्रच्छर्दनविधारणाभ्यां वा प्राणस्य ।३४।

I.34 pracchardana vidhāraṇābhyāṁ vā prāṇasya

pracchardana	emitting, sending forth, discharging, expelling, exhalation
vidhāraṇābhyāṁ	restraining, maintaining, supporting, executing
vā	or, an option, also the power of choosing correctly, selection, alternatively
prāṇasya	of breath

Or, by maintaining the pensive state felt at the time of soft and steady exhalation and during passive retention after exhalation.

Another possibility of diffusing consciousness is the attainment of that serene state by retention of the breath after exhalation.

In this and the following five sūtras (I:34–39) several alternative methods of calming the mind and preparing it for spiritual evolution are described.

One should inhale and exhale slowly and pause, maintaining the retention for as long as is comfortable. This practice ensures a state of consciousness which is like a calm lake.

(For breath control, see *Light on Prāṇāyāma*.)

विषयवती वा प्रवृत्तिरुत्पन्ना मनसः स्थितिनिबन्धनी ।३५।

I.35 viṣayavatī vā pravṛttiḥ utpannā manasaḥ sthiti nibandhanī

viṣayavatī	related to, attached to object, that which is perceived
vā	or
pravṛttiḥ	moving onwards, advancing, progressing, contemplating, devoting, applying
utpannā	born, produced, acquired, accomplished
manasaḥ	mind
sthiti	state
nibandhanī	origin, basis, foundation, binding together

Or, by contemplating an object that helps to maintain steadiness of mind and consciousness.

One may equally attain an exalted state of consciousness by becoming totally engrossed, with dedication and devotion, in an object of interest.

The practice of contemplating upon an object is the foundation of mental stability. Total absorption in the object brings about direct perception of its essence.

This sūtra shows how to develop awareness and sensitivity in intelligence. In so doing, one may gain insight into the phenomena of nature (*prakṛti*), as well as into the nature of the seer (*puruṣa*).

विशोका वा ज्योतिष्मती ।३६।

I.36 viśokā vā jyotiṣmatī

viśokā	free from grief, sorrowless effulgent light
vā	or
jyotiṣmatī	luminous, bright, shining, possessed of luminous bodies, a tranquil state of mind

Or, inner stability is gained by contemplating a luminous, sorrowless, effulgent light.

Here, the concentration is on the innermost core of the heart, wherein alone the sorrowless, effulgent light glows. That is the seat of the soul. The mind is guided in such a way that it becomes engrossed, and penetrates towards its source. Movements in the form of thoughts in the mind are the waves, and *citta*, or the seat of consciousness, is the ocean. The *sādhaka* must learn to keep the *citta* motionless and thoughtfully silent, without creating waves of thought. This effort of stilling and silencing the *citta* brings forth the sorrowless effulgent light of the soul (see I.45).

वीतरागविषयं वा चित्तम् ।३७।

I.37 vītarāga viṣayaṁ vā cittam

vīta	devoid of, free from
rāga	desire, passion, love, affection
viṣayaṁ	an object
vā	or
cittam	consciousness

Or, by contemplating on enlightened sages who are free from desires and attachments, calm and tranquil, or by contemplating divine objects.

Vyāsa, Śuka, Śaṅkara, Rāmānūja, Mādhva, Vallabha, Caitanya, Śrī Aurobindo, Rāmaṇa Māharṣi and Śri Rāmakṛṣṇa, are examples of men of illumination. If the *sādhaka* reflects on the serene, pure state of such divine persons and emulates their practices, he gains confidence, attains stability and develops a desireless state of mind.

In the same way, one can also contemplate each stage of an *āsana* or each movement of breath in order to bring the *citta* to a state of desirelessness. If consciousness is kept free from desire, it becomes pure. Mere withdrawal from the world does not in itself achieve this aim.

स्वप्ननिद्राज्ञानालम्बनं वा ।३८।

I.38 svapna nidrā jñāna ālambanaṁ vā

svapna	dream state, a state of delusion
nidrā	sleep state
jñāna	wakeful state, awareness, intelligent state
ālambanaṁ	support, base, dependence or resting upon, assistance, help, distinguishing the gross from the eternal
vā	or

Or, by recollecting and contemplating the experiences of dream-filled or dreamless sleep during a watchful, waking state.

Citta has four planes: the unconscious, subconscious, conscious and superconscious. The unconscious plane is the state of dreamless sleep (*nidrā*). The subconscious plane is the dream-filled (*svapna*) state. The conscious plane is the waking (*jāgratā*) state. The superconscious plane is the fourth state known as *turyā*. *Turyā* is *samādhi*, the final state wherein the individual soul (*jīvātman*) is merged with the Universal Soul (*Paramātman*).

By close examination of dream-filled and dreamless sleep, the *sādhaka* comes to distinguish the various levels of consciousness, and learns to transform them into a single state of consciousness.

The *sādhaka* should also contemplate on the thought of the soul before going to sleep, so that the same thought flows uninterruptedly whether he is awake, dreaming or asleep. This supports progress towards the attainment of spiritual bliss.

In III.11–12 Patañjali explains *kṣaya* (waning) *citta*, *śānta* (calm) *citta* and *udaya* (rising) *citta*. These may be compared to *svapna*, *nidrā* and *jāgratā* states. Normally, declining thoughts lead to quietness; but strong rising thoughts keep one awake. A yogi maintains passive alertness without allowing thoughts to spring forth, or strives to restrain them. This is reflective contemplation (see III.13, table 13).

The *sādhaka* begins his *sādhana* dreaming of the pros and cons of each *āsana*. This is a *svapna* state. He stabilizes his ideas and rests on them. This is *nidrā* state. Later he learns to distinguish the subtle points and perform them with awareness. This is the state of *jñāna*.

यथाभिमतध्यानाद्वा ।३९।

I.39 yathābhimata dhyānāt vā

yathābhimata	that which is desirable, a selected thing, a pleasing thing, according to one's wish or taste
dhyānāt	by meditation
vā	or

Or, by meditating on any desired object conducive to steadiness of consciousness.

The final method is to choose an object conducive to meditation: not one which is externally pleasing, but auspicious and spiritually uplifting.

Practising this simple method of one-pointed attention, the *sādhaka* gradually develops the art of contemplation. Later, when a degree of mental stability is attained, he will be able to meditate on any object at will.

The perfect performance of an *āsana* is pleasing, and through it, too, one can gain serenity.

On the face of it this sūtra is simple: it describes meditation on a pleasing object. Its deeper, hidden meaning is harder to comprehend. Having explained various methods of meditation with support, Patañjali now comes to subjective meditation. The most 'pleasing' object of meditation is in fact one's very existence, the core of the being. Patañjali advises us to trace the seed of that core, the living spirit that pervades everything from the most infinitesimal particle to the infinitely greatest. This is the most difficult subject to meditate upon.

This is the last of the six alternative methods of stilling the mind and consciousness. This group of sūtras shows that Patañjali's teaching was broad-based, enabling people of all creeds and all walks of life to aspire to life's spiritual goal. (See Table 4.)

परमाणुपरममहत्त्वान्तोऽस्य वशीकारः ।४०।

I.40 paramāṇu paramamahattvāntaḥ asya vaśīkāraḥ

paramāṇu	an infinitesimal particle, an atom
paramamahattvāntaḥ	most distant, most excellent, highest, best, greatest
asya	of this
vaśīkāraḥ	bringing into subjugation, having mastery over passions, or in one's power

Mastery of contemplation brings the power to extend from the finest particle to the greatest.

By following the various alternative methods of contemplation described above, the *sādhaka* develops the power to penetrate from the most infinitesimal particles to infinity.

The *sādhaka* is not only freed from all disturbances of the mind; he has also subjugated his consciousness and mastered his passions. His consciousness

Table 4: *Stages in the purification of* citta

Sūtra	Method	Limbs of yoga	Elements of *prakṛti*
		TYPES OF MEDITATION	
1.33	Cultivating appropriate attitudes	*Yama*	Behaviour (*Ācāra*) Character (*Śīlam*)
		Niyama	Organs of action (*Karmendriyas*) Organs of perception (*Jñanendrias*)
		Āsana	Mind (*Manas*)
1.34	Breath control	*Prāṇāyāma*	Breath (*Prāna*)
1.35	Absorption in object	*Pratyāhāra*	Senses of perception Mind
1.36	Contemplation of inner light	*Dhāraṇā*	Mind (*Manas*)
1.37	Contemplation of sages	*Dhāraṇā*	Ego, 'I' consciousness (*Ahaṁkāra*)
		OBJECTIVE MEDITATION	
		SUBJECTIVE MEDITATION	
1.38	Recollection of dreams and sleep	*Dhāraṇā*	(consciousness) *Citta*
1.39	Meditation on any desired object	*Dhyāna*	(soul) *Antaḥkaraṇa*

reaches a height of purity in which it develops the power of penetrating objects from the minutest atoms to the mighty cosmos.

This sūtra describes how the ordinary mind is transformed into a super-mind, able to penetrate the boundless regions of space, and the deepest regions within (see I.45).

क्षीणवृत्तेरभिजातस्येव मणेर्ग्रहीतृग्रहणग्राह्येषु तत्स्थतदञ्जनता समापत्तिः ।४१।

I.41 kṣīṇavṛtteḥ abhijātasya iva maṇeḥ grahītṛ grahaṇa grāhyeṣu tatstha tadañjanatā samāpattiḥ

kṣīṇa	dissolving of the *sattva-*, *rajo-* and *tamo- guṇas*
vṛtteḥ	modifications, fluctuations
abhijātasya	inborn, noble, courteous, polite, worthy, learned, distinguished, wise, transparent
iva	like
maṇeḥ	a gem, a flawless crystal
grahītṛ	knower, taker, perceiver, one who has comprehended
grahaṇa	act of seizing, catching, accepting, grasping, instrument of cognition
grāhyeṣu	to be known
tatstha	becoming stable
tadañjanatā	acquiring or taking the shape of the seen or known
samāpattiḥ	transformation, assuming the original form, consummation, completion, conclusion

The yogi realizes that the knower, the instrument of knowing and the known are one, himself, the seer. Like a pure transparent jewel, he reflects an unsullied purity.

With refinement, the consciousness becomes highly sensitive, choiceless, stainless and pure. The perceiver, the instrument of perception and the perceived object, clearly reflected, are nothing but the seer. Like an object reflected flawlessly in a clean mirror, the perceiver, the perceived and the instrument are reflected as one. This transparent reflecting quality of consciousness is termed *samāpatti*, which means assumption of the original form of the seer.

Patañjali's description of *samāpatti* underlines the subtle distinction between yoga, *samādhi* and *samāpatti*. Yoga is the employment of the means to reach *samādhi*. *Samādhi* is profound meditation, total absorption. *Samāpatti* is the balanced state of mind of the seer who, having attained *samādhi*, radiates his own pure state. Yoga and *samādhi*, in other words, can be regarded as practices; *samāpatti* the state towards which they lead.

When all the fluctuations of mind's *sāttvic*, *rājasic* and *tāmasic* nature reach an end, mind ceases to gather and transmit information, and *citta* is like the still, clear water of a calm lake. It transforms itself to the level of the seer, and reflects its purity without refraction. Like a transparent jewel, it becomes at once the knower, the instrument of knowing and the object known. Thus the *sādhaka* experiences the true state of the soul.

Samāpatti is enshrined in *abhijātamaṇi*, which means flawless jewel. *Citta* is now a flawless jewel. A hungry or a thirsty person needs only food or water. Hunger and thirst are necessities of life: their demands are instinctive and instantaneous. Emotions such as lust, anger, greed, infatuation, pride and hatred are not instinctive but are imbibed through contact with the external world; yet, in man they are reflected in their totality. Truthfulness, purity and a loving nature are intuitive and are also fully expressed in man. By yogic discipline and contemplation, the *sādhaka* develops these intuitive qualities of purity and truthfulness and realizes the flawless quality of consciousness. Through it, he becomes the seer and transmits rays of wisdom through his words, thoughts and actions.

तत्र शब्दार्थज्ञानविकल्पैः संकीर्णा सवितर्का समापत्तिः ।४२।

I.42 tatra śabda artha jñāna vikalpaiḥ saṅkīrṇā savitarkā samāpattiḥ

tatra	there
śabda	word
artha	purpose, aim, meaning
jñāna	knowing, knowledge, intelligence
vikalpaiḥ	an option, imagination, the act of allowing a rule to be observed or not as one pleases, surmise, the carrying out of a transaction upon stipulated terms
saṅkīrṇā	poured together, mixed together, strewn, intermingled
savitarkā	becoming totally engrossed, thoughtful
samāpattiḥ	transformation

At this stage, called savitarkā samāpatti, *the word, meaning and content are blended, and become special knowledge.*

In the refined state of consciousness, words and their meanings are simultaneously and harmoniously blended with understanding, so that consciousness becomes engrossed in a new kind of knowledge. This is *savitarkā samāpatti.*

स्मृतिपरिशुध्दौ स्वरुपशून्येवार्थमात्रनिर्भासा निर्वितर्का ।४३।

I.43 smṛtipariśuddhau svarūpaśūnya iva arthamātranirbhāsā nirvitarka

smṛti	memory
pariśuddhau	completely cleansed, purest of minds
svarūpaśūnya	devoid of one's nature
iva	as it were
arthamātranirbhāsā	shining alone in its purest form
nirvitarka	unreflecting, unconsidered, without analysis or logic

In nirvitarka samāpatti, *the difference between memory and intellectual illumination is disclosed; memory is cleansed and consciousness shines without reflection.*

When memory is completely cleansed and purified, mind too is purified. Both cease to function as distinct entites; a no-mind state is experienced, and consciousness alone manifests itself, shining unblemished without reflection of external objects. This is called *nirvitarka samāpatti*.

Memory is the recollection of past thoughts and experiences. It is the storehouse of past impressions. Its knowledge is reflected knowledge. The *sādhaka* should be aware that memory has tremendous impact on intelligence. By perseverance in yoga practices and persistent self-discipline, new experiences surface. These new experiences, free from the memories of the past, are fresh, direct and subjective; they expunge what is remembered. Then memory ceases to function as a separate entity. It either merges with consciousness or takes a back seat, giving predominance to new experiences and bringing clarity in intelligence. For the average person memory is a past mind. For the enlightened man, memory is a present mind. As memory is purified, intelligence becomes illuminative and moves closer to the seer, losing its identity. This is *nirvitarka samāpatti*.

Even for the unripe mind, there is a right and a wrong use of memory. It is not for recollecting pleasure, but for establishing a fund of experience as a basis for further correct action and perception.

In *āsana*, for example, we start with trial and error. The fruits of these experiments are graded by the discriminating intelligence and stored in the memory. As we progress, trial and error decreases, and correct perception increases. So memory provides foresight against error. In the headstand, for example, something that usually goes wrong is that the upper arm shortens.

Memory warns us, 'be aware before it happens'. Discriminating experiment awakens consciousness. Awareness, with discrimination and memory, breaks down bad habits, which are repeated actions based on wrong perception, and replaces them with their opposite. In this process the brain must be creative, not mechanical. The mechanical brain questions only the external phenomena, bringing objective knowledge. The creative brain calls into question the inner and outer, bringing subjective and spiritual knowledge. In *āsana* understanding begins with the inner skin; in *prāṇāyāma*, with the inner membrane of the nose. These are the starting points of the spiritual quest in *āsana* and *prāṇāyāma*.

In this way, a virtuous character is built up. When awareness is linked to intelligence, honesty comes into being; when brain and body move in harmony, there is integrity. In all this long process of *tapas*, memory supports the building-up process. When memory functions perfectly, it becomes one with the intelligence. At this point, memory, which had originally dug for us so many pits, has transformed itself into our true *guru*.

एतयैव सविचारा निर्विचारा च सूक्ष्मविषया व्याख्याता ।४४।

I.44 etayaiva savicāra nirvicāra ca sūkṣmaviṣayā vyākhyātā

etaya	by this
eva	also
savicāra	reflection, deliberation, consideration, investigation
nirvicāra	without reflection, not needing any consideration
ca	and
sūkṣmaviṣayā	subtle object, subtle thing
vyākhyātā	related, explained, expounded, commented upon

The contemplation of subtle aspects is similarly explained as deliberate (savicāra samāpatti) *or non-deliberate* (nirvicāra samāpatti).

Transformation of the consciousness by contemplation on subtle objects such as the ego (*ahaṁkāra*), intelligence (*buddhi*) or the counterpart of the elements (sound, touch, sight, taste and smell), or the qualities of luminosity, vibrancy and dormancy of nature, conditioned by space, time and causation, is *savicāra samāpatti*. Without these reflections it becomes *nirvicāra samāpatti*.

In *nirvicāra samāpatti*, the *sādhaka* experiences a state without verbal deliberation. All the subtle objects reflected in *savicāra* are extinguished. He is free from memory, free from past experiences, devoid of all past impressions. This new state of contemplation is without cause and effect, place or time. The inexpressible states of pure bliss (*ānanda*) and pure self (*sāsmitā*) rise to the surface and are experienced by the *sādhaka* (see I.41).

सूक्ष्मविषयत्वं चालिङ्गपर्यवसानम् ।४५।

I.45 sūkṣmaviṣayatvaṁ ca aliṅga paryavasānam

sūkṣmaviṣayatvaṁ	subtle object
ca	and
aliṅga	having no characteristic mark, unmanifested form
paryavasānam	ending

The subtlest level of nature (prakṛti) *is consciousness. When consciousness dissolves in nature, it loses all marks and becomes pure.*

By exploring the subtle particles of nature, the consciousness reaches its goal. It is a state of complete cessation of the fluctuations of the mind. That is the subtle, infinitesimal intelligence (*mahat*) of nature (*prakṛti*).

Prakṛti and *pradhāna*:

Prakṛti	original or natural form of anything, nature; *aliṅga*, unmanifested form
Pradhāna	primary or original matter, the first evolved or source of the material world, that which is placed or set before, chief or principal thing (these are all susceptible to change, whereas the soul (*puruṣa*) is changeless)

The subtlest of the infinitesimal principles of nature is the cosmic intelligence (*mahat*), which in an individual is transformed as the 'I' in a dynamic, minute form, called *asmitā* or the small self. Though the Self does not change, the small self brings about changes in a human being due to the influence of nature's qualities. The body is made up of the particles of *prakṛti* – from its outermost sheath, the body, to its innermost core, the deep Self. When the individual self, the 'I' is quietened by yogic practices, *prakṛti* has reached its end and merges into the Self. This is subjective experience, or subjective knowledge.

The *sādhaka* attains purity in *buddhi* and *ahaṁkāra*, the infinitesimal source or apex of nature, *mūla-prakṛti*.

Here, the *sādhaka* has reached the crossroads of Self-Realization (see II.19).

ता एव सबीजः समाधिः ।४६।

I.46 tā eva sabījaḥ samādhiḥ

tā	they
eva	only
sabījaḥ	with seed
samādhiḥ	profound meditation or absorption

The states of samādhi described in the previous sūtras are dependent upon a support or seed, and are termed sabīja.

The *savitarka*, *nirvitarka*, *savicāra*, *nirvicāra*, *sānanda* and *sāsmitā samādhis* are known as *sabīja* (seeded or with seed) *samādhis*.

All the states of *samāpatti* described in I.17–19 and I.42–45 are seeded *samādhis*. All these *samādhis* are dependent upon an object which includes the intelligence (*buddhi*) and the 'I' principle (*asmitā*). Their seed is the core of the being, the only seedless seat in each individual.

It is interesting to note that the six *samāpattis* mentioned so far belong to the functions of the brain. The source of analysis (*savitarka*) or absence of analysis (*nirvitarka*) is the frontal brain. For investigation and examination (*savicāra*) or absence of them (*nirvicāra*), the source is the back brain. The source of joy (*ānanda*) is the base of the brain, and of individuality (*asmitā*), the top of the brain.

Through the disciplines of yoga, the *sādhaka* transforms his attention from the gross to the subtle. When he reaches the apex of nature, the brain being a part of nature, he attains perfection in controlling the modes of consciousness. He is able to stop all functions of the brain (see IV. 4), deliberate and non-deliberate, at will. That is why it is termed *samādhi* with seed.

Whatever is dependent on nature for contemplation is seeded *samāpatti*. The contemplation of the seer, who is the source of all seeds, is without support. Though both seer and nature are eternal, nature is changeable while the seer remains the same, immutable, not dependent on any support except his own self. That is why contemplation of the seer is seedless or supportless (*nirbīja*) *samādhi*. Another state of *samādhi*, coming between *sabīja* and *nirbīja* has been discussed by Patañjali in I.18.

Like the petals of the lotus, which unfold as the sun rises, and close as it sets, the petals of the brain retreat from the periphery to its source, its stem, or bud, and all its functions cease. This is commonly called *asaṁprajñāta samādhi*. It is the threshold between *sabīja* and *nirbīja samādhi*. If the *sādhaka* remains on the threshold, he merely conquers the elements. If he falls back, he is caught in pleasures and pains. If he crosses over, he attains freedom and beatitude.

निर्विचारवैशारद्येऽध्यात्मप्रसादः ।४७।

I.47 nirvicāra vaiśāradye adhyātmaprasādaḥ

nirvicāra	non-reflection, or reflection without seeds
vaiśāradye	skilfulness, profound knowledge, undisturbed pure flow
adhyātma	supreme soul (manifested as an individual soul); the relation between the supreme and the individual soul
prasādaḥ	clearness, brightness, pellucidity, serenity of disposition

From proficiency in nirvicāra samāpatti *comes purity.* Sattva *or luminosity flows undisturbed, kindling the spiritual light of the self.*

When intelligence and consciousness, the essence of man, remain nonreflective, profound and unconditioned, the vehicles of the soul – the anatomical body, the organs of action, the senses of perception, the mind, intelligence and consciousness – are illumined. Knowledge and understanding of the real state of the soul manifest in luminosity (see I.3).

Table 5: *The stages of* samādhi

Stages of *samādhi*		Evolutionary growth	Refinement of body and consciousness	Sheaths of body	Connected to	Associated elements GROSS	SUBTLE
Vitarka	*Savitarka* *Nirvitarka*	Five gross elements Organs of action Senses of perception Mind Intellect	Frontal brain (seat of logic)	1 *Annamaya kośa* 2 *Prāṇamaya kośa*	Anatomical Physiological	Earth (*pṛthvī*) Water (*āp*)	Smell (*gandha*) Taste (*rasa*)
Vicāra	*Savicāra* *Nirvicāra*	Mind Intellect Five subtle elements	Back brain (seat of reasoning)	3 *Manomaya kośa*	Psychological	Fire (*tej*)	Shape (*rūpa*)
Ānanda-Sānanda		Intellect transforming into intelligence (*buddhi*) Wisdom	Base of brain (seat of imprints of pleasure and pain)	4 *Vijñānamaya kośa*	Intellectual	Air (*vāyu*)	Touch (*sparśa*)
Asmitā-Sāsmitā		'I' consciousness Intelligence	Top brain	5 *Ānandamaya kośa*	Ethereal	Ether (*ākāśa*)	Sound (*śabda*)
Aṇya or *Virāma Pratyaya*		Between consciousness (*citta*) and *mahat*		6 *Cittamaya kośa*	Consciousness	*Mahat*	
Nirbīja-Dharmamegha		*Mahat* *Mūla prakṛti* *Puruṣa*		7 *Ātmamaya kośa*	Causal		

ऋतंभरा तत्र प्रज्ञा ।४८।

I.48 ṛtaṁbharā tatra prajñā

ṛtaṁbharā	upholding truth, full of truth, full of intellectual essence
tatra	therein
prajñā	faculty of insight, wisdom

When consciousness dwells in wisdom, a truth-bearing state of direct spiritual perception dawns.

This earned spiritual illumination is filled with unalloyed wisdom, glowing with truth and reality. This luminosity of the soul manifests, shining with full fragrance.

Ṛtaṁbharā prajñā is a state of seasoned intelligence or mature wisdom accompanied with intense insight.

श्रुतानुमानप्रज्ञाभ्यामन्यविषया विशेषार्थत्वात् ।४९।

I.49 śruta anumāna prajñābhyām anyaviṣayā viśeṣārthatvāt

śruta	heard, listened, ascertained
anumāna	inference, conjecture
prajñābhyām	from the wisdom of insight
anyaviṣayā	other object
viśeṣa	peculiar, distinguishing between, special property
arthatvāt	object, purpose, aim, end

This truth-bearing knowledge and wisdom is distinct from and beyond the knowledge gleaned from books, testimony, or inference.

Truth-bearing knowledge is first-hand, intuitive knowledge.

This wisdom is gained through insight. It is a special, direct knowledge arising from the soul, not from the perception of the senses or from the ordinary intellect. Hence, it has a peculiar property of its own. The knowledge that springs from one's inner self is intuitive knowledge. It is also known as 'listening to the inner voice'.

It is instructive to compare this sūtra with I.7, in which Patañjali says that one's perception should be verified by logic and measured by traditional and spiritual lore. Now, approaching the end of this chapter, the *sādhaka* may be judged to be of a ripe and cultured mind; his perceptions have an independent validity requiring no verification from other sources. An ordinary man has free will in the sense that he experiences choice and must find his way by discrimination. The enlightened *sādhaka*, having left duality behind him, experiences only his own will, which transcends the hesitations of choice. This is the intelligence of *sattva* in *sattva*.

तज्जः संस्कारोऽन्यसंस्कारप्रतिबन्धी ।५०।

I.50 tajjaḥ saṁskāraḥ anyasaṁskāra pratibandhī

tajjaḥ	born or sprung from *ṛtaṁbharā prajñā*
saṁskāraḥ	conception, instinct, formation in the mind; impressions acquired by effort are subliminal (*saṁskāra*), and recollecting them is an impression or memory
anyasaṁskāra	other conceptions, other impressions or formations
pratibandhī	contradicting, objecting, impeding

A new life begins with this truth-bearing light. Previous impressions are left behind and new ones are prevented.

When the power of the intellect springs from intense insight, that insight negates all previous residues of action, movement and impression.

As explained in I.45, the *sādhaka* is again at a crossroads. New *saṁskāras* may continue to emerge due to the oscillations of the mind, and this may impede real knowledge. These mental impressions must be superseded by the power of discrimination, and then all doubts dissolve. When doubts are cleared, the *sādhaka* has to discard even this discriminative knowledge. The new illuminating wisdom is free from doubts and discriminations; it blazes forth, a glowing beacon of knowledge.

तस्यापि निरोधे सर्वनिरोधान्निर्बीजः समाधिः ।५१।

I.51 tasyāpi nirodhe sarvanirodhāt nirbījaḥ samādhiḥ

tasyāpi	that too
nirodhe	by shutting, closing, restraining, destroying, by cessation
sarva	all
nirodhāt	checking, suppressing, destroying
nirbījaḥ	seedless
samādhiḥ	profound meditation

When that new light of wisdom is also relinquished, seedless samādhi *dawns.*

The *sādhaka* must learn to restrain even this new impression of truth-bearing light. When both old and new impressions are dissolved, a state of seedless enlightenment arises, in which all illusions and delusions terminate. This is *nirbīja samādhi*: the state of absolute identity with the seer.

Even this distinctive knowledge of insight (I.50) has to be restrained, subdued and contained. Then, as a flame is extinguished when the wood is burnt out, or as rivers lose their existence on joining the sea, all volitions and impressions of the unconscious, subconscious, conscious and superconscious mind cease to exist. All these rivers of consciousness merge in the ocean of the seer.

Nirbīja samādhi is the conquest of the *citta* wherein the root mind is one with the seer (see III.56). As all invading thoughts are brought to an end by practice and detachment, the soul is freed from the shackles of earthly vehicles: the body, senses, mind, intelligence and consciousness. The seer is in the *amanaskatva* state.

When *citta* is dependent upon an object, idea or symbol, the state is called *sabīja samādhi*. In *nirbīja samādhi, citta* dissolves and no residue of impressions remains. All residual impressions, the thinking faculty and the feelings of 'I' are extinguished without trace and become universal. The soul alone manifests and blazes without form, in pristine clarity.

Here ends the exposition on *samādhi*, the first *pāda* of Patañjali's *Yoga Sūtras*.

part two

साधनपादः ।
Sādhana Pāda

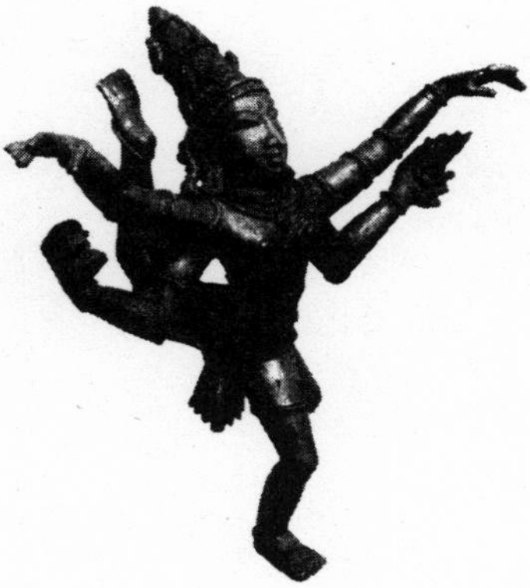

Sādhana means practice. By the practice of yogic discipline, one is led towards spiritual illumination. A *sādhaka* is one who practises, applying his mind and intelligence with skill, dedication and devotion.

Samādhi pāda prescribes a certain level of *sādhana* for those of balanced mind and stable spiritual attainment. Nevertheless, Patañjali does not neglect beginners. In *sādhana pāda*, they too are told how to begin their *sādhana* and work towards spiritual emancipation. Here, the art of practice, *abhyāsa* is fully laid out to uphold the *sādhaka* in the uninterrupted maintenance of his *sādhana*, to guide him around pitfalls so that he may gain great clarity by acute observation and reflection and immaculate precision in practice.

This development was outlined in I.12 when Patañjali described *abhyāsa* and *vairāgya* as the twin uprights of the ladder of spiritual evolution. In I.18, Patañjali hints how the aspirant who has reached a certain level of development but is doubtful of his further direction, may reorientate his *sādhana* from the very first sūtra of this second *pāda*.

Sādhana pāda therefore carries the torch for both the spiritually evolved and the uninitiated. It teaches the complete beginner, who knows no yoga, how he may rise, through his *sādhana*, to the level of high aspirants.

तपःस्वाध्यायेश्वरप्रणिधानानि क्रियायोगः ।१।

II.1 tapaḥ svādhyāya Īśvarapraṇidhānāni kriyāyogaḥ

tapaḥ	heat, burning, shining, ascetic devotion, a burning desire to reach perfection, that which burns all impurities, self-discipline
svādhyāya	Self-study, reflection of one's own self, understanding oneself from the outer sheath, the body, inwards towards the inner self
Īśvara	God, Lord of all
praṇidhānāni	laying on, imposing, turning on, directing upon; profound religious meditation; surrender
kriyāyogaḥ	yoga of action

Burning zeal in practice, self-study and study of scriptures, and surrender to God are the acts of yoga.

For Patañjali, the practice of yoga is the 'yoga of action', *kriyāyoga**, composed of *tapas*, self-discipline, *svādhyāya*, self-study and *Īśvara praṇidhāna*, surrender to God.

Tapas is the blazing desire to burn away the impurities of body, senses and mind. *Svādhyāya* is the repetition of sacred mantras and the study of spiritual sacred texts in order to comprehend one's own self. *Īśvara praṇidhāna* is surrender of one's body, mind and soul to God through love for Him.

Most commentators consider that this *pāda* is intended for novices, and not for those who have already reached a high level of spiritual evolution. This is surely untrue, as *sādhana* is meant for both. The argument that it is only for those still roaming aimlessly in the world of pleasure does not take account of the fact that this wandering is merely a sign of a fluctuating consciousness, which may remain a problem even for evolved souls. By following the precepts of *kriyāyoga*, all aspirants may learn to live in unshakeable serenity regardless of circumstances.

* *Kriyāyoga* has come to have a wider connotation than the path of action, the path of knowledge, or even the dedication of all actions to the Divine (*karma, jñāna*, and *bhakti-mārga* respectively).

This is because *Īśvara praṇidhāna* means not only the surrender of the fruits of actions, but of all actions themselves to the Divinity. Love of God and the act of surrender to Him, is the path of *bhakti*. Hence, *bhaktimārga* too is encompassed by *kriyāyoga*.

From this *pāda* onwards, both beginner and evolved soul learn how to stabilize the mind. Its instructions enable the evolved soul to progress more rapidly towards the goal of purity and emancipation.

The disciplines of purifying man's three constituents, body, speech and mind constitute *kriyāyoga*, the path to perfection. Our bodies are purified by self-discipline (*tapas*), our words by Self-study (*svādhyāya*) and our minds by love and surrender to Him (*Īśvara praṇidhāna*).

This sūtra represents the three great paths: *karma*, *jñāna* and *bhakti*. The path of action (*karma-mārga*) is the discipline (*tapas*) of body, senses and mind. The path of knowledge (*jñāna-mārga*) is the study of the self (*svādhyāya*) from the skin to the core and back again. The path of love of God (*bhakti-mārga*) is surrender (*praṇidhāna*) of all to God.

Sādhana pāda identifies the source of all these paths. The first represents life, the second wisdom. The third, through the surrender of ego, brings the humility that leads to the effulgent, sorrowless light of *Īśvara*, God.

समाधिभावनार्थः क्लेशतनूकरणार्थश्च ।२।

II.2 samādhi bhāvanārthaḥ kleśa tanūkaraṇārthaśca

samādhi	absorption, profound meditation
bhāvana	for bringing about
arthaḥ	contemplating with meaning and feeling, for the purpose of
kleśa	afflictions
tanūkaraṇār-thaḥ	for the purpose of thinning, reducing, making slender, fine, weakening, attenuating
ca	and, both, as well as

The practice of yoga reduces afflictions and leads to samādhi.

By reducing afflictions to a minimum or even eradicating them, *kriyāyoga* promotes profound meditation, which is a precursor to *samādhi*. The purpose of this yoga is to minimize all impediments to meditation and thus bring the intelligence to full, vibrant life.

Table 6: *The acts of* kriyāyoga *and the paths of the* Bhagavad Gītā

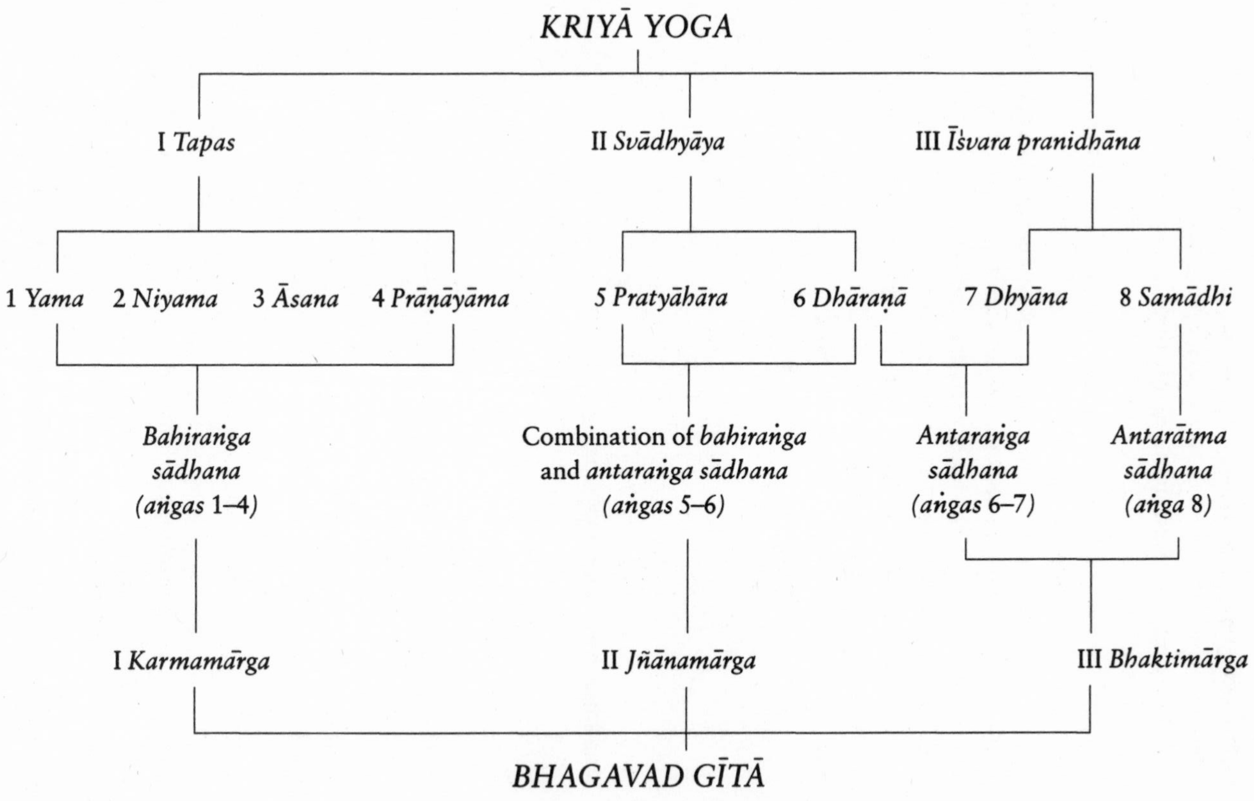

अविद्याऽस्मितारागद्वेषाभिनिवेशाः क्लेशाः ।३।

II.3 avidyā asmitā rāga dveṣa abhiniveśaḥ kleśāḥ

avidyā	lack of spiritual knowledge, spiritual ignorance
asmitā	ego, pride, 'I' or 'me'
rāga	desire, attachment, love, passion, affection, joy, pleasure, musical mode, order of sound
dveṣa	hate, dislike, abhorrence, enmity
abhiniveśaḥ	love of life, fear of death, clinging to life, application, leaning towards attachment, intent, affection, devotion, determination, adherence, tenacity
kleśaḥ	affliction, pain, distress, sorrow, trouble

The five afflictions which disturb the equilibrium of consciousness are: ignorance or lack of wisdom, ego, pride of the ego or the sense of 'I', attachment to pleasure, aversion to pain, fear of death and clinging to life.

Afflictions are of three levels, intellectual, emotional and instinctive. *Avidyā* and *asmitā* belong to the field of intelligence; here lack of spiritual knowledge combined with pride or arrogance inflates the ego, causing conceit and the loss of one's sense of balance. *Rāga* and *dveṣa* belong to emotions and feelings. *Rāga* is desire and attachment, *dveṣa* is hatred and aversion. Succumbing to excessive desires and attachments or allowing oneself to be carried away by expressions of hatred, creates disharmony between body and mind, which may lead to psychosomatic disorders. *Abhiniveśa* is instinctive: the desire to prolong one's life, and concern for one's own survival. Clinging to life makes one suspicious in dealings with others, and causes one to become selfish and self-centred.

The root causes of these five afflictions are the behavioural functions and thoughts of the various spheres of the brain. *Avidyā* and *asmitā* are connected with the conscious front brain, and the top brain is considered the seat of the 'I' consciousness. *Rāga* and *dveṣa* are connected with the base of the brain, the hypothalamus. *Abhiniveśa* is connected with the 'old' brain or back brain which is also known as the unconscious brain, as it retains past subliminal impressions, *saṁskāras**.

* According to Patañjali the five fluctuations (*vṛttis*), the five afflictions (*kleśas*) as well as the maturity of intelligence through *savitarka*, *nirvitarka*, *savicāra*, *nirvicāra*, *ānanda* and *asmitā* are all functions of the four lobes of the brain. The seat of logic is in the front brain, the seat of reasoning in the back brain, the imprinting of pleasure and pain takes place in the base and the seat of individuality, the 'I' or 'Me' is in the top. When all four lobes of the brain are cultured and blended together, the brain becomes superconscious (see I.17).

Table 7: *The five kleśas (afflictions) and the brain*

Level	Kleśas	Functions of four lobes	Location	
I Intellectual	1 Avidyā	→ the seat of logic	front brain = conscious brain	⎫
	2 Asmitā	→ the seat of the individual self	top brain	⎬ the four lobes combined = super-conscious brain
II Emotional	3 Rāga	the seat of imprints of pleasures and pains	base of the brain (hypothalamus) = subconscious brain	
	4 Dveṣa			⎭
III Instinctive	5 Abhiniveśa	→ the seat of reasoning	back brain or old brain = unconscious brain	

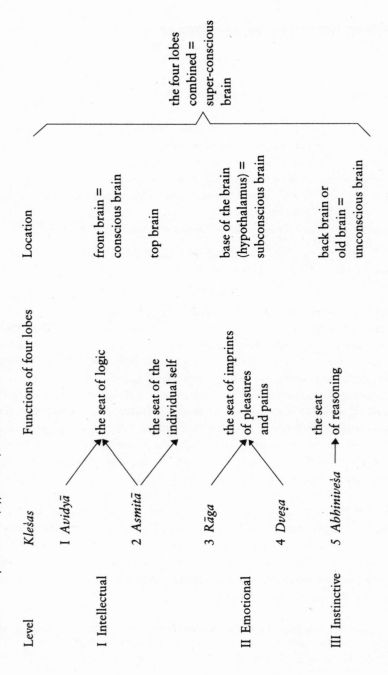

The *sādhaka* must learn to locate the sources of the afflictions, in order to be able to nip them in the bud through his yogic principles and disciplines (see I.8 *viparyaya*).

अविद्या क्षेत्रमुत्तरेषां प्रसुप्ततनुविच्छिन्नोदाराणाम् ।४।

II.4 avidyā kṣetram uttareṣāṁ prasupta tanu vicchinna udārāṇām

avidyā	lack of knowledge, ignorance, nescience
kṣetram	a place, a field, fertile soil, a region, the origin
uttareṣāṁ	that which follows, is followed by, subsequent, consequent
prasupta	asleep, sleepy, dormant
tanu	thin, lean, emaciated, delicate, slender, attenuated
vicchinna	interrupted, hidden, alternated
udārāṇām	fully active

Lack of true knowledge is the source of all pains and sorrows whether dormant, attenuated, interrupted or fully active.

Avidyā, spiritual ignorance, is the source of all the other obstacles: arrogance, desire, aversion and thirst to survive. These afflictions, whether dormant, attenuated or alternating between hidden and fully active, are hindrances to self-enlightenment. Patañjali designates *avidyā* as the breeding-ground of all affliction, whatever its nature.

अनित्याशुचिदुःखानात्मसु नित्यशुचिसुखात्मख्यातिरविद्या ।५।

II.5 anitya aśuci duḥkha anātmasu nitya śuci sukha ātma khyātiḥ avidyā

anitya	not eternal, impermanent
aśuci	impure
duḥkha	sorrow, grief, distress, pain

anātmasu	not spiritual, corporeal, something different from the soul
nitya	eternal, everlasting, constant
śuci	pure
sukha	joy, pleasure
ātma	soul
khyātiḥ	opinion, view, idea, assertion
avidyā	ignorance, nescience

Mistaking the transient for the permanent, the impure for the pure, pain for pleasure, and that which is not the self for the self: all this is called lack of spiritual knowledge, avidyā*.

Naturally we make mistakes, but when, through want of understanding, we fail to reappraise or reflect, error becomes a habit. As the processes of thought and action have existed from the beginning of civilization, so has trial and error been used in the search for knowledge. But when all doubts have been resolved in the pursuit of *sādhana*, the discriminative power of intelligence comes to an end and pure wisdom alone remains, in which perception and action are simultaneous. Experimental and experiential knowledge concur. Objective knowledge and subjective knowledge become one. This is pure *vidyā*, the highest knowledge.

दृग्दर्शनशक्त्योरेकात्मतेवास्मिता ।६।

II.6 dṛk darśanaśaktyoḥ ekātmatā iva asmitā

dṛk	power of vision, cause to see, power of consciousness
darśana	power of seeing, looking, displaying, inspecting, perceiving
śaktyoḥ	ability, capability, strength, power
ekātmatā	having the same nature, in the same manner
iva	as if, appearance
asmitā	egoism

Egoism is the identification of the seer with the instrumental power of seeing.

* Here is an example of *avidyā*. Iron and coal are two different entities, but when iron is heated, it becomes red hot and looks like live coal. Similarly, though the body and the eternal Self are distinct entities, lack of knowledge makes one believe that they are one. Taking pride in the body as the Self is also *avidyā*.

Identifying the instruments of cognition – the senses of perception, intelligence and ego or the sense of the individual self – with the pure seer is egoism, or the conception of individuality.

Though there is a distinction between the seer (*ātmā*) and the seen, during the act of seeing the seen (the mind itself) appears to be the pure seer. This appearance of merging or 'oneness' is due to *asmitā*.

One must be aware of the difference between the seer (*ātmā*) and the instrument that sees (*buddhi*). If they blend and work together, that experience is reality. But if the mind and senses, the seer's agents, take it upon themselves to identify with the true seer, as if the seer were manifest or apparent, then polarities are created and seer and seen become separated or split. This is *asmitā*.

(To understand these polarities, see II.17, II.21–23, III.36. For *asmitā*, see IV.4.)

सुखानुशयी रागः ।७।

II.7 sukha anuśayī rāgaḥ

sukha	happiness, delight, sweetness, pleasure
anuśayī	close connection, close attachment, succeeded by, followed by
rāgaḥ	love, affection, musical mode

Pleasure leads to desire and emotional attachment.

Dwelling on pleasurable experiences ignites desire and a sense of attraction, which creates attachment. Pleasurable experiences generate greed and lust, which strengthen attachment and stimulate a greater craving, as one always wants more and more. One becomes absorbed by the pursuit of pleasure, and addicted to gratification of the senses. The aspirant may thus forget his chosen path and allow himself to be caught up in sorrow and sickness.

दुःखानुशयी द्वेषः ।८।

II.8 duḥkha anuśayī dveṣaḥ

duḥka	unpleasantness, sorrow, grief, unhappiness, pain, distress, agony
anuśayī	followed by, close connection, subsequent
dveṣaḥ	aversion, hate, dislike, abhorrence, distaste

Unhappiness leads to hatred.

Pain, sorrow and misery trigger a chain of hate or aversion. Recollecting lost pleasures, tormented by desires unfulfilled, man is led to sorrow. In extreme distress he comes to hate himself, his family, neighbours and surroundings, and feels a sense of worthlessness.

A discriminating person strives to acquire knowledge so that he may strike a balance between *sukha* and *duḥkha* and live at the mercy of neither pleasure nor pain.

स्वरसवाही विदुषोऽपि तथा रूढोऽभिनिवेशः ।९।

II.9 svarasavāhī viduṣaḥ api tatha ārūḍhaḥ abhiniveśaḥ

svarasavāhī	current of love of life
viduṣaḥ	a wise man, a learned man, a scholar
api	even, likely
tatha	all the same
ārūḍhaḥ	having ascended, advanced
abhiniveśaḥ	intentness of affection, leaning towards, attachment to life

Self-preservation or attachment to life is the subtlest of all afflictions. It is found even in wise men.

Love of life is sustained by life's own force. This urge for self-perpetuation is so strong that it does not spare even the wise, and is an affliction for them and the ignorant alike. If even a highly educated, scholarly person cannot easily remain unattached to life, it is not difficult to gauge the feelings of an average individual.

Patañjali indicates that each human being has had a taste of death, which lingers. This imprint is the seed of fear.

Abhiniveśa is an instinctive defect which can be transformed into intuitive knowledge and insight by practising yoga.

While practising *āsana, prāṇāyāma* or *dhyāna*, the *sādhaka* penetrates deep within himself. He experiences unity in the flow of intelligence, and the current of self-energy. In this state, he perceives that there is no difference between life and death, that they are simply two sides of the same coin. He understands that the current of self, the life-force, active while he is alive, merges with the universe when it leaves his body at death. Through this understanding, he loses his attachment to life and conquers the fear of death. This frees him from afflictions and sorrows and leads him towards *kaivalya*.

If *avidyā* is the root cause of afflictions, so *abhiniveśa* results in pain. In realizing the oneness of life and death there is an end to ignorance in the aspirant, and he lives forever in the flow of tranquillity (see III.10 and IV.10).

ते प्रतिप्रसवहेयाः सूक्ष्माः ।१०।

II.10 te pratiprasavaheyāḥ sūkṣmāḥ

te	these
prati	in opposition, against
prasava	procreation, generation (*prati prasava* = involution)
heyāḥ	to abandon, desert, relinquish, emit, renounce, abstain
sūkṣmāḥ	subtle, minute, delicate

Subtle afflictions are to be minimized and eradicated by a process of involution.

Afflictions may be gross or subtle; both must be counteracted and eliminated, silenced at their very source.

The five afflictions – ignorance, egoism, lust, malice and attachment to life (II.3) appear gross (*sthūla*) on the surface, but their subtle nature may be either dormant or highly active, or may alternate between the two (II.4). Meditation helps to eradicate them (II.2, 11).

The subtle afflictions begin with attachment to life, move in the reverse order, contrary to spiritual evolution of II.3 and end with the gross affliction, ignorance. Subtle afflictions should be overcome before they lead to worse trouble.

How does one overcome them? If a seed becomes parched, it cannot germinate; so one must render an affliction sterile by tracing it back to its source. The father of subtle afflictions is the mind, whose movements should be directed towards the seer by the yogic process of involution (*prati prasava*). (See the detailed explanation given under *pratyāhāra*, II.54.) In this way, subtle afflictions are vanquished and an unpolarized state of pure knowledge is attained (II.48).

ध्यानहेयास्तद्वृत्तयः ।११।

II.11 dhyānaheyāḥ tadvṛttayaḥ

dhyāna meditation, reflection, attention, observation
heyāḥ annihilated, rejected, quietened, avoided, silenced
tad their
vṛttayaḥ fluctuations, movements, operations

The fluctuations of consciousness created by gross and subtle afflictions are to be silenced through meditation.

Both II.10 and II.11 point to a way of controlling the modifications of thought-waves. In II.10, the mind is stilled through involution, the practice of renunciation or folding-in of the mind. Here, Patañjali offers meditation as another method to quieten the mind. By these means, the mind's impulses are reduced to their subtlest point and it is compelled to rest silently in its source, the soul.

Afflictions are of three intensities: gross (*sthūla*), subtle (*sūkṣma*), and the subtlest of the subtle (*sūkṣmatama*). *Tapas*, *svādhyāya* and *Īśvara praṇidhāna* eradicate the gross, the subtle and the subtlest afflictions respectively (see I.17).

क्लेशमूलः कर्माशयो दृष्टादृष्टजन्मवेदनीयः ।१२।

II.12 kleśamūlaḥ karmāśayaḥ dṛṣṭa adṛṣṭa janma vedanīyaḥ

kleśa	affliction, pain, distress, sorrow
mūlaḥ	root, origin, source
karma	action, deed, work, performance
āśayaḥ	resting place, abode, asylum, reservoir
dṛṣṭa	visible, capable of being seen, perceivable
adṛṣṭa	not capable of being seen, unperceivable, unobservable, invisible, fate
janma	birth, life
vedanīyaḥ	to be known, to be experienced

The accumulated imprints of past lives, rooted in afflictions, will be experienced in present and future lives.

The imprints or residual impressions of one's actions, whether good or bad, afflict one according to their degree of merit and demerit. They are the seed of future sorrows and pleasures which we experience both in this life and in lives to come.

Past actions are the seeds of affliction which in turn give rise to other actions, necessitating further lives, or reincarnation. This is known as *karma*, or the universal law of cause and effect. Afflictions and actions intermingle and interact, and the cycles of birth and death roll on. Actions rooted in desire, greed, anger, lust, pride and malice invite affliction, just as those which are free from the spokes of the wheel of desire lead towards the state of bliss. The effects of both types of action may be visible or invisible, manifest or latent; they may surface in this life or in future lives. According to Śrī Hariharānanda* 'one's reservoir of *karma* is analogous to a seed; desire, greed and lust are shoots from the field; life is the plant and life's pain and pleasure are the flowers and fruits'. Through the practices of *kriyāyoga* – *tapas*, *svādhyāya* and *Īśvara praṇidhāna* – we try to expunge in this life our residual *karma*. This is the accumulated fruit of our actions, gathered over our past lives and in this life, in the form of visible and invisible or predetermined effects which we regard as destiny or fate.

Hindu lore is full of examples of the work of *karmāśaya*; there is

* Patañjali's *Yoga Sūtra*, Calcutta University Press.

Nandīśvara who became the vehicle of Lord Śiva, Viśvāmitra, a warrior king who became a pure and true brahmin, Ūrvaṣi, a nymph who became a creeper; and Nahūṣa, king of heaven who became a snake.

Nahūṣa, a king of Bhārata (India) was a virtuous king. When Lord Indra, King of heaven, killed the demon Vṛtra, he had to do penance for having killed a brahmin, leaving heaven temporarily without its king. For his virtue Nahūṣa was invited by the Gods to rule heaven in Indra's stead until his return from the penance. Reluctantly Nahūṣa agreed. But while there, he fell in love with Śachi, Indra's wife. Nahūṣa made it known to Śachi that as Lord of heaven he considered he had a right to share her favours. To safeguard herself, Śachi asked her preceptor, Bṛhaspati, how she should protect herself. On his advice, she acquiesced on one condition; Nahūṣa was to come to their tryst borne on a most extraordinary palanquin, carried by the seven sages (*saptarṣis* – the constellation known as the Great Bear). Lust overruled his reflective thoughts and at once he summoned the seven sages and ordered them to bear his palanquin to Śachi's house. In his infatuation and anxiety to reach her quickly, Nahūṣa ordered them to move fast. The Sanskrit word for 'move fast' is *sarpa* which also means 'snake'. He lost his self-control and kicked sage Agastya. Agastya lost his temper and in his anger cursed the king with the word *sarpobhava* meaning 'become a snake'. Nahūṣa fell to earth in the form of a serpent (see I.5). Nahūṣa remained a snake until Yudhiṣṭira washed off his *karma*. Nahūṣa had entwined himself around Bhīma, son of Pāṇḍu of Mahābhārata fame, promising his release only if he answered all his questions. Bhīma failed to do so, but was rescued by Yudhiṣṭira, his elder brother, who had gone out in search of him. Yudhiṣṭira was alarmed to discover Bhīma in the coils of a large snake, but the serpent gave his word to set Bhīma free unharmed provided all his questions were answered. This Yudhiṣṭira willingly fulfilled and regained Bhīma. Soon the snake returned to a human form, realized his folly and resumed his penance.

There is another example of a good *karma* which elevated a young bull called Nandi to reach God. Nandi, the child of Kāmadhenu, the cow of plenty who yields all desires, reached the highest state of emancipation through *sādhana* to become the attendant of Lord Śiva on which He rides.

सति मूले तद्विपाको जात्यायुर्भोगाः ।१३।

II.13 sati mūle tadvipākaḥ jāti āyuḥ bhogāḥ

sati	being, existing, real, essential, tone
mūle	root
tat	its
vipākaḥ	fruit, ripening
jāti	rank, class, birth
āyuḥ	span of life
bhogāḥ	experiencing, enjoying

As long as the root of actions exists, it will give rise to class of birth, span of life and experiences.

Life itself springs from the admixture of good and bad actions, favourable and unfavourable imprints. These form one's birth, rank in life, span of life and the kind of experiences one has to undergo.

According to the law of *karma*, all conditions in the nature of our birth and life stem from our past actions, and are responsible for the experiences, pleasant or otherwise, which we meet in life.

The fruits of the actions gathered in this life are called *saṁskāras*, which become residual imprints or impressions. The fruits of actions committed in all previous lives are called *vāsanas* (knowledge derived from memory, or the present consciousness of past perceptions). *Vāsanas* are impressions remaining unconsciously in the mind from past good or bad actions, producing pleasure or pain.

ते ह्लादपरितापफलाः पुण्यापुण्यहेतुत्वात् ।१४।

II.14 te hlāda paritāpa phalāḥ puṇya apuṇya hetutvāt

te	they
hlāda	pleasant, to be glad, delighted, to rejoice
paritāpa	pain, anguish, grief, lamentation

phalāḥ	fruits
puṇyāpuṇya	virtues and vices, or assets and liabilities
hetutvāt	being caused by, on account of

According to our good, bad or mixed actions, the quality of our life, its span, and the nature of birth are experienced as being pleasant or painful.

In this sūtra, the karmic law of cause and effect is further considered.

Sūtras 12–14 indicate *sādhaka* should plan a yogic, disciplined way of life to minimize the imprints of action.

(To understand the nature of right actions, see I.33, II.30, II.32–33.)

परिणामतापसंस्कारदुःखैर्गुणवृत्तिविरोधाच्च दुःखमेव सर्वं विवेकिनः ।१५।

II.15 pariṇāma tāpa saṁskāra duḥkaiḥ guṇavṛtti virodhāt ca duḥkham eva sarvaṁ vivekinaḥ

pariṇāma	change, alteration, transformation, consequence, result
tāpa	heat, torment, pain, sorrow, afflictions, distress
saṁskāra	impressions, refinement, conception, faculty of recollection, instinct
duḥkhaiḥ	unhappiness, pain, sorrow, grief, misery
guṇa	qualities, characteristics
vṛtti	fluctuations
virodhāt	on account of opposition, obstruction, restraint, contrast
ca	and
duḥkham	pain, sorrow
eva	indeed
sarvaṁ	all, whole
vivekinaḥ	the enlightened, man of discrimination

The wise man knows that owing to fluctuations, the qualities of nature, and subliminal impressions, even pleasant experiences are tinged with sorrow, and he keeps aloof from them.

This sūtra explains that the wise man knowing that all pleasure leads to pain, remains apart from the laws and the machinery of *karma*. Owing to past impressions, obstructions and anguish, the quality of any action is adulterated by its contact with the *guṇas* of nature, so he treats even pleasant experiences as inherently painful, and holds himself aloof from them.

There are three types of characteristics of the intelligence: luminosity (*sattva*), vibrancy (*rajas*) and inertia (*tamas*). The wise person knows that thought transformations, afflictions, instincts and even pleasures end sooner or later in pain, so he shuns the causes of both pain and pleasure (see II.7–8).

The eyelids, being very sensitive, resist extraneous light or matter immediately, and protect the eyes by shutting. Similarly, if we are intellectually sensitive, we will be able to discriminate quickly between the pleasant and unpleasant, the mixed and unmixed, and reject unsuitable thought and action.

This sūtra states that pure inner peace can be reached by acquiring the right knowledge that will weed out the roots of pain and pleasure.

हेयं दुःखमनागतम् ।१६।

II.16 heyaṁ duḥkham anāgatam

heyaṁ	to be avoided, to be rejected, to be prevented
duḥkham	sorrow, agony
anāgatam	not yet come, future, unknown

The pains which are yet to come can be and are to be avoided.

Past pain is finished. Pain that we are in the process of experiencing cannot be avoided, but can be reduced to some extent by yogic practice and discriminative knowledge. Unknown future pains can be prevented by adhering now to yogic discipline.

Patañjali is saying that yoga is a preventive healing art, science and philosophy, by which we build up robust health in body and mind and construct a defensive strength with which to deflect or counteract afflictions that are as yet unperceived afflictions.

Furthermore, strong health and a stable mind will enable us to face the wonder of wonders – the spiritual bliss – if and when, thanks to our good actions in former lives, the spiritual gate is set open.

One should remember that even Arjuna, hero of the Mahābhārata, had to beg Lord Kṛṣṇa to grace him with divine perception in order to face the divine light which his ordinary eyes would not be able to bear. Patañjali warns us here of the pitfalls in spiritual growth, and advises us to stabilize the body and mind so that we may not be shattered when spiritual light dawns.

द्रष्टृदृश्ययोः संयोगो हेयहेतुः ।१७।

II.17 draṣṭṛdṛśyayoḥ saṁyogaḥ heyahetuḥ

draṣṭṛa	seer, self, *puruṣa*
dṛśyayoḥ	the seen, the known, nature
saṁyogaḥ	union, association, conjunction, connection, junction, mingling
heyaḥ	to be relinquished, to be avoided
hetuḥ	cause, ground, reason, purpose

The cause of pain is the association or identification of the seer (ātmā) *with the seen* (prakṛti) *and the remedy lies in their dissociation.*

A wise person notices that inner harmony is disturbed when the mind lets itself be lured into indiscriminately sampling the world of phenomena. He tries to remain free by avoiding material attachment, in which objects draw the intelligence like a magnet and the self is enticed into an illusory relationship with the external, seen world, provoking pleasures and pains. The intelligence is the vehicle closest to the soul, which must be wary of its influence if the seer is to remain free. Otherwise intelligence enmeshes the seer in a painful relationship with external objects. As long as intelligence is undiscriminating, there is suffering. The moment it develops discriminative power, it realizes its source, and mingles with the seer. Then there is transparency between the seer and seen, allowing free, uncontaminated passage between them.

The seat of the ego or small self is the seat of the brain, and the seat of the great Self is in the spiritual heart. Though intelligence connects the head and the heart, it oscillates between the two. This oscillation ceases through right knowledge and understanding. Intelligence is then transformed: free from polarity, pure and unbiased. This is true meditation, in which ego dissolves, allowing the great Self (*puruṣa*) to shine in its own glory (IV.4).

प्रकाशक्रियास्थितिशीलं भूतेन्द्रियात्मकं भोगापवर्गार्थं दृश्यम् ।१८।

II.18 prakāśa kriyā sthiti śīlaṁ bhūtendriyātmakaṁ bhogāpavargārthaṁ dṛśyam

prakāśa	brightness, brilliance, clearness, splendour, elucidation, lustre
kriyā	action, study, investigation
sthiti	steadiness, firmness, steadfastness, being
śīlaṁ	disposition, virtue, character, piety
bhūtam	elements
indriya	the eleven senses: mind, five senses of perception, five organs of action
ātmakaṁ	the nature or essence of a thing, being composed of
bhoga	enjoyment of pleasures
apavarga	emancipation, liberation
arthaṁ	means, purpose
dṛśyam	knowable, seen

Nature, its three qualities, sattva, rajas *and* tamas, *and its evolutes, the elements, mind, senses of perception and organs of action, exist eternally to serve the seer, for enjoyment or emancipation.*

The visible objective world consists of elements of nature and senses of perception comprising three qualities or attributes (*guṇas*), which are illumination, motion or action, and inertia or dormancy. All these exist eternally to serve the seer (the subject) for the purpose of experiencing the pleasures and infatuations (objects) of the world, or for emancipation.

This sūtra describes the characteristics, actions and uses of nature (*prakṛti*).

The three attributes of nature are *sattva*, *rajas* and *tamas*. When one mixes with another, it is subdivided into *sattva* in *sattva* (*sattvo-sattva*), *sattva* in *rajas* (*sattva-rajas*) and *sattva* in *tamas* (*sattva-tamas*). Similarly, *rajas* is divided into *rajo-sattva*, *rajo-rajas* and *rajo-tamas* and *tamas* into *tamo-sattva*, *tamo-rajas* and *tamo-tamas*. According to Patañjali, *sattva*, *rajas* and *tamas* represent *prakāśa*, *kriyā* and *sthiti*. These attributes have their own virtues for example, *prakāśa* or brilliance or splendour is *sattva*; *kriyā* or study, investigation and action is *rajas*; and the essence of the being resting as *sthiti* or dormancy is *tamas*.

All these attributes and virtues are established in the elements of nature, senses, mind, intelligence and ego. Together they function harmoniously in the form of illumination, action and inertia, allowing the seer to enjoy the world's pleasures (*bhoga*); or by divesting himself of them, to experience liberation.

The seer is clothed with five sheaths (*kośas*), by the elements of nature: earth, water, fire, air and ether. Earth represents the anatomical, water the physiological, fire the mental, air the intellectual and ether the spiritual sheaths. The organs of action and senses of perception aid the *sādhaka* in purifying the anatomical and physiological sheaths through *yama* and *niyama*. *Āsana*, *prāṇāyāma* and *pratyāhāra* divest the seer of the mental sheath; *dhāraṇā* and *dhyāna* cleanse the intellectual sheath. *Samādhi* brings the seer out through the prison-gates of all the sheaths to experience freedom and beatitude. (See Table 8.)

विशेषाविशेषलिङ्गमात्रालिङ्गानि गुणपर्वाणि ।१९।

II.19 viśeṣa aviśeṣa liṅgamātra aliṅgāni guṇaparvāṇi

viśeṣa	the art of distinguishing or discriminating, a state of being especial, a mark
aviśeṣa	uniform, alike, without any difference, unspecified state
liṅgamātra	indicator, mark, sign (chief mark or indication of *prakṛti*, that is, the cosmic intelligence – *mahat*), phenomenal, directly apprehended, observed
aliṅgāni	without mark, without sign, non-primary matter or unevolved matter, unknown and unknowable substance or thing as it is in itself, the noumenal
guṇaparvāṇi	changes in qualities

The guṇas *generate their characteristic divisions and energies in the seer. Their stages are distinguishable and non-distinguishable, differentiable and non-differentiable.*

This sūtra analyses nature (*prakṛti*) by identifying the progressive layers of its manifestation, from the most specific and definable up through the non-specific and non-distinguished and back to the undifferentiated or universal.

Table 8: *The evolution of* citta

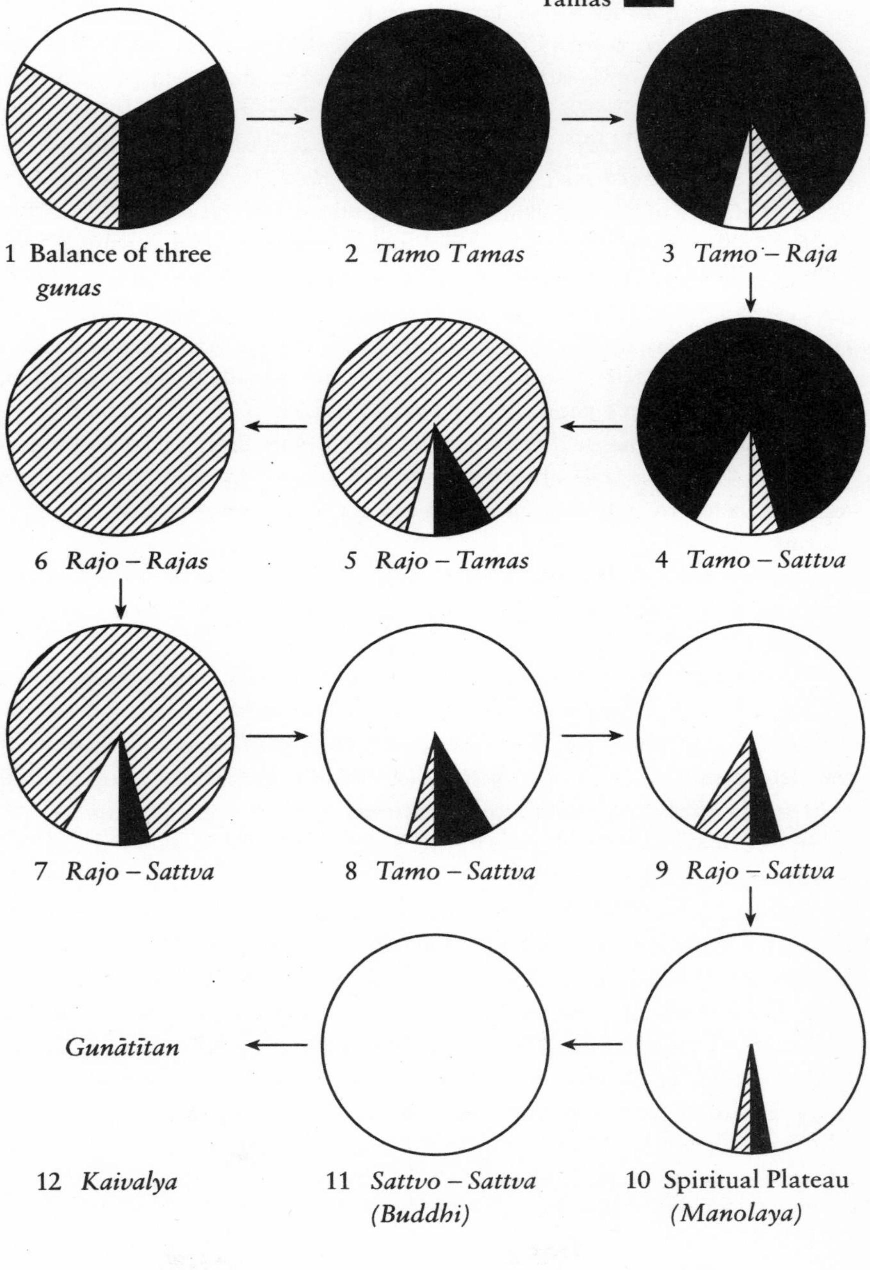

To release ourselves from the confines of nature, we have to be familiar with its geography and its divisions, and with how these are affected and changed by the *guṇas*, so that we can understand the internal rules that govern nature in all its forms, however subtle.

Nature (*prakṛti*) consists of cosmic intelligence (*mahat*), which has the three qualities of luminosity (*sattva*), action and motion (*rajas*) and inertia (*tamas*). It is the changing influence of these qualities that gives form to our life in its cycle of births and shapes our characteristics according to the nature of our past actions and experiences. *Prakṛti* also manifests its energy in the character of the five elements: earth, water, fire, air and ether; and in the five subtle manifestations of smell, taste, shape, touch and sound.

The individual counterpart of cosmic intelligence (*mahat*) is consciousness, or *citta*. *Citta* consists of mind (*manas*), which reviews sensory and vibrational stimuli; intelligence (*buddhi*), which is the discriminative faculty; and ego or small self (*ahaṁkāra*) which is the individual 'I'. In addition, hidden deep in man's nature is a powerful hidden spiritual weapon: 'conscience' (*antaḥkaraṇa* or *dharmendriya*) which embodies ethical and moral principles. *Antaḥkaraṇa* observes right and wrong in one's conduct and motives, helps to cultivate *citta* and directs it to perform only the right actions.

There are also the five senses of perception – ears, tongue, eyes, nose and skin, and five organs of action – legs, arms, speech, genital and excretory organs.

These are the principles of *prakṛti*. The five elements, intelligence, senses of perception and organs of action are distinguishable, that is, physically manifest in concrete form. The other parts, the five subtle manifestations of the elements and the 'I' consciousness (*ahaṁkāra*, *antaḥkaraṇa* and *asmitā*) exist in a non-distinguishable or vibrational form, being non-primary and unevolved matter. Yet, all these revolve around the three *guṇas* of nature: *tamas*, *rajas* and *sattva*.

The principles (*tattvas*) of distinguishable elements (*viśeṣa*) produce changes which may be pleasant, unpleasant or stuporous (a state of suspended or deadened sensibility). The unspecified principles (*aviśeṣa tattvas*) are unevolved matter, and when such matter is transformed into a specified state, creation takes place. This is called *pravṛttimārga*. The reverse process, *nivṛtti mārga*, is the merging of the specified in the unspecified, of the non-specified in and of nature (see I.45) into the universal spirit (*puruṣa*). The merging of nature into spirit is a divine marriage, which becomes possible through the work of yoga.

(See III.13 and Table 9.)

द्रष्टा दृशिमात्रः शुद्धोऽपि प्रत्ययानुपश्यः ।२०।

II.20 draṣṭā dṛśimātraḥ śuddhaḥ api
pratyayānupaśyaḥ

draṣṭā	seer, *puruṣa*, one who sees
dṛśimātraḥ	awareness only, consciousness only
śuddhaḥ	pure
api	even though
pratyayaḥ	conviction, trust, reliance, faith, cognition, confidence
anupaśyaḥ	one who sees, seeing along with, cognizing ideas

The seer is pure consciousness. He witnesses nature without being reliant on it.

This sūtra moves on from nature to soul, the Supreme Seer, the absolute knower. It is the pure essence of consciousness beyond words. Though the soul is pure, it tends to see through its agent, the intelligence (*buddhi*) and being carried away by the influence of nature, it loses its identity.

The previous sūtra dealt with nature (*prakṛti*) and discernible objects. Here, the nature of the seer, the soul (*puruṣa*) is described. *Ātmā*, *draṣṭa* and *dṛśimātraḥ* are terms which show the innate nature of the seer.

Intelligence clouds consciousness in such a way that it comes to identify itself as the true seer and forgets the soul. But if intelligence can keep its power of discernment, consciousness too will remain uncoloured. If consciousness is clear, the seer is unobscured.

Intelligence, belonging as it does to manifest nature, is constantly changing, sometimes conscious and often unconscious. It is subject to *sattva*, *rajas* and *tamas*, whereas the seer, *puruṣa*, is beyond all these, immutable and ever-conscious (see I.3, IV.22).

तदर्थ एव दृश्यस्यात्मा ।२१।

II.21 tadarthaḥ eva dṛśyasya ātmā

tadarthaḥ	for that purpose, for that sake
eva	alone
dṛśyasya	of the seen, of the knowable, nature (*prakṛti*)
ātmā	seer (*puruṣa*), soul, principle of life, awareness, witnesser

Nature and intelligence exist solely to serve the seer's true purpose, emancipation.

Intelligence exists to serve as the seer's agent, to free the consciousness from *avidyā*. The natural tendency of all the soul's agents – mind, senses of perception and organs of action – to be drawn to and identify with the sensory and phenomenal world is to be avoided by discrimination, a faculty of intelligence. Uninterrupted yogic *sādhana* will help us overcome these obstacles and allow the soul to reveal itself.

If the *sādhaka* slackens in his *sādhana* and becomes inattentive, the senses disturb the seer and he is caught again in the pleasures of the senses. This study of mind and investigation through intelligence is the innermost quest: *antarātma sādhana*.

This sūtra conveys that consciousness, the essence of nature, which is cognizable, exists for the sake of the seer who sees to see.

कृतार्थं प्रति नष्टमप्यनष्टं तदन्यसाधारणत्वात् ।२२।

II.22 kṛtārthaṁ prati naṣṭam api anaṣṭaṁ tadanya sādhāraṇatvāt

kṛtārthaṁ	whose purpose has been fulfilled, who has attained an end, successful, satisfied
prati	against, in opposition to
naṣṭam	destroyed, disappeared, lost sight of
api	although
anaṣṭaṁ	not disappeared, not destroyed, not lost

tat	that
anya	to others
sādhāraṇatvāt	average, being normal

The relationship with nature ceases for emancipated beings, its purpose having been fulfilled, but its processes continue to affect others.

As soon as the vehicles of nature which act as agents of the seer accomplish their task of freeing him from his mental and sensory prison, they are quietened, having accomplished their purpose. The bond between the seer and nature comes to an end. Nature ceases to exist for him. He is able to perceive his own form (*svarūpa*).

However, the vehicles of nature, elements, their subtle qualities, cosmic intelligence, individual self, ego, intelligence, senses of perception and organs of action are common to all, so for others, who remain caught up in the world's turmoils, the bondage endures.

स्वस्वामिशक्त्योः स्वरूपोपलब्धिहेतुः संयोगः ।२३।

II.23 sva svāmiśaktyoḥ svarūpopalabdhi hetuḥ saṁyogaḥ

sva	one's own, of being, owned, nature
svāmi	owner, master, lord, seer
śaktyoḥ	strength of *prakṛti* and *puruṣa*, power of the two
svarūpa	form, one's own
upalabdhi	to find, obtain, perceive, to see, recognize, to experience
hetuḥ	cause, reason, purpose
saṁyogaḥ	union, conjunction

The conjunction of the seer with the seen is for the seer to discover his own true nature.

The powers of *puruṣa* and *prakṛti* are intended for Self-Realization. The purpose of their contact is the unfolding of their inherent powers, and the seer's discovery of his own essential nature.

This sūtra makes clear that a desire for fusion or a close association or

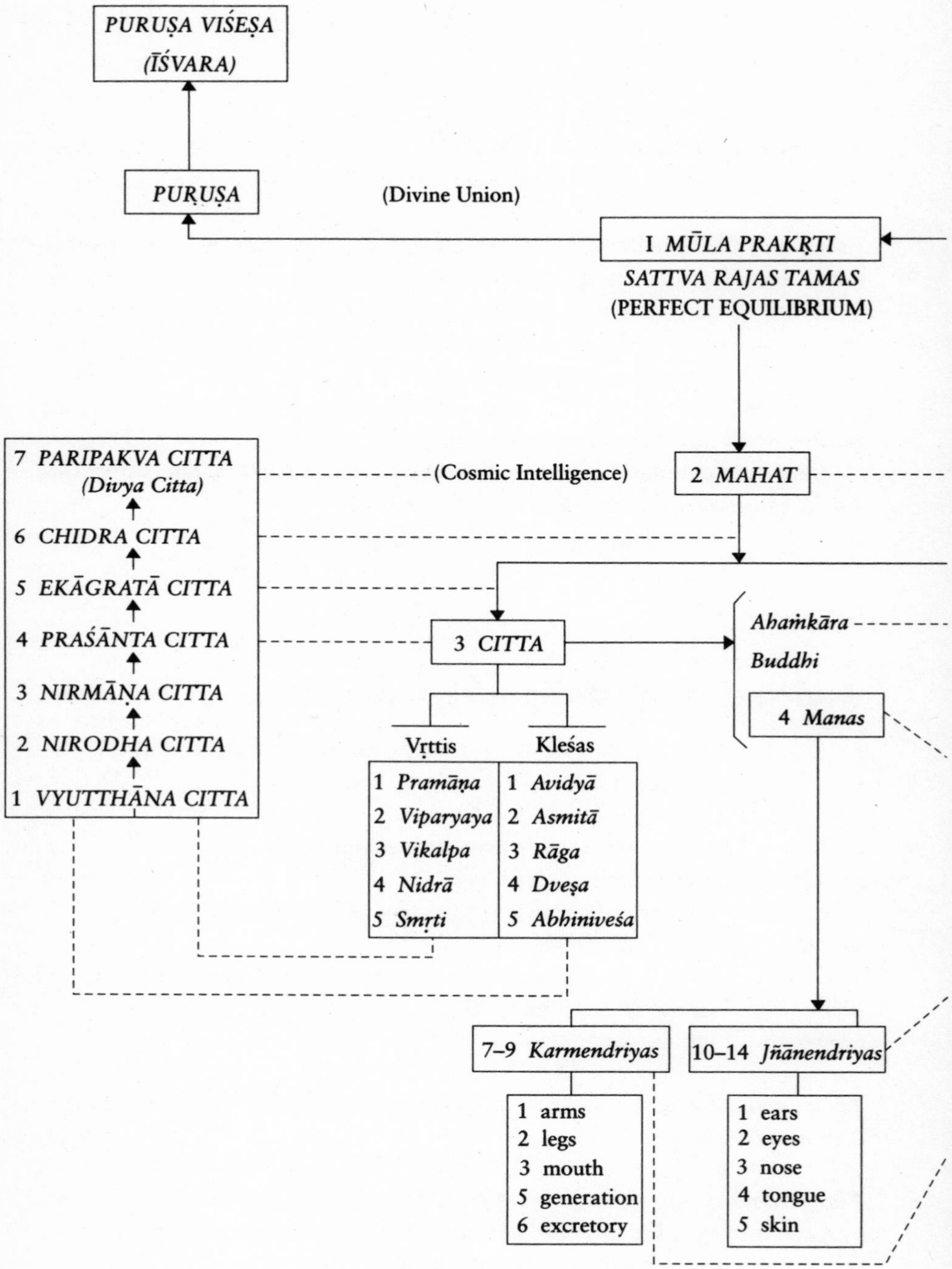

PURUṢA VIŚEṢA
(ĪŚVARA)
PURUṢA
(Divine Union)
I MŪLA PRAKṚTI
SATTVA RAJAS TAMAS
(PERFECT EQUILIBRIUM)
7 PARIPAKVA CITTA
(Divya Citta)
6 CHIDRA CITTA
5 EKĀGRATĀ CITTA
4 PRAŚĀNTA CITTA
3 NIRMĀṆA CITTA
2 NIRODHA CITTA
1 VYUTTHĀNA CITTA
(Cosmic Intelligence)
2 MAHAT
3 CITTA
Ahaṁkāra
Buddhi
4 Manas
Vṛttis
1 Pramāṇa
2 Viparyaya
3 Vikalpa
4 Nidrā
5 Smṛti
Kleśas
1 Avidyā
2 Asmitā
3 Rāga
4 Dveṣa
5 Abhiniveśa
7–9 Karmendriyas
1 arms
2 legs
3 mouth
5 generation
6 excretory
10–14 Jñānendriyas
1 ears
2 eyes
3 nose
4 tongue
5 skin

Table 9: *The evolution and involution of* prakṛti

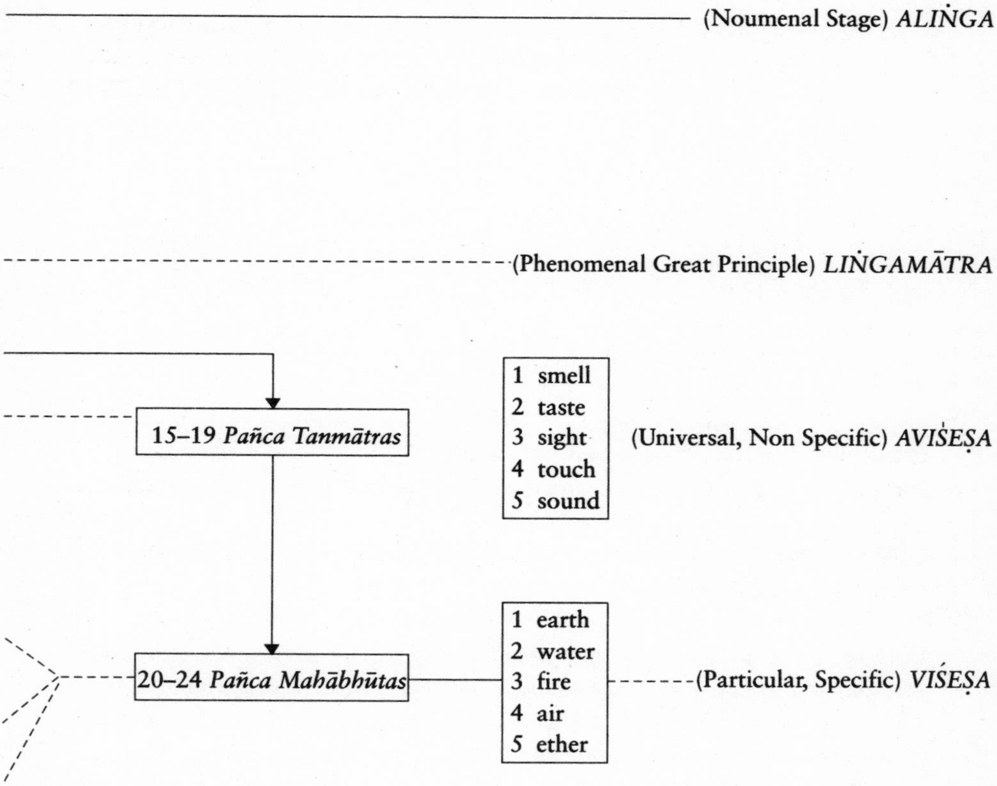

integration between the owner, the 'owning' and the owned has existed since the beginning of civilization.

By the light of pure knowledge, the owner, the seer, perceives and cognizes whatever is to be perceived or cognized through his association with nature. If this association is fed by ignorance, it leads the master towards enjoyment, desire, and ailments, and binds him. But if non-attachment is developed, it leads to detachment or renunciation, *vairāgya*.

If the master maintains constant watchful awareness of his consciousness, associates with nature without attachment and remains a witness, nature (*prakṛti*) leads its owner, the soul, to freedom, *mokṣa*.

तस्य हेतुरविद्या ।२४।

II.24 tasya hetuḥ avidyā

tasya	its conjunction
hetuḥ	cause, ground, purpose
avidyā	ignorance, lack of awareness, lack of spiritual knowledge

Lack of spiritual understanding (avidyā) *is the cause of the false identification of the seer with the seen.*

In II.18, it was said that the mingling of *prakṛti* with *puruṣa* can either lead to emancipation or stop our progress by involving us in desires and emotions. This sūtra underlines the fact that *avidyā*, ignorance or lack of awareness, is at the root of the confusion that brings us suffering as well as pleasure. *Vidyā* (discriminative knowledge) destroys ignorance, for a fire will burn only as long as fuel lasts (see I.4, 8, 30, 31 and II.5).

What is right knowledge? When discernment banishes doubt, pure understanding begins the process of disownment and detachment which releases us from the shackles of possessing and being possessed.

तदभावात् संयोगाभावो हानं तद्दृशेः कैवल्यम् ॥२५॥

II.25 tad abhāvāt saṁyogābhāvaḥ hānaṁ taddṛśeḥ kaivalyam

tad	its
abhāvāt	from non-existence, from non-occurrence, from absence, from non-entity
saṁyogaḥ	union, association, conjunction
abhāvaḥ	absence, disappearance
hānaṁ	act of leaving, stopping, removing, remedying
tad	that
dṛśeḥ	of the knower, seer
kaivalyam	absolute freedom, emancipation, absorption in the supreme soul

The destruction of ignorance through right knowledge breaks the link binding the seer to the seen. This is kaivalya, *emancipation.*

Sūtra II.16 deals with the avoidance of pain; sūtras II.17–24 with how to control pleasure and pain, and attain freedom by dissociating the seer and the seen. This sūtra explains the effect of snapping the link that binds the knower to the known.

At this point, the seen loses its hold and influence on the seer, miseries terminate and the soul is elevated to experience perfect freedom (see I.3 and IV.34).

Without doubt, sūtras II.17–25 are terse and many have groped for a precise and clear explanation of them. We must read and re-read them in order to grasp their meaning.

The kernel of Patañjali's message in these difficult sūtras is this: yoga is specifically designed to help us avoid the sort of slips and errors in our conduct which store up future sorrows, and it builds up our strength, vigour and courage to deal with the inevitable problems of life (see I.5).

We know that our mind turns more readily to the world's pleasures than to the vision of the soul. It is a bridge between the senses and the spirit; it is a secret enemy, and a treacherous friend, which can change our conduct without giving us time to consider. Patañjali advises the *sādhaka* to train the mind and cultivate discrimination, so that objects and events are seen only for what they are: then they cannot gain power over us. This is extremely difficult but an understanding of nature will help. We are matter (temporarily) and we live surrounded by matter. Interaction with matter or nature is the condition of our life. Without discrimination we cannot break free, but with understanding and practice we can use this interaction to reach the highest peace and bliss.

If we want to experience heaven on earth, we have to grasp the qualities of nature, the *guṇas*, that is to say the polarity of *rajas* and *tamas*, the eternal pulse of nature between movement and stillness, and the higher balancing state of *sattva*. Nature has degrees of subtlety. Sometimes it is more densely or clearly manifest than at others, and Patañjali analyses as follows. The four parts are: distinguishable (*viśeṣa*), unspecified or universal (*aviśeṣa*), phenomenal (*liṅga*) and, beyond this, noumenal (*aliṅga*). The five energetic qualities of nature, the elements, are, with the senses of perception and organs of action, distinguishable; while the five counterparts of the elements, sound, touch, taste, sight and smell are without specific signs (*aliṅga*); so also is the ego (*asmitā*).

All these are subject to the *guṇas*, which blend the behavioural patterns of an individual. If we understand the flow of these forces, we can reach balance, and from balance go on to true freedom. If not, we are swayed from one extreme to another, between pleasure and another pain. Yoga, says Patañjali, is the way to harmonize ourselves at every level with the natural order of the universe, from the physical to the most subtle, to reach the total state of health which brings stability, to cultivate the mind with real understanding, and to reach out ultimately to undifferentiated infinity.

The seer is an absolute knower – awareness personified. Though pure, it becomes entangled in the tricks of the mind, which are part of nature. Yet the vehicles of nature are all there to help the seer to experience serene, pristine, divine purity. Then, the elements of nature and their counterparts recede and merge in the root of nature, *mūla-prakṛti*.

(See I.45.)

विवेकख्यातिरविप्लवा हानोपायः ।२६।

II.26 vivekakhyātiḥ aviplavā hānopāyaḥ

vivekakhyātiḥ (*viveka* = discrimination, judgement, true knowledge, discretion; *khyāti* = the faculty of discriminating objects by an appropriate designation) awareness of knowledge, fame, celebrity

aviplavā undisturbed, unbroken, unfluctuating, unfailing

hānopāyaḥ the means for removal, the means for dispersion

The ceaseless flow of discriminative knowledge in thought, word and deed destroys ignorance, the source of pain.

Unfluctuating sound judgement with uninterrupted awareness is the essence of true knowledge, the sole means to eradicate ignorance and free the seer from the seen. It should always be kept in the highest state of awareness and attentiveness known as *vivekakhyāti*, the crown of wisdom.

The seeds of false knowledge are to be burnt up through uninterrupted yogic practices to maintain an unbroken flow of discriminative intelligence.

तस्य सप्तधा प्रान्तभूमिः प्रज्ञा ।२७।

II.27 tasya saptadhā prāntabhūmiḥ prajñā

tasya	its
saptadhā	sevenfold, of seven stages
prāntabhūmiḥ	territory, province, resting place
prajñā	perfect knowledge, supreme knowledge, awareness, consciousness

Through this unbroken flow of discriminative awareness, one gains perfect knowledge which has seven spheres.

There are seven frontiers to be integrated between the seen (*prakṛti*) and the seer (*puruṣa*). They are: integration of the body (*śarīra saṁyama*), the senses (*indriya saṁyama*), energy (*prāṇa saṁyama*), mind (*mano saṁyama*), intellect (*buddhi saṁyama*), consciousness (*citta saṁyama*) and soul (*ātma saṁyama*), each realizing its own individual identity. Proficiency in yoga will bring this sevenfold knowledge.

According to Patañjali, the seven states of conscious awareness are: emerging consciousness (*vyutthāna citta*), restraining consciousness (*nirodha citta*), sprouted or individualized consciousness (*nirmāṇa citta*), tranquil consciousness (*praśānta citta*), attentive consciousness (*ekāgratā citta*), fissured or rent consciousness (*chidra citta*) and ripe or pure consciousness (*paripakva* or *divya citta*). Though this sevenfold knowledge is explained differently in

Table 10: *The seven states of consciousness* as described by Patañjali, Vyāsa and the Yoga Vasiṣṭa and corresponding levels of knowledge and integration as described by the author*

Seven States of Consciousness as described by:			Corresponding levels of knowledge and integration as described by the author	
Patañjali	*Vyāsa*	*Yoga Vasiṣṭa*	*Knowledge*	*Stage of Integration*
1 *Vyutthāna citta* emerging consciousness	*Parijñāta prajñā* the knowable is known	*Śubhecchā* right desire	*Śarīra jñāna* knowledge of body	*Śarīra saṁyama* integration of body
2 *Nirodha citta* restraining consciousness	*Heya kśīna prajñā* that which should be discarded is discarded	*Vicaraṇā* right reflection	*Prāṇa jñāna* knowledge of energy	*Indriya saṁyama* integration of senses
3 *Nirmāṇa citta* individualized consciousness	*Prāpya prāpti prajñā* the attainable is attained	*Tanumānasā* disappearance of the mind	*Mano jñāna* control of mind	*Prāṇa saṁyama* integration of energy
4 *Prasānta citta* tranquil consciousness	*Kārya śuddhi prajñā* what must be done is done	*Sattvāpatti* self realization	*Vijñāna jñāna* stability in intelligence	*Mano saṁyama* integration of mind
5 *Ekāgratā citta* attentive consciousness	*Caritādhikāra prajñā* the aim to be reached is reached	*Asaṁsakta* non-attachment	*Ānubhāvika jñāna* knowledge from experience	*Buddhi saṁyama* integration of intellect
6 *Chidra citta* fissured consciousness	*Guṇātīta prajñā* untainted intelligence	*Parārthabhāvana* non-perception of objects	*Rasātmaka jñāna* absorption of the flavours of life	*Citta saṁyama* integration of consciousness
7 *Paripakva citta* (*Divya citta*) pure consciousness	*Svarūpa mātra jyoti prajñā* self -illumined consciousness	*Brahmavidvariṣṭha* experience of state beyond words	*Ātma jñāna* knowledge of the self	*Ātma saṁyama* integration of soul

*The four known states, *jagrata* (wakeful), *svapnā* (dream), *nidrā* (sleep) and *turyā* (union with supreme soul) and the three states between them classify as seven states of awareness.

various texts, I feel that this explanation of the seven states of awareness correctly represents Patañjali's thought (see II.9–11; IV.27 and 29).

The seven states of awareness are variously described by different commentators. According to one version they are: what has to be known is known (*parijñāta prajñā*), what has to be discarded (*heya kṣīna prajñā*), what has to be attained is attained (*prāpya prāpti prajñā*), what has to be done is done (*kārya śuddhi prajñā*), the aim which has to be reached is reached (*caritādhikāra prajñā*), no qualities (*guṇas*) can taint the intelligence (*guṇātīta prajñā*), and the knower is Self-illumined and maintains his inner light while attending to his wordly duties (*svarūpa mātra jyoti prajñā*).

According to another version, they are: right desire (*śubhecchā*), right reflection (*vicāraṇā*), disappearance of the mind (*tanumānasā*), Self-Realization (*sattvāpatti*), non-attachment (*asaṁsakta*), non-perception of objects (*parārthabhāvana*), and the experiencing of a state beyond words (*brahmavidvariṣṭa*).

The seven states can also be correlated with the wakeful (*jāgrata*), dreamy (*svapnā*), and sleepy (*nidrā*) states, and the state of oneness with the Supreme Soul (*turyā*); and the three intermediate states between them.

To simplify the meaning of this sūtra for yoga practitioners, I would like to offer the following interpretation: knowledge of the body (*śarīra jñāna*), knowledge of energy (*prāṇa jñāna*), control of the mind (*mano jñāna*), stability in intelligence (*vijñāna jñāna*), knowledge gained by experience (*ānubhavika jñāna*), absorption of the various flavours that life offers (*rasātmaka jñāna*), knowledge of the self (*ātma jñāna*).

In other words, by yogic practices, the *sādhaka* conquers his body, controls his energy, restrains the movements of the mind and develops sound judgement, from which he acts rightly and becomes luminous. From this luminosity he develops total awareness of the very core of his being, achieves supreme knowledge, and surrenders his self to the Supreme Soul, *Paramātman*. (See Tables 10 and 11.)

योगाङ्गानुष्ठानादशुद्धिक्षये ज्ञानदीप्तिराविवेकख्याते: ।२८।

II.28 yogāṅgānuṣṭhānāt aśuddhikṣaye
jñānadīptiḥ āvivekakhyāteḥ

yoga	to yoke, to join, to associate, to unite
aṅga	components, accessories, aspects

anuṣṭhānāt	by devoted practice
aśuddhiḥ	impurities
kśaye	diminish, destroy
jñana	knowledge, wisdom
dīptiḥ	shines forth, radiates
āvivekakhyāteḥ	the essence of knowledge, the glory of knowledge

By dedicated practice of the various aspects of yoga impurities are destroyed: the crown of wisdom radiates in glory.

Patañjali sums up the effects of yoga in this one sūtra. He says that by regular and devoted practice, the impurities of the *sādhaka*'s body and mind are consumed, the causes of afflictions removed and the crown of wisdom is acquired. This wisdom and achievement keep the *sādhaka* innocent and free of pride.

Here, instead of the usual word *abhyāsa* (repeated practice), *anuṣṭhāna* is used. It is a dignified and noble word with a spiritual import, implying practice with dedication or religious fervour. The former brings stability; the latter develops maturity of intelligence.

Yoga can cure or lessen our physical, mental, moral and spiritual sufferings. Perfection and success are certain only if one practises with love and whole-hearted dedication.

यमनियमासनप्राणायामप्रत्याहारधारणाध्यानसमाधयोऽष्टावङ्गानि ।२९।

II.29 yama niyama āsana prāṇāyāma pratyāhāra dhāraṇā dhyāna samādhayaḥ aṣṭau aṅgāni

yama	self-restraint, vows of abstention, control
niyama	fixed observance, fixed rules, precepts, established order, law
āsana	sitting in various postures, seat in general, a posture
prāṇāyāma	regulation of breath, restraint of breath
pratyāhāra	retreat, withdrawal of the senses
dhāraṇā	the act of concentration, act of holding, keeping the mind collected
dhyāna	meditation, contemplation, reflection, attention

Table 11: *The seven* kośas *(body sheaths) and corresponding states of consciousness*

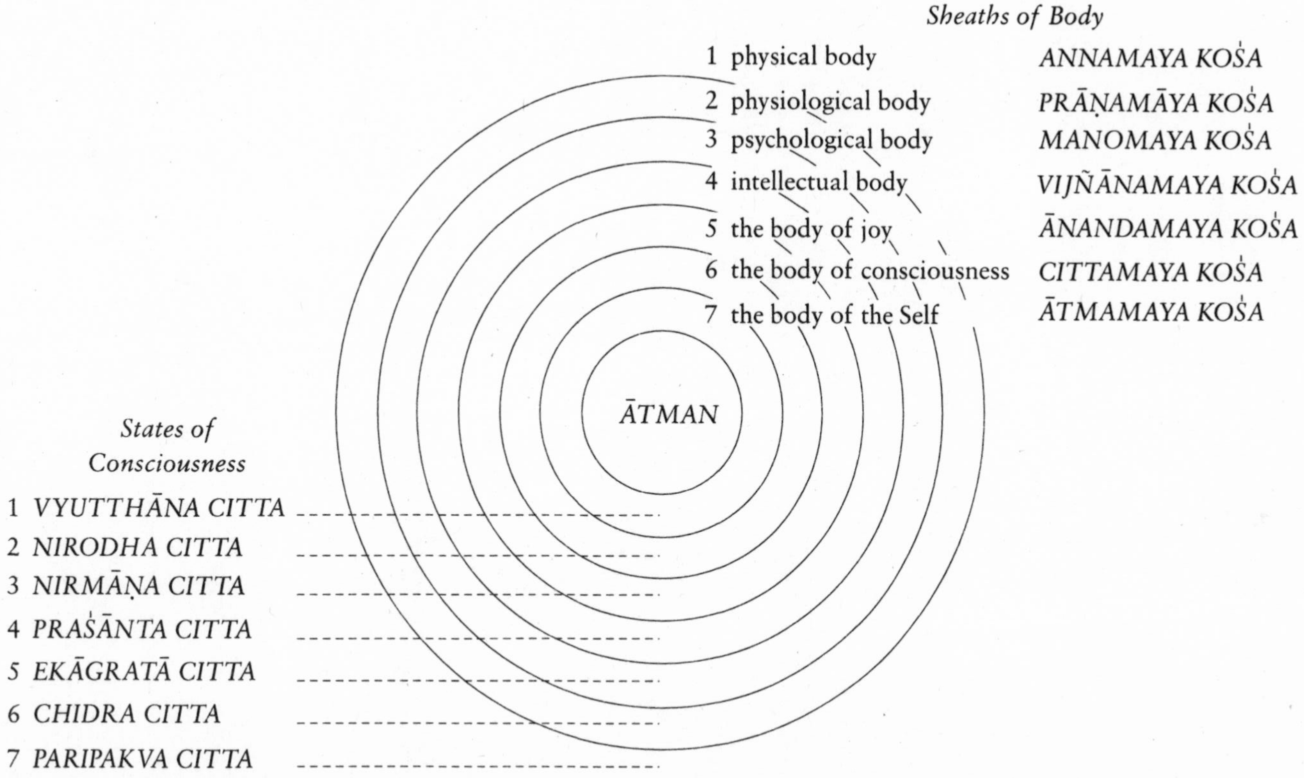

samādhayaḥ	putting together, collection, composition, profound meditation, absorption, superconsciousness
aṣṭau	eight
aṅgāni	constituent parts, members or divisions, limbs

Moral injunctions (yama), *fixed observances* (niyama), *posture* (āsana), *regulation of breath* (prāṇāyāma), *internalization of the senses towards their source* (pratyāhāra), *concentration* (dhāraṇā), *meditation* (dhyāna) *and absorption of consciousness in the self* (samādhi), *are the eight constituents of yoga.*

This sūtra sets out the eightfold path of yoga (*aṣṭāṅga yoga*), which Patañjali proceeds to describe in detail in the remaining sūtras of *sādhana pāda* and in the first three sūtras of *vibhūti pāda.*

Restraints and observances that are bound by tradition and lineage follow uninterruptedly in the practice of yoga. Although *āsana, prāṇāyāma* and *pratyāhāra* are separate entities, they depend upon one another for expressing the hidden facets of yoga. These stages, which enable the seeker to rise in the art of yoga, are called progressive *sādhana.* Through them we reach higher and higher. The first five aspects of yoga are individual efforts for the evolution of the consciousness, while *dhāraṇā, dhyāna* and *samādhi* are the universal manifestation or the natural states of yoga (*yoga svarūpa*).

अहिंसासत्यास्तेयब्रह्मचर्यापरिग्रहा यमाः ।३०।

II.30 ahiṁsā satya asteya brahmacarya aparigrahāḥ yamāḥ

ahiṁsā	harmlessness, non-violence
satya	real, genuine, honest, virtuous, truthful
asteya	non-stealing, non-misappropriating
brahmacarya	continence, chastity, religious studentship
aparigrahāḥ	without possessions, without belongings, non-acceptance of gifts
yamāḥ	self-restraint

Non-violence, truth, abstention from stealing, continence, and absence of greed for possessions beyond one's need are the five pillars of yama.

The principle of *yama* involves wishing no harm in word, thought or deed; being sincere, truthful and honest; not stealing or misappropriating another's wealth or possessions; chastity; and not accepting gifts or possessing only what one needs, without being greedy.

These rules and restraints are clearly laid down for us to live in society whilst remaining a yoga practitioner.

जातिदेशकालसमयानवच्छिन्नाः सार्वभौमा महाव्रतम् ।३१।

II.31 jāti deśa kāla samaya anavacchinnāḥ sārvabhaumāḥ mahāvratam

jāti	class of birth, type of birth, rank, lineage
deśa	place, spot, country
kāla	time
samaya	condition, circumstance
anavacchinnāḥ	not limited, not bound
sārvabhaumāḥ	relating to or consisting of the whole world, universal
mahāvratam	mighty vow, great obligation

Yamas *are the great, mighty, universal vows, unconditioned by place, time and class.*

The five components of *yama* are called 'mighty universal vows', as they are not confined to class, place, time or concept of duty. They should be followed unconditionally by everyone, and by students of yoga in particular, irrespective of origin and situation, with a reservation concerning cultural phenomena such as religious ceremonies, vows and vocations of certain people. They form the framework of rules on which society is based.

I believe that this universal approach should be applied to all the other component stages of yoga, without distinction of time, place or circumstances, to lay down the precepts of a universal culture.

शौचसंतोषतपःस्वाध्यायेश्वरप्रणिधानानि नियमाः ॥३२॥

II.32 śauca santoṣa tapaḥ svādhyāya Īśvarapraṇidhānāni niyamāḥ

śauca	cleanliness, purity
santoṣa	contentment
tapaḥ	religious fervour, a burning desire
svādhyāya	study which leads to the knowledge of the self
Īśvara praṇidhānāni	resignation to God, surrender to God (*pra* = fullness; *ni* = under; *dhāna* = placement); making God the target of concentration
niyamāḥ	established observance

Cleanliness, contentment, religious zeal, self-study and surrender of the self to the supreme Self or God are the niyamas.

As *yama* is universal social practice, *niyama* evolves from individual practices necessary to build up the *sādhaka*'s own character.

These five observations accord with the five sheaths of man and the elements of nature: the anatomical (earth), physiological (water), psychological (fire), intellectual (air) and spiritual (ether) layers. As ether (*mahat ākāśa*) is considered as an empty space, outside, so the soul is an empty space within and is called *cit-ākāśa*.

The principles of *niyama* that are encompassed by *kriyāyoga* emphasize the importance of self-discipline. Mastery of yoga would be unrealizable without the observance of the ethical principles of *yama* and *niyama*.

Cleanliness or purification is of two types, external and internal. Both are necessary. Taking a bath is external purification; performing *āsanas* and *prāṇāyāma* is internal. Observance of *niyama* develops friendliness, compassion and indifference, and is a further aid in cleansing the body, mind and intelligence. *Svādhyāya* is checking oneself to see if the principles of yoga are being followed. In order to follow these principles one has first to decide whether one's own pattern of behaviour is aligned with them or not. If not, one has to prepare one's thoughts and actions in accordance with them, and remove those faults which hinder one's *sādhana*.

Owing to desires, anger, greed, infatuation, arrogance and jealousy, the mind is engulfed in pain. Misled by these emotions, the *sādhaka* loses his balance of mind and behaves unethically. Re-examination of his thoughts reduces the tendency to go wrong. The ethical disciplines of *yama* and *niyama* transform the *sādhaka*'s alloyed or tainted mind and enable his consciousness to radiate in its own unalloyed purity. Therefore, yoga stresses that discipline is religion and in discipline is not religion.

What in fact is true religion? It is eternal, and has no denominations or boundaries. It is a method knowingly designed to lift each individual's awareness so that he may experience the vision of the core of his being, *ātma darśana*. It sustains the *sādhaka*'s development and prevents his downfall; it lifts him when he slips. In short, religion is the means to Self-Realization.

वितर्कबाधने प्रतिपक्षभावनम् ।३३।

II.33 vitarkabādhane pratipakṣabhāvanam

vitarka	questionable or dubious matter, doubt, uncertainty, supposition
bādhane	pain, suffering, grief, obstruction, obstacles
pratipakṣa	the opposite side, to the contrary
bhāvanam	affecting, creating, promoting, manifesting, feeling

Principles which run contrary to yama *and* niyama *are to be countered with the knowledge of discrimination.*

This sūtra stresses that *yama* and *niyama* are an integral part of yoga. Sūtras II.30 and 32, explain what one should avoid doing and what one has to do.

Now the *sādhaka* is counselled to cultivate a temperament which can resist the current of violence, falsehood, stealing, non-chastity and venality, which is *pratipakṣa bhāvana*; and to go with the current of cleanliness, contentment, fervour, self-study and surrender to the Universal Spirit, which is *pakṣa bhāvana*.

The principles that prevent *yama* and *niyama* are to be countered with right knowledge and awareness.

When the mind is caught up in dubious ideas and actions, right perception is obstructed. The *sādhaka* has to analyse and investigate these ideas and actions and their opposites; then he learns to balance his thoughts by repeated experimentation.

Some people give an objective interpretation to this sūtra and maintain that if one is violent, one should think of the opposite, or, if one is attached, then non-attachment should be developed. This is the opposite thought or *pratipakṣabhāvana*. If a person is violent, he is violent. If he is angry, he is angry. The state is not different from the fact; but instead of trying to cultivate the opposite condition, he should go deep into the cause of his anger or violence. This is *pakṣabhāva*. One should also study the opposite forces with calmness and patience. Then one develops equipoise.

Pakṣa means to take one side (in an argument), to espouse one view; while *pratipakṣa* conveys the idea of taking the opposite position. Let me turn to the physical plane to help the reader understand and experience the sense of these two words.

Each *āsana* acts and reacts in its own way, cultivating health on a physical level, helping the organic systems (such as the lungs, liver, spleen, pancreas, intestines and cells) to function rhythmically at a physiological level, which effects changes in the senses, mind and intellect at a mental level. While practising the *āsana*, the *sādhaka* must carefully and minutely observe and adjust the position of the muscles, muscle fibres and cells, measuring lightness or heaviness, *pakṣa* or *pratipakṣa*, as required for the performance of a healthy and well balanced *āsana*. He adjusts harmoniously the right and left sides of the body, the front and the back. Learning to interchange or counterbalance the weaker with the intelligent side brings about changes in the *sādhaka*: he grows, able to observe equipoise in the body cells and the lobes of the brain; and calmness and sobriety in the mind. Thus the qualities of both *pakṣa* and *pratipakṣa* are attended to. By raising the weak or dull to the level of the intelligent or strong, the *sādhaka* learns compassion in action.

In *prāṇāyāma*, too, we focus the consciousness on the various vibrations of the nerves with the controlled flow of inbreath and outbreath, between the right and left sides of the lungs and also between the right and left nostrils. This adjustment and observation in the practice of yoga fuses *pakṣa* and *pratipakṣa*, freeing us from the upheavals of anger and depression, which are replaced with hope and emotional stability.

The internal measuring and balancing process which we call *pakṣa pratipakṣa* is in some respects the key to why yoga practice actually works, why it has mechanical power to revolutionize our whole being. It is why *āsana* is not gymnastics, why *prāṇāyāma* is not deep breathing, why *dhyāna* is not self-induced trance, why *yama* is not just morality. In *āsana* for example, the pose first brings inner balance and harmony, but in the end it is merely the outer expression of the inner harmony.

We are taught nowadays that the miracle of the world's ecosystem is its balance, a balance which modern man is fast destroying by deforestation, pollution, over-consumption. This is because when man becomes unbalanced, he seeks to change not himself but his environment, in order to create the illusion that he is enjoying health and harmony. In winter he overheats his house, in summer he freezes it with air-conditioning. This is not stability but arrogance. Some people take tablets to go to sleep and tablets to wake up. Their life has the rhythm of a pingpong ball. The student of yoga who learns to balance himself internally at every level, physical, emotional, mental, by observation of *pakṣa* and *pratipakṣa*, frees himself from this hellish to-ing and fro-ing and lives in harmony with the natural world. Because he is stable, he can adapt to outside changes. The flexibility we gain in *āsana* is the living symbol of the suppleness we gain in relation to life's problems and challenges.

Through *pakṣa* and *pratipakṣa* we can balance the three energetic currents of *iḍā*, *piṅgalā* and *suṣumnā*, the three principal *nāḍīs*, or channels of energy. Imagine the calf muscle as it is extended in *Trikoṇāsana*, the Triangle Posture. Initially the outer calf surface may be active or awake on one side, dull on the other, and its absolute centre completely unaware. Then we learn to stretch in such a way as to bring the excess energy of *iḍā* equally to *piṅgalā* and *suṣumnā* or vice versa. So there is an equal and harmonious flow of energy in the three channels.

Similarly, learning to maintain clarity and equanimity of intelligence in body, mind, intellect and consciousness through meditation is the remedy for uncertain knowledge. To gain this state in meditation, *yama* and *niyama* must be cultivated. Success or failure at higher levels of consciousness depend on *yama* and *niyama*. This blending of *pakṣa* and *pratipakṣa* in all aspects of yoga is true yoga.

I should like to emphasize here that *yama* and *niyama* are not only the foundation of yoga, but the reflection of our success or failure at its higher levels. Take, for example, a successful 'godman' who is an adept in meditation: if he carelessly lets himself down in *yama* and *niyama*, he invalidates his claim to spirituality.

वितर्का हिंसादयः कृतकारितानुमोदिता लोभक्रोधमोहपूर्वका
मृदुमध्याधिमात्रा दुःखाज्ञानानन्तफला इति प्रतिपक्षभावनम् ।३४।

II.34 vitarkaḥ hiṁsādayaḥ kṛta kārita anumoditāḥ lobha krodha moha pūrvakaḥ mṛdu madhya adhimātraḥ duḥkha ajñāna anantaphalāḥ iti pratipakṣabhāvanam

vitarkaḥ	dubious knowledge
hiṁsa	of violence, injuries
ādayaḥ	and so forth
kṛta	done
kārita	caused to be done, induced, aroused
anumoditāḥ	abetted, permitted to be done
lobha	desire, greed
krodha	anger
moha	delusion, infatuation
pūrvakaḥ	preceded by, caused by
mṛdu	mild, slight
madhya	moderate, medium
adhimātraḥ	intense, sharp
duḥkha	pain, sorrow, grief
ajñāna	ignorance
ananta	endless, infinite
phalāḥ	fruit, result
iti	thus
pratipakṣa	contrary thoughts
bhāvanam	feeling, resting place

Uncertain knowledge giving rise to violence, whether done directly or indirectly, or condoned, is caused by greed, anger or delusion in mild, moderate or intense degree. It results in endless pain and ignorance. Through introspection comes the end of pain and ignorance.

Improper or perverse actions and thoughts result in endless pain. These thoughts, emotions and actions are of three types and vary in intensity, being mild, medium or acute. They are caused by direct indulgence, unconsciously induced, or externally abetted. Violence, for example, committed directly, caused, or condoned results in endless ignorance, physical pain and mental distress. Such behaviour is motivated by greed, anger and delusion, and may be corrected by its opposites, i.e., introspection, proper thinking and action.

This sūtra elaborates the dissensions and misguided efforts that hinder progress in yoga.

Disease, pain and distress are of three types. One comes through deliberate over-indulgence in pleasures through desire, lust and pride. This is known as *ādhyātmika roga* or self-inflicted disease. The second comes from non-deliberate habits and behaviour, which arise from the imbalance of the five elements in the body and their sensory counterparts. These are *ādhibhautika rogas*. The last type, *ādhidaivika roga*, is often a disease of genetic or hereditary origin that appears without obvious cause. All three types may be experienced in mild, moderate or intense form.

Patañjali stresses that it is by the exercise of the discriminative faculty that dubious, wavering or uncertain knowledge, *vitarka*, is curtailed.

अहिंसाप्रतिष्ठायां तत्संनिधौ वैरत्यागः ।३५।

II.35 ahiṁsāpratiṣṭhāyāṁ tatsannidhau vairatyāgaḥ

ahiṁsā	non-violence, harmlessness, non-injury
pratiṣṭhāyāṁ	standing firmly, firmly established
tat	his
sannidhau	presence, vicinity
vaira	animosity, hostility
tyāgaḥ	forsaking, abandoning, deserting

When non-violence in speech, thought and action is established, one's aggressive nature is relinquished and others abandon hostility in one's presence.

Sūtras II.35–39 describe the effects of observing the five *yamas*.

When the yogi has thoroughly understood the nature of violence, he is established firmly in the practice of non-violence. Peace in words, thoughts and deeds, whether awake or dreaming, is a sign of goodwill and love towards all.

In the vicinity of a yogi, men and animals who are otherwise violent and antipathetic towards each other, abandon their hostility and exhibit friendliness and mutual tolerance.

सत्यप्रतिष्ठायां क्रियाफलाश्रयत्वम् ।३६।

II.36 satyapratiṣṭhāyāṁ kriyāphalāśrayatvam

satya	truth, sincerity, genuineness, honesty
pratiṣṭhāyāṁ	firmly established
kriyā	action
phalāḥ	results
āśrayatvam	substratum, foundation, dependence

When the sādhaka *is firmly established in the practice of truth, his words become so potent that whatever he says comes to realization.*

Most of us think we tell the truth, but truth is causal, not integrated and cellular. For instance, if we say 'I will never eat chocolates again', as long as one cell of our body holds back and disagrees with the others, our success is not assured. If the stated intention is totally whole-hearted, not one cell dissembling, then we create the reality we desire. It is not our mind, but the inner voice of our cells which has the power to implement our intentions.

अस्तेयप्रतिष्ठायां सर्वरत्नोपस्थानम् ।३७।

II.37 asteyapratiṣṭhāyāṁ sarvaratnopasthānam

asteya	non-stealing, non-misappropriation, desirelessness, non-covetousness
pratiṣṭhāyāṁ	well established
sarva	all
ratna	gems, precious things
upasthānam	approaching, coming up

When abstention from stealing is firmly established, precious jewels come.

Upon the man who does not take what does not belong to him, all riches are showered. Being without desire, he effortlessly attracts what is precious, materially and figuratively, including the gem of all jewels, virtue.

ब्रह्मचर्यप्रतिष्ठायां वीर्यलाभः ॥३८॥

II.38 brahmacaryapratiṣṭhāyāṁ vīryalābhaḥ

brahmacarya	continence, chastity
pratiṣṭhāyāṁ	well established
vīrya	energy, vigour, potency, valour
lābhaḥ	gained, obtained, acquired

When the sādhaka *is firmly established in continence, knowledge, vigour, valour and energy flow to him.*

The celibate transforms the energy of procreation into spiritual energy (*ojas*), creating lustre.

Brahmacarya, in its sense of sexual control or celibacy is often misunderstood.

Sexual energy is the most basic expression of the life force. It is immensely powerful, and it is essential to control and channel it. In no way should we despise it. On the contrary, we must respect and esteem it. He who seeks merely to suppress or stamp down his sexual energy is in effect denigrating his own origins. Of course there is a moral aspect to sexual behaviour, but cultural differences permit vastly different behaviour. Some cultures allow one wife, some three, some many. In parts of the Himālayās a woman may have several husbands. Often what we call sexual immorality offends less against the code of *brahmacarya* than against the other injunctions of *yama*. Imagine the case of a married man who commits adultery with a married woman, and lies when he is suspected. Has he not offended, by the pain he gives, against *ahiṁsā*? By his lies, against *satya*? By taking another man's wife, against *asteya*? By his greed, against *aparigraha*? The sexual misdemeanour in itself shrinks in comparison.

A yogi may or may not practise total abstinence; the great yogi Vasiṣṭa had one hundred children, yet he was called a *brahmacāri*. Ancient yogis studied the conjunction of stars and planets to discover the most auspicious moment for procreation. Continence or control in no way belies or contradicts the enjoyment of pleasure. Assuredly they enhance it. It is when sensory pleasure is the sole motivating factor that *brahmacarya* is infringed.

The life-force which finds sexual expression also serves to find the warmth of our emotions, the passions of our intellect, and our idealism. As our physical essence is sperm or egg, so our spiritual essence is the soul. Their relationship should be based on co-operation. It is the creative relationship of *puruṣa* and *prakṛti* which leads to freedom. Renunciation is a positive process of disengagement, not a sterile rejection. In the past, most great yogis were householders. We must learn to husband and control the life-force because it provides the energy which carries us to goals other than procreation. Also we should remember that procreation by those practising *brahmacarya* will tend to be of a higher order than that which is carried out thoughtlessly or promiscuously.

The religious or educational studentship of adolescence is also termed *brahmacarya*. That is because the enormous outburst of energy which is released by puberty needs to be contained and channelled for the child's all-round growth. If a child were to indulge in sexual activity the moment he or she was biologically ripe, a large part of his or her human potential would be thrown away.

We need application, study and idealistic motivation if we are to achieve anything. If, by youthful profligacy, the concentrated source of our energy has already been squandered, we will rediscover it later in life only with enormous difficulty. Lack of control can lead to despair, dejection and depression. But if energy is abundant and controlled we have hope and confidence, and our mind turns automatically to higher thoughts.

अपरिग्रहस्थैर्ये जन्मकथंतासंबोधः ।३९।

II.39 aparigrahasthairye janmakathaṁtā saṁbodhaḥ

aparigraha	without possessions, without belongings, non-acceptance of gifts
sthairye	by becoming steady, stable
janma	birth
kathaṁtā	how, in what way, in what manner, whence
saṁbodhaḥ	knowledge, illusion

Knowledge of past and future lives unfolds when one is free from greed for possessions.

When one is steady in living without surplus possessions and without greed, one realizes the true meaning of one's life, and all life unfolds before one.

Perseverance in this austerity leads to knowledge of one's past and future lives which appear like reflections in a mirror. When the *sādhaka* is free of worldly aspirations, he is a *kṛtārthan* (a happy and satisfied person).

Aparigraha means not only non-possession and non-acceptance of gifts, but also freedom from rigidity of thought. Holding on to one's thoughts is also a form of possessiveness, and thoughts, as well as material possessions, should be shunned. Otherwise they leave strong impressions on the consciousness and become seeds to manifest in future lives. These cycles of life continue until the *sādhaka* is totally clean and clear in thoughts, words and deeds.

Aparigraha is the subtlest aspect of *yama*, and difficult to master. Yet, repeated attempts must be made to gain pure knowledge of 'what I am' and 'what I am meant for'.

This discriminative thinking helps one to plan one's future lives from this present life. This is what Patañjali intends when he says that the pattern of future lives unfolds to an *aparigrahin*.

शौचात् स्वाङ्गजुगुप्सा परैरसंसर्गः ।४०।

II.40 śaucāt svāṅgajugupsā paraiḥ asaṁsargaḥ

śaucāt	by cleanliness, by purity
sva	self
aṅga	limbs, body
jugupsā	censure, dislike, aversion, being on one's guard, abhorrence, disgust
paraiḥ	with others
asaṁsargaḥ	non-contact, non-intercourse

Cleanliness of body and mind develops disinterest in contact with others for self-gratification.

Purity and cleanliness protect the body and make it a fit home for the seer. Consequently it no longer leans towards sensual pleasures and tends to refrain from contact with other bodies.

Sūtras II.40–45 describe the effects of practising the five *niyamas*.

Although he recognizes that the body is perishable, the *sādhaka* does not regard it with disgust or distaste, but keeps it clean and pure out of respect for the dweller, *puruṣa*, within. To that extent, he respects the body as a temple (see II.43).

As a temple or a church is kept clean each day, the inner body, the temple of the soul, should be bathed with a copious supply of blood through *āsanas* and *prāṇāyāma*. They cleanse the body physically, physiologically and intellectually. The body, having its own intelligence, develops its potential to change its behavioural patterns. It helps the *sādhaka* to detach himself from sensual desires, and guides him towards the holder of the body, the soul. Thus, *śauca* makes the body a fit instrument for the pursuit of spiritual knowledge.

सत्त्वशुद्धिसौमनस्यैकाग्र्येन्द्रियजयात्मदर्शनयोग्यत्वानि च ।४१।

II.41 sattvaśuddhi saumanasya aikāgrya indriyajaya ātmadarśana yogyatvāni ca

sattvaśuddhi	purity in the essence of consciousness
sau	cheerful, pleasing, benevolent
manasya	mind
ekāgra	concentration, fixity
indriya	senses of perception and organs of action
jaya	controlled, conquered
ātma	self, soul
darśana	knowledge, vision
yogyatvāni	fitness to see
ca	and also

When the body is cleansed, the mind purified and the senses controlled, joyful awareness needed to realize the inner self, also comes.

With cleanliness the body becomes the temple of the seer and feels the joy of self-awareness.

When the consciousness is cheerful and benevolent, the seeker becomes ready to receive the knowledge and vision of the soul.

संतोषादनुत्तमः सुखलाभः ।४२।

II.42 saṁtoṣāt anuttamaḥ sukhalābhaḥ

saṁtoṣāt	from contentment
anuttamaḥ	unexcelled, unsurpassed, supreme, excellent
sukha	delight, happiness
lābhaḥ	gain

From contentment and benevolence of consciousness comes supreme happiness.

Through cleanliness of the body, contentment is achieved. Together they ignite the flame of *tapas*, propelling the *sādhaka* towards the fire of knowledge. This transformation, which indicates that the *sādhaka* is on the right path of concentration, enables him to look inwards through Self-study (*svādhyāya*) and then towards Godliness.

कायेन्द्रियसिद्धिरशुद्धिक्षयात्तपसः ।४३।

II.43 kāya indriya siddhiḥ aśuddhikṣayāt tapasaḥ

kāya	body
indriya	senses
siddhiḥ	attainment, power
aśuddhi	impurities
kṣayāt	destruction
tapasaḥ	ascetic devotion, a burning desire to reach perfection, that which burns all impurities, self-discipline

Self-discipline (tapas) *burns away impurities and kindles the sparks of divinity.*

Self-discipline destroys all impurities, perfecting the body, mind and senses, so that consciousness functions freely and attains divinity.

Ahiṁsā cannot be properly understood without reference to *tapas*. *Tapas* is the inner *hiṁsā* (violence) by which we create the possibility of outer *ahiṁsā*. *Ahiṁsā* cannot exist alone. A complementary force must necessarily exist. Mahātma Gāndhi would never have been able to summon up the implacable peacefulness which moved an empire, without his ruthless attitude towards his own self. Violence is perhaps too strong a word for *tapas*, but it is a burning inner zeal and austerity, a sort of unflagging hardness of attitude towards oneself which makes possible compassion and forgiveness towards others.

स्वाध्यायादिष्टदेवतासंप्रयोगः ।४४।

II.44 svādhyāyāt iṣṭadevatā saṁprayogaḥ

svādhyāyāt	by study which leads to the knowledge of the Self, Self-study or reading the scriptures
iṣṭadevatā	the desired deity
saṁprayogaḥ	union, communion, coming in contact with the divine

Self-study leads towards the realization of God or communion with one's desired deity.

Study of the Self has two paths. One is for communicating from the skin, through the inner sheaths towards the seer; the other from the seer to the outer layer of his abode. Though consciousness exists in the body, it needs to be tapped through the practice of *āsana* and *prāṇāyāma*, in which the intelligence acts as a bridge to connect awareness of the body with the core and vice versa. This connecting intelligence alone brings harmony of body, mind and soul, and intimacy with the Supreme Soul (*Iṣṭadevatā*).

Traditionally, *svādhyāya* has been explained as the study of the sacred scriptures and recitation of *mantra*, preceded by the syllable *ĀUṀ* (see I.27–28), through which the *sādhaka* gains a vision of his tutelary or chosen deity, who fulfils all his desires.

समाधिसिद्धिरीश्वरप्रणिधानात् ।४५।

II.45 samādhisiddhiḥ Īśvarapraṇidhānāt

samādhi	absorption, profound meditation, superconsciousness
siddhiḥ	accomplishment, success
Īśvara	God
praṇidhānāt	by surrender, by resignation, by application

Surrender to God brings perfection in samādhi.

Samādhi is attained through clarity of intelligence and intensity in thought to surrender to God. The power of *samādhi* comes to him who takes refuge in God.

Surrender to God releases the *sādhaka* from the bondage of earthly desires, leads to the renunciation of sensuous desires, and nurtures in him the most intense form of application (see I.16 and IV.29).

स्थिरसुखमासनम् ।४६।

II.46 sthira sukham āsanam

sthira	firm, fixed, steady, steadfast, lasting
sukham	happiness, delight
āsanam	postures, poses

Āsana *is perfect firmness of body, steadiness of intelligence and benevolence of spirit.*

Sūtras II.46–48 define *āsana* and the effects of its practice.

The definition of *āsana* is given as follows: whatever *āsana* is performed, it should be done with a feeling of firmness, steadiness and endurance in the body; goodwill in the intelligence of the head, and awareness and delight in the intelligence of the heart. This is how each *āsana* should be understood, practised and experienced. Performance of the *āsana* should be nourishing and illuminative.

Some have taken this *sūtra* to mean that any comfortable posture is suitable. If that were so, these would be *āsanas* of pleasure (*bhogāsanas*) not *yogāsanas*. This sūtra defines the perfected *āsana*. From the very first sūtra Patañjali demands the highest quality of attention to perfection. This discipline and attention must be applied to the practice of each *āsana*, to penetrate to its very depths in the remotest parts of the body. Even the meditational *āsana* has to be cultivated by the fibres, cells, joints and muscles in cooperation with the mind. If *āsanas* are not performed in this way they become stale and the performer becomes diseased (a *rogi*) rather than a yogi.

Nor does *āsana* refer exclusively to the sitting poses used for meditation. Some divide *āsanas* into those which cultivate the body and those which are used in meditation. But in any *āsana* the body has to be toned and the mind tuned so that one can stay longer with a firm body and a serene mind. *Āsanas* should be performed without creating aggressiveness in the muscle spindles or the skin cells. Space must be created between muscle and skin so that the skin receives the actions of the muscles, joints and ligaments. The skin then sends messages to the brain, mind and intelligence which judge the appropriateness of those actions. In this way, the principles of *yama* and *niyama* are involved and action and reflection harmonize. In addition the practice of a variety of *āsanas* clears the nervous system, causes the energy to flow in the system without obstruction and ensures an even distribution of that energy during *prāṇāyāma*.

Usually the mind is closer to the body and to the organs of action and perception than to the soul. As *āsanas* are refined they automatically become meditative as the intelligence is made to penetrate towards the core of being.

Each *āsana* has five functions to perform. These are conative, cognitive, mental, intellectual and spiritual. Conative action is the exertion of the organs of action. Cognitive action is the perception of the results of that action. When the two are fused together the discriminative faculty of the mind acts to guide the organs of action and perception to perform the *āsanas* more correctly; the rhythmic flow of energy and awareness is experienced evenly and without interruption both centripetally and centrifugally throughout the channels of the body. A pure state of joy is felt in the cells and the mind. The body, mind and soul are one. This is the manifestation of *dhāraṇā* and *dhyāna* in the practice of an *āsana*.

Patañjali's explanation of *dhāraṇā* and *dhyāna* in sūtras III.1–2 beautifully describes the correct performance of an *āsana*. He says 'the focusing of attention on a chosen point or area within the body as well as outside is concentration (*dhāraṇā*). Maintaining this intensity of awareness leads from one-pointed attention to non-specific attentiveness. When the attentive awareness between the consciousness of the practitioner and his practice is unbroken, this is *dhyāna*.' In II.48, when Patañjali says that the pairs of opposites do not exist in the correct performance of an *āsana* he clearly implies the involvement of *dhāraṇā* and *dhyāna*.

(See I.20 and also *Light on Yoga* for further details.)

प्रयत्नशैथिल्यानन्तसमापत्तिभ्याम् ।४७।

II.47 prayatna śaithilya ananta samāpattibhyām

prayatna	persevering effort, continued exertion, endeavour
śaithilya	laxity, relaxation
ananta	endless, boundless, eternal, infinite
samāpattibhyām	assuming original form, completion, conclusion

Perfection in an āsana *is achieved when the effort to perform it becomes effortless and the infinite being within is reached.*

Perfection in *āsana* is reached only when effort ceases, instilling infinite poise and allowing the finite vehicle, the body, to merge in the seer.

The *sādhaka* can be considered firm in his postures when persevering effort is no longer needed. In this stability, he grasps the physiology of each *āsana* and penetrates within, reaching the minutest parts of the body. Then he gains the art of relaxation, maintaining the firmness and extension of the body and consciousness. In this way he develops a sensitive mind. With this sensitivity, he trains his thinking faculty to read, study and penetrate the infinite. He is immersed in the boundless state of oneness which is indivisible and universal.

Some say that it is possible to acquire mastery of *āsana* merely by surrendering to God. How can this be so? In yoga we are on a razor's edge and in *āsana* perfection must be attained through perseverance, alertness and insight. Without these we remain dull and make no progress. Surrender to God alone does not make us perfect, although it helps us to forget the stresses of life and of our efforts, and guides us towards humility even when perfection in *āsana* has been attained.

When the *sādhaka* has reached that state of balance, attention, extension, diffusion and relaxation take place simultaneously in body and intelligence, and they merge in the seat of the soul. This is a sign of release from the dualities of pleasure and pain, contraction and extension, heat and cold, honour and dishonour, etc.

Perfection in *āsana* brings unalloyed happiness, blessedness and beatitude.

ततो द्वन्द्वानभिघातः ।४८।

II.48 tataḥ dvandvāḥ anabhighātaḥ

tataḥ	from that, then
dvandvāḥ	dualities, opposites
anabhighātaḥ	cessation of disturbance

From then on, the sādhaka *is undisturbed by dualities.*

The effect of *āsana* is to put an end to the dualities or differentiation between the body and mind, mind and soul. None of the pairs of opposites can exist for the *sādhaka* who is one with body, mind and soul.

When body, mind and soul unite in a perfect posture, the *sādhaka* is in a state of beatitude. In that exalted position, the mind, which is at the root of dualistic perception, loses its identity and ceases to disturb him. Unity is achieved between body and mind and mind and soul. There is no longer joy or sorrow, heat or cold, honour or dishonour, pain or pleasure. This is perfection in action and freedom in consciousness.

तस्मिन्सति श्वासप्रश्वासयोर्गतिविच्छेदः प्राणायामः ।४९।

II.49 tasmin satiśvāsa praśvāsayoḥ gativicchedaḥ prāṇāyāmaḥ

tasmin	on this
sati	being accomplished
śvāsa	inbreath, inhalation
praśvāsayoḥ	outbreath, exhalation

gati	movement, motion, path, course, way
vicchedaḥ	cessation, stoppage, interruption
prāṇāyāmaḥ	(*prāṇa* = breath, vital force; *āyāmaḥ* = ascension, extension and expansion or length, breadth and circumference) regulation of breath, expansion of the life force or vital energy by regulation of breath

Prāṇāyāma *is the regulation of the incoming and outgoing flow of breath with retention. It is to be practised only after perfection in* āsana *is attained.*

Sūtras II.49–53 describe *prāṇāyāma* and its effects.

Prāṇāyāma, the fourth constituent of yoga, is what the heart is to the human body.

It is interesting to note that Patañjali expressly advises the *sādhaka* to do *prāṇāyāma* only after attaining perfection in *āsana*. For the first time, he shows a distinct step in the ascent of the ladder of yoga, whereas he has not stipulated progression for the other aspects.

Normally the flow of breath is unrestrained and irregular. Observing these variations, and conditioning the mind to control the inflow, outflow and retention of the breath in a regular, rhythmic pattern, is *prāṇāyāma*.

Prāṇa is an auto-energizing force which creates a magnetic field in the form of the Universe and plays with it, both to maintain, and to destroy for further creation. It permeates each individual as well as the Universe at all levels. It acts as physical energy; as mental energy, where the mind gathers information; and as intellectual energy with a discriminative faculty, where information is examined and filtered. This same *prāṇa* acts as sexual energy, spiritual energy and cosmic energy. All that vibrates in the Universe is *prāṇa*: heat, light, gravity, magnetism, vigour, power, vitality, electricity, life and spirit are all forms of *prāṇa*. It is the cosmic personality, potent in all beings and non-beings. It is the prime mover of all activity. It is the wealth of life.

This self-energizing force is the principle of life and of consciousness. It is the creation of all beings in the Universe. All beings are born through it and live by it. When they die, their individual breath dissolves into the cosmic breath. *Prāṇa* is not only the hub of the wheel of life, but also of yoga. Everything is established in it. It permeates life, creating the sun, the moon, the clouds, the wind, the rain, the earth and all forms of matter. It is both being (*sat*) and non-being (*asat*). Each and every thing, or being, including man, takes shelter under it. *Prāṇa* is the fundamental energy and the source of all knowledge.

Prāṇa (energy) and *citta* (consciousness) are in constant contact with each other. They are like twins. Prāṇa becomes focussed where *citta* is, and *citta* where *prāṇa* is. In yogic texts, it is said that as long as the breath is still, *prāṇa* is still, and hence *citta* is still. All types of vibrations and fluctuations come to a standstill when *prāṇa* and *citta* are steady and silent.

The wise yogis studied this connection between breath and consciousness and advocated the practice of *prāṇāyāma* to stabilize energy and consciousness.

The word *prāṇāyāma* consists of two components, *prāṇa* and *āyāma*. *Prāṇa* is energy, when the self-energizing force embraces the body. *Āyāma* means stretch, extension, expansion, length, breadth, regulation, prolongation, restraint and control. When this self-energizing force embraces the body with extension, expansion and control, it is *prāṇāyāma*.

In the *Śrīmad Bhāgavatam*, the story is told of how 'the nectar of immortality' was produced through the churning of the ocean. This story, as will be understood from the interwoven explanation, symbolizes what takes place in the human body in the practice of *prāṇāyāma*.

The strength of the *asuras* (demons) alarmed the *devas* (angels), who, fearing that vice would dominate virtue, approached Lord Śiva, Lord Brahma and Lord Indra, who in turn approached Lord Viṣṇu, the protector of the Universe, for help.

Lord Viṣṇu suggested the churning of the ocean to bring out the nectar (*amṛta*) of immortality hidden in it. He advised the *devas* to discuss with the demons the effects of the nectar, and to persuade them to jointly churn the ocean. Lord Viṣṇu said that he would do the rest.

The angels and demons decided to use Mount Meru as the churn-staff for the churning, and Lord Ādiśeṣa, the serpent, the couch of Lord Viṣṇu, as the rope for whirling the mountain.

Plants, creepers, various grasses and herbs were gathered together and thrown into the ocean as raw materials so that they might be churned to produce the nectar of life.

According to *āyurveda*, the body is made up of seven constituents (*dhātus*) and three permeating humours (*doṣas*). The seven elements are so-called because they sustain the body. They are chyle (*rasa*), blood (*rakta*), flesh (*māṁsa*), fat (*meda*), bones (*asthi*), marrow (*majjā*), semen (*śukra*). They keep the body immune from infection and diseases. They are churned together in *prāṇāyāma* for the production of the nectar of life.

Mount Meru represents the spinal column, it acts as a whisk to churn the breath to produce energy. Lord Ādiśeṣa represents *suṣumna*: it is the rope which dashes or controls the spine in respiration. The head and tail of Ādiśeṣa represent the *piṅgalā* and *iḍā nāḍīs* (energy channels) or the upward and downward course of the in- and outbreath.

Iḍā also corresponds to the parasympathetic nervous system in western medical terminology, *piṅgalā* with the sympathetic nervous system and *suṣumna* with the central nervous system. As Ādiśeṣa was used as a rope for churning, so inhalation and exhalation are the two ends of the central nervous system, the rod that churns to create the energy that is then stored in the seven chambers (*cakras*) of the spine. Together they churn the inbreath and outbreath to generate the vital energy known as *prāṇa*.

To return to our story: as the churning began, Mount Meru sank deep into the ocean. Lord Viṣṇu incarnated as *Kūrma* (tortoise), crept underneath the mountain and lifted it from the floor of the seabed so that it might float and the churning could continue. Several gems were generated as a result of the churning. The last to spring out of the ocean was the *amṛta*, the nectar of immortality.

Puruṣa or the soul represents Lord Viṣṇu and the body represents *prakṛti*, or nature. The body becomes the fountain for production and the Lord of the body is its generative force. *Ātman* acts as a tortoise to lift and keep the diaphragm floating upwards, allowing the breath to come in contact with the inner elements of the body (earth, water, fire, air and ether) and its seven constituents (chyle, blood, flesh, fat, bones, marrow, semen), as well as the ten types of vital energy: *prāṇa*, *apāna*, *samāna*, *udāna*, *vyāna*, *nāga*, *kūrma*, *kṛkara*, *devadatta* and *dhanaṁjaya*.

Through the contact of these seven constituents and ten vital energies, and with the help of the seer, the spine and the breath, the elixir of life-force is produced in the body. This *prāṇa* is now known as bio-energy. As *prāṇa* is a self-energizing force, it generates more power through the process of *prāṇāyāma*.

The first thing to spring from the ocean was the poison called *halāhala*. This was swallowed by Lord Śiva, who alone was capable of absorbing it. This *halāhala* represents the toxic output of exhalation.

The life elixir is produced by the five primary elements, which are its raw material. Earth is the base for production and ether acts as a distributor of energy. Air is active in the processes of breathing in and out. This stirs and creates a fusion of the elements of water and fire, which by nature are opposed to one another, resulting in the production of electrical energy known as life-force. In Sanskrit, this is called *ojas*, spiritual lustre.

The generation and distribution of *prāṇa* in the human system may be compared to the production and functioning of electrical energy. Stored water is stale; running water has a dynamic life-giving force. Water running with minimal force cannot generate electricity. Through the construction of a reservoir, water falls on turbines which whirl with speed and force for the production of energy. The energy of falling water or rising steam is made to rotate turbines within a magnetic field to generate electricity. The power is stepped up or down by transformers which regulate the voltage or current.

It is then transmitted along cables to light cities and run machinery. *Prāṇa* is like the falling water or the rising steam.

The thoracic area is the magnetic field. The practice of *prāṇāyāma* makes the spindles act as turbines and transmits the drawn-in energy to the remotest cells of the lungs for generating energy. The energy is accumulated in the *cakras* which are situated in the spinal column and act as transformers. This energy generated in the thoracic cavity is like electricity. It is stepped up or down by the *cakras* and is distributed throughout the body through the transmission lines of the circulatory and nervous systems.

The yogis discovered *prāṇāyāma* for making full use of this drawn-in energy so that it might maintain the entire human system, comprising the respiratory, circulatory, nervous, digestive, excretory and reproductive systems with optimum efficiency and harmony.

In *prāṇāyāma*, the carpet of the mucous membrane of the nostrils filters and cleanses the breath as it enters in inhalation. Upon exhalation, sufficient time is given for the system to absorb the drawn-in energy so that the breath may mingle with the blood. This purified blood, filled with chemical properties and hormones, is called 'a constituent full of jewels' or 'the jewel of blood' (*ratna pūrita dhātu*).

Full use of this absorption and re-absorption of energy will allow one to live a hundred years with perfect health of body, clarity of mind, and equipoise of spirit. That is why the practice of *prāṇāyāma* is considered to be a great science and art.

(See notes on III.40 and also *Light on Yoga, Light on Prāṇāyāma* and *Tree of Yoga.*)

बाह्याभ्यन्तरस्तम्भवृत्तिर्देशकालसंख्याभि : परिदृष्टो दीर्घसूक्ष्मः ।५०।

II.50 bāhya ābhyantara stambha vṛttiḥ deśa kāla saṁkhyābhiḥ paridṛṣṭaḥ dīrgha sūkṣmaḥ

bāhya	external
ābhyantara	internal
stambha	restraint, suspension, a pause
vṛttiḥ	movement
deśa	place
kāla	time, duration
saṁkhyābhiḥ	number, precision, minuteness, reflection, deliberation

paridṛṣṭaḥ	regulated, measured
dīrgha	long in place and time, expansion, high
sūkṣmaḥ	subtle, soft, minute, fine, exquisite

Prāṇāyāma *has three movements: prolonged and fine inhalation, exhalation and retention; all regulated with precision according to duration and place.*

The first three components of *prāṇāyāma* are regulated inhalation, exhalation and retention; all are to be performed, prolonged and refined according to the capacity of the aspirant. The components are to be observed with regard to place (*deśa*), here meaning the torso, *kāla* indicating length of breath and *saṁkhyā*, indicating precision.

There are two types of retention in *prāṇāyāma*. They are the interruption of the breath flow following either the in- or outbreath. The movements of the breath and the pauses between them are regulated and prolonged according to the capacity of the lungs (*deśa*), the duration and measured regulation of the breath (*kāla*) and the degree of refinement and subtlety (*saṁkhyā*) of the *sādhaka*. Mastery is attained by practising in harmony, with rhythmic regulation (*paridṛṣṭa*).

Focus on the regulation of breath (*prāṇa vṛtti*), exhalation (*bāhya vṛtti*), inhalation (*antara vṛtti*) and retention (*stambha vṛtti*) is called *sabīja* (seed) *prāṇāyāma* as attention is on the breath itself.

Inhalation moves from the core of being – the seer – towards the consciousness. As *mahat* or cosmic intelligence is the first principle for nature's activity, its individual counterpart, *citta*, acts to stir the soul to activity. The inbreath is made to touch the five sheaths of the body: *ānandamaya*, *vijñānamaya*, *manomaya*, *prāṇamaya* and *annamaya*, or the elements: *ākāśa*, *vāyu*, *tej*, *āp* and *pṛthvi*; while the outbreath touches in the reverse order.

Bracing of the inbreath is the evolution of the soul or the ascending order of the *puruṣa*. When the self comes in contact with the physical body, inhalation is complete. Here, the *puruṣa* embraces *prakṛti*. The outbreath moves from the external body towards the seer, layer after layer. It is involution, or the descending order of *prakṛti* to meet its Lord, *puruṣa*. If the inbreath is the divine union of *puruṣa* with *prakṛti*, the outbreath is the union of *prakṛti* with *puruṣa*. Retention of the former is *antara kumbhaka*, retention of the latter is *bāhya kumbhaka*. If *antara kumbhaka* establishes consecration of the seer (*svarūpa pratiṣṭha*), *bāhya kumbhaka* frees one from the four aims of life (*puruṣārtha śūnya*). (See IV.34).

बाह्याभ्यन्तरविषयाक्षेपी चतुर्थः ।५१।

II.51 bāhya ābhyantara viṣaya ākṣepī caturthaḥ

bāhya	external
ābhyantara	internal
viṣaya	region, sphere, an object, reference, aim, realm
ākṣepī	passing over, gaining over, overcoming, transcending
caturthaḥ	the fourth

The fourth type of prāṇāyāma *transcends the external and internal* prāṇāyāmas, *and appears effortless and non-deliberate.*

The fourth type of *prāṇāyāma* goes beyond the regulation or modulation of breath flow and retention, transcending the methodology given in the previous sūtra. It is a state similar to *kevala kumbhaka*, which is mentioned in the *haṭhayoga* texts and in the *yoga upaniṣads*.

When the movement of the breath functions without one's volition or effort, the fourth stage of *prāṇāyāma* has been reached. The movements of the mind and consciousness cease. The flows of vital energy, intelligence and consciousness come to a standstill except for subliminal impressions. This is like *virāma pratyaya*, as explained in I.18. A state of pause is experienced, in both the breath and the mind. From this springs forth a new awakening and the light of intelligence vigorously penetrates the *sādhaka*'s innermost being.

Since this fourth stage contains no restrictions, it transcends the range of movements described in the *prāṇāyāmas* of II.50. It is therefore a 'seedless' (*nirbīja*) *prāṇāyāma*.

ततः क्षीयते प्रकाशावरणम् ।५२।

II.52 tataḥ kṣīyate prakāśa āvaraṇam

tataḥ	from that, then
kṣīyate	destroyed, dissolved
prakāśa	light
āvaraṇam	covering

Prāṇāyāma *removes the veil covering the light of knowledge and heralds the dawn of wisdom.*

Its practice destroys illusion, consisting of ignorance, desire and delusion which obscure the intelligence; and allows the inner light of wisdom to shine. As the breeze disperses the clouds that cover the sun, *prāṇāyāma* wafts away the clouds that hide the light of the intelligence.

In the *Yoga Chuḍāmaṇi Upaniṣad*, it is said that there is no discipline higher than *prāṇāyāma*. It is called an exalted knowledge (*mahāvidyā*), a royal road to well-being, freedom and bliss.

धारणासु च योग्यता मनसः ।५३।

II.53 dhāraṇāsu ca yogyatā manasaḥ

dhāraṇāsu	for concentration
ca	and
yogyatā	fitness, suitability, propriety, ability, capability, appropriateness
manasaḥ	of the mind

The mind also becomes fit for concentration.

Prāṇāyāma is not only an instrument to steady the mind, but also the gateway to concentration, *dhāraṇā*.

Once the new light of knowledge has dawned through the practice of *prāṇāyāma*, the mind is fit and competent to move on towards the realization of the soul.

The implication here is clear that the *sādhaka* who had to struggle initially to cultivate a yogic way of life by self-discipline and study, now finds his efforts transformed into a natural zeal to proceed in his *sādhana*.

स्वविषयासंप्रयोगे चित्तस्यस्वरूपानुकार इवेन्द्रियाणां प्रत्याहारः ।५४।

II.54 svaviṣaya asaṁprayoge cittasya svarūpānukāraḥ iva indriyāṇāṁ pratyāhāraḥ

sva	their own
viṣaya	objects
asaṁprayoge	not coming in contact with
cittasya	of the thinking faculty, of the conscious faculty
svarūpa	own form, natural form
anukāraḥ	imitation, following
iva	as if, as it were
indriyāṇāṁ	senses
pratyāhāraḥ	(*prati* + *aṅg* + *hṛ* = *pratyāhāra*, i.e., to drawn towards the opposite. *Prati* = opposite, against, in return; *aṅg* = near, near to, towards, strength; *hṛ* = to take, bear, carry; *hṛ* is the root of *pratyāhāra*) drawing back, marching back, retreating, restraining, withholding, withdrawal of the senses

Withdrawing the senses, mind and consciousness from contact with external objects, and then drawing them inwards towards the seer, is pratyāhāra.

Now the mind is able to concentrate and the senses no longer importune the mind for their gratification. They lose interest in the tastes and flavours of their respective objects, and are drawn back from the external world in order to help the mind in its inner quest. This is *pratyāhāra.*

This is the foundation of the path of renunciation. As a bird cannot fly if one of its wings is cut off, so is it in the case of the *sādhaka*. The two wings of yoga are practice, from *yama* to *prāṇāyāma*, and renunciation, from *pratyāhāra* to *samādhi*. For flight, both are necessary. Then the yogi dwells in his soul, perceiving all things directly, without the intervention of *citta*, the conscious faculty.

In normal daily life, consciousness helps the senses see the objects of the world with thoughts of acquisition, rejection and resignation. They become hypnotized by them, and are drawn outwards, towards pleasure. In *pratyāhāra*, the senses are directed inwards, towards the realization of the soul. *Pratyāhāra* is the withdrawal of the mind from its contact with the senses of perception and organs of action; then its direction is towards the soul.

The relationship between the mind and the senses is aptly compared to that of bees following the queen bee. If the queen bee moves, the others follow. When she rests, the others rest. They do not function independently of their queen. Similarly, when the mind stops, the senses, too, stop functioning. This is *pratyāhāra*. It is the beginning of man's return journey towards his Maker. It is the science of restraining the senses by depriving them of that which feeds them, the external objective world. It frees them, by withdrawing the supply of nourishment in the form of desires and their satisfactions.

By controlling the senses and mind, the *sādhaka* draws *citta* towards its source – the soul, *ātma*, and through *ātma* to *Paramātma*, God. For example, while performing an *āsana* the intelligence of the body extends outwards, and the senses of perception, mind and intelligence are drawn inwards. It is the same in the performance of *prāṇāyāma*. This is *pratyāhāra*.

Here, in order to understand the characteristics and components of nature, the reader should refer again to II.19, in which the basic elements of the universe according to *sāṁkhya* philosophy are fully described. To summarize: Nature consists of five gross elements, earth, water, fire, air and ether with their five subtle counterparts, smell, taste, shape, touch and sound. These interact with the three *guṇas* – *sattva*, *rajas* and *tamas*. *Citta*, comprised of ego, intelligence and mind is the individual counterpart of *mahat*, cosmic intelligence. This cosmic intelligence is the unevolved primary germ of nature, or the productive principle, for creation of all phenomena of the material world. There are also the five senses of perception – ears, nose, tongue, eyes and skin – and five organs of action – legs, arms, speech and the organs of generation and excretion.

The five senses of perception come in contact with sound, smell, taste, sight and touch, send their impressions to the mind and are stored in the memory. Memory longs for further experiences and incites the mind to bypass intelligence and solicit the senses for yet more sense gratification. This in turn incites the mind to seek further experiences through the organs of action. Throughout this process, intelligence measures advantages and disadvantages in order to counterbalance memory, mind and senses which, recalling the taste of past pleasures, are avid for more. Almost inevitably, intelligence remains unheeded. Through over-stimulation and misuse, the organs of action lose their potency and are no longer capable of exciting the organs of perception or the mind.

Owing to the force of past impressions, one continues to hanker after renewed sensation. But one can never be satisfied. This breeds unhappiness and frustration. Here lies the true role of *pratyāhāra*, the fifth aspect of yoga. It is the friend who releases you from the snares of the external world, and leads you towards happiness in the delight of the soul.

The practice of *pratyāhāra* modifies the mechanism described above in the following manner. The mind, which until now had bypassed intelligence, now approaches it for guidance. Intelligence employs its discriminative faculty to weigh right and wrong, the appropriate and inappropriate, and supports the mind in its struggle to free itself from the vociferous claims of memory and imprints. This act of going against the current of memory and mind is *pratyāhāra*. *Pratyāhāra* is called an external quest (*bahiraṅga sādhana*), because the senses are disciplined by intelligence so that they may begin a journey in reverse, and return to their points of origin.

This process of weighing one's instincts, thoughts and actions is the practice of detachment or renunciation (*vairāgya*). Energy is conserved and used only when necessary; the continual longing to repeat old sensations is gradually curbed. Memory collects new and fresh impressions and is subdued: it becomes subservient to intelligence and consciousness. It is consciousness which grasps intelligence, and brings it to rest at the source of conscience. Then the impulses of nature end and intuitive insight flows freely. This is the effect of *pratyāhāra*.

It has already been mentioned that *prāṇāyāma* removes the clouds that obscure intelligence and allows it to shine forth. The mind is now fit for meditation. Earlier, consciousness was always willing to oblige by listening to the senses, and even went out of its way to help them to find gratification. Now the senses take a reverse turn, and help consciousness fulfil its desire to experience Self-Realization.

This is *pratyāhāra*. It can be divided into four stages, physical, mental, intellectual and spiritual. Withdrawing energy from the organs of action and senses of perception towards the brain is physical *pratyāhāra*. Quietening the fluctuations in the four lobes of the brain is mental *pratyāhāra*; drawing intelligence towards the stem of the brain is intellectual *pratyāhāra*. Directing the energies of intelligence and consciousness towards the seat of conscience is spiritual *pratyāhāra*. It culminates in the vision of the seer, *ātmasākṣātkāra*.

ततः परमा वश्यतेन्द्रियाणाम् ।५५।

II.55 tataḥ paramā vaśyatā indriyāṇām

tataḥ	then, from that
paramā	the highest

vaśyatā subdued, controlled, governed
indriyāṇām of the senses

Pratyāhāra *results in the absolute control of the sense organs.*

The effect of *pratyāhāra* is felt when the senses are mastered, and the mind is ripe and avid for its spiritual quest.

When the senses have ceased to run after pleasures obtained from the phenomenal world, they can be yoked to serve the soul.

Sādhana pāda instructs the *sādhaka* how to survey his own weaknesses in each domain – moral, physical, physiological and intellectual – and how to eliminate them, since they are not conducive to yogic discipline and spiritual emancipation.

Yama develops the art of living in society honestly; *niyama*, that of cleansing one's impurities. *Āsana* eliminates physical and mental perturbations, and *prāṇāyāma* maintains harmony and prevents dissipation of the flow of vital energy, making the mind a fit instrument for meditation. *Pratyāhāra* sublimates both senses and mind.

Thus ends the external quest (*bahiraṅga sādhana*). Now the *sādhaka* crosses the threshold of the internal quest (*antaraṅga sādhana*) of yoga.

Here ends the exposition on *sādhana*, the second *pāda* of Patañjali's *Yoga Sūtras*.

part three

विभूति पादः ।

Vibhūti Pāda

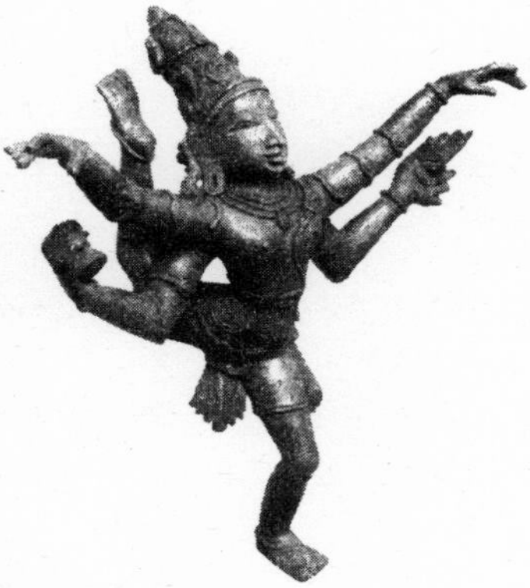

In this *pāda* Patañjali speaks of the properties of yoga and the art of integration (*saṁyama*) through concentration, meditation and profound absorption.

On this innermost quest, supernatural powers or accomplishments (*vibhūtis*) come naturally to a yogi who has integrated his body, mind and soul. There is a danger that he will be seduced by these powers. He should bypass them in order to pursue his *sādhana* as far as *kaivalya*, the height of indivisible existence.

Samādhi pāda concerned evolved beings and their practice in relation to achieving seedless *samādhi*. *Sādhana pāda* dealt with the external quest (*bahiraṅga sādhana*), through which beginners and advanced practitioners alike learn to maintain their mental poise under any stress. *Vibhūti pāda* moves on to the inner quest (*antaraṅga sādhana*), comprising concentration (*dhāraṇā*), meditation (*dhyāna*) and total absorption (*samādhi*). Patañjali coins the expression *saṁyama yoga* to link them.

Saṁyama explains the disciplines necessary both to live in the natural grace of yoga, and to accrue supernatural powers, or *siddhis*.

The idea of the supernatural or supernormal powers presents a problem to the modern reader, who is probably of a rational and scientific bent. That is because we feel obliged to believe or disbelieve in them. If we disbelieve, and consider them to be a fantasy left over from a mythical and superstitious culture, this can lead us to have serious doubts about the validity of Patañjali's other chapters.

In feeling that we must make up our minds on this subject,

we are underestimating the subtlety of Patañjali's intentions. The *Yoga Sūtras* are addressed to everyone: those who are spiritually evolved and those who are not. The extraordinary point is that they are addressed to both, *all the time*. Nothing Patañjali says is inappropriate to anyone. All levels are present, and trouble often comes from where we least expect it. Has not a failure to observe the basics of *yama/niyama* brought many a modern God-man's reputation crashing? Does not even a criminal in sleep and on the moment of waking experience a feeling akin to *samādhi*? So we can be sure that Patañjali, when discussing the dangers engendered by *siddhis*, was talking equally to ordinary as well as to advanced *sādhakas*, and not just indulging in flights of fancy.

The essence of what he is saying is this: when we strive mightily for a goal on our path, gratifying rewards and results incidentally come in our way. We can easily become so enamoured of what we have accidentally acquired, that we mistake it for the goal itself.

Imagine a young person who wants to be a great actor, a worthwhile goal. On the way he acquires fame, and if he is not steadfast in his purpose, he makes fame alone his new goal. The *siddhi* of renown has beguiled and swallowed him up.

Or an ambitious young businessman sets off on his career to provide for his family, and on the way becomes rich. He now has more than enough. But riches and their pursuit now possess him: he neglects his wife and children who live in sterile luxury while he pursues money and more money for its own sake.

Imagine a man who through merit of past lives is born into a royal household. Instead of regarding his good fortune as a sign that he must humbly serve his people, he becomes seized by pride of birth and behaves tyrannically.

In all these cases the protagonist has let himself be side-tracked, has substituted an agreeable and merited by-product of his efforts for the real goal. At best his progress is stopped, at worst he is consumed; and in all cases illusion has displaced reality. The lesson of *siddhis* for all of us is not to allow ourselves to be side-tracked, but to be steadfast. A man who has let himself become ensnared by the glamour of *siddhis* is like one who believes that the bricks and mortar of the temple are God Himself. This is known as spiritual materialism.

The Aṣṭa (eight) Siddhis

1 *aṇimā* = to become as minute as an atom
2 *mahimā* = to wax in magnitude
3 *laghimā* = to become light
4 *garimā* = to become heavy
5 *prāpti* = the power to dominate and obtain what one wants
6 *prākāmya* = the freedom of will and attainment of wishes
7 *īśatva* = supremacy over all
8 *vaśitva* = the power to subjugate anyone or anything

These are the eight powers which come unbidden to the yogi. Although they indicate that his *sādhana* is on the right path, they are also capable of catching him up with the force of a whirlwind to bring his *sādhana* crashing down. Such *siddhis* must be ignored and the ultimate goal of freedom and beatitude maintained. Pride in *siddhis* and preoccupation with them lead to disaster and chaos. They create attachment and affliction, and that is why Patañjali (III.38) holds them to be obstacles to *dhyāna* and *samādhi*. They are only of use if one has forgotten the aim of yoga. 'Discard them', he says, 'and devote all energies to the realization of God.'

देशबन्धश्चित्तस्य धारणा ॥१॥

III.1 deśa bandhaḥ cittasya dhāraṇā

deśa	place, spot, region
bandhaḥ	binding, combining, connecting, uniting, fixing
cittasya	of mind, of consciousness
dhāraṇā	the act of holding, keeping the mind collected, concentration

Fixing the consciousness on one point or region is concentration (dhāraṇā).

Dhāraṇā means focus of attention. Focusing the attention on a chosen point or area, within or outside the body, is concentration. By it the functions of the mind are controlled and brought to one focal point.

Once mastery of the five stages of yoga from *yama* to *pratyāhāra* is achieved, the art of focusing the mind and consciousness is undertaken. *Dhāraṇā* is established when the mind learns to remain steady on its own, or hold on to an unmoving object.

Through the practice of *yama* and *niyama*, the *sādhaka* develops emotional stability. Through *āsana*, he keeps his body, the abode of the soul, free from disease. In *prāṇāyāma*, he learns to stop the dissipation of energy by regulating its flow for proper distribution throughout his body and mind. Through *pratyāhāra*, he develops willpower, detaches himself from the organs of senses and acquires clarity of thought. This is the beginning of culturing the brain. Once he has become indifferent to worldly matters, he is fit to proceed on the inner quest, enriching the mind through *dhāraṇā*. *Dhyāna* and *samādhi* lead the consciousness on the innermost quest (*antarātmā sādhana*), to the soul itself.

The eight components of *aṣṭāṅga yoga* are interwoven, though each is described individually for the sake of convenience. They are subdivided into the external quest (*bahiraṅga sādhana*), the internal quest (*antaraṅga sādhana*) and the innermost quest (*antarātmā sādhana*) which enable even the uninitiated to learn to concentrate, step by step, on concrete forms through systematic practice. Having reached maturity and refinement they are able to penetrate their inmost thoughts and feelings (see II.53).

For example, most people, even most yoga practitioners, are under the impression that *āsanas* are merely external and physical. This sūtra removes that misconception. Patañjali defines concentration as the focusing of attention either within or outside the body. If, in performing an *āsana*, one directs the organs of action and senses of perception towards the mind, and the mind towards the core, the external *sādhana* is transformed into internal *sādhana*. If the limbs, the senses of perception, the mind and the discriminative intelligence are then yoked and fused with the energy of the soul, this becomes the innermost *sādhana*. If one performs each *āsana* zealously, fusing with integrated attention the parts of the body, the wandering mind and the discriminative intelligence with the soul, is this not a spiritual practice?

Who has not noticed something of this process in watching children? Has not one seen a little boy with a passion for aeroplanes building his own model? His passionate interest fuels his concentration and he becomes totally absorbed in his task, oblivious of his surroundings. In *āsana*, our initial commitment or passion lifts itself, through concentration, to the level of total absorption. Such practice brings humility, without which penetration of the subtle levels is impossible.

Dhāraṇā is the art of reducing the interruptions of the mind and ultimately eliminating them completely, so that the knower and the known become one (I.41).

Dhāraṇā may be focused on external or internal objects. External objects should be auspicious and associated with purity. Internally, the mind penetrates to the soul, the core of one's being: the object is, in reality, pure existence.

Śrī Vyāsa's commentary on this sūtra indicates certain parts of the body as being suitable for concentration. They are the sphere of the navel (*nābhicakra*), the lotus of the heart (*hṛdaya puṇḍarīka*), the centre of the head (*mūrdhani*), the shining light (*jyotiṣi* or *ājñācakra*), the tip of the nose (*nāsikāgra*) and the root of the tongue (*jihvāgra*). As attention is fixed on these inner points, one gradually becomes engrossed first in oneself (*sāsmitā*) and then in one's soul, *ātman*.

तत्र प्रत्ययैकतानता ध्यानम् ।२।

III.2 tatra pratyaya ekatānatā dhyānam

tatra	there (in those places of concentration)
pratyaya	base, content, belief, going towards, firm conviction, device
ekatānatā	continuous, uninterrupted flow of attentive awareness
dhyānam	meditation, reflection, profound contemplation

A steady, continuous flow of attention directed towards the same point or region is meditation (dhyāna).

The characteristic feature of meditation (*dhyāna*) is the maintenance of an uninterrupted flow of attention on a fixed point or region, without intervention or interruption. In *dhyāna*, psychological and chronological time come to a standstill as the mind observes its own behaviour. The intensity of attention in the field of consciousness neither alters nor wavers, remaining as stable, smooth and constant as oil pouring from a jug. Maintaining the same intensity of awareness, the attentive awareness moves from one-pointed concentration to no-pointed attentiveness.

The difference between *dhāraṇā* and *dhyāna* is that *dhāraṇā* is more concerned with the elimination of fluctuating thought-waves in order to achieve single-pointed concentration; in *dhyāna*, the emphasis is on the maintenance of steady and profound contemplative observation.

Ekatānatā implies an unbroken flow of contact between the *sādhaka*'s consciousness and his *sādhana*. We can see, therefore, that *dhyāna* may be achieved in both *āsana* and *prāṇāyāma*. In *āsana*, there is a centrifugal movement of consciousness to the frontiers of the body, whether extended vertically, horizontally or circumferentially, and a centripetal movement as the whole body is brought into single focus. If the attention is steadily maintained in this manner, meditation takes place. Similarly, in *prāṇāyāma*, the flow of in- or outbreath is sensitively measured and sustained, resulting in total involvement with the self. During retention, when the breath, cells of the torso, consciousness and soul are brought into unison, meditation occurs. In short, when attention, reflection and contemplation in action and observation are steadily sustained, *dhāraṇā* evolves into *dhyāna* (see I.2).

तदेवार्थमात्रनिर्भासं स्वरूपशून्यमिव समाधिः ॥३॥

III.3 tadeva arthamātranirbhāsaṁ svarūpaśūnyam iva samādhiḥ

tadeva	the same (*dhyāna*)
artha	object, purpose, aim, end, wish, desire
mātra	alone, only
nirbhāsaṁ	appearing, shining
svarūpa	essential form, by itself
śūnyam	empty, void
iva	as if, as it were

samādhiḥ perfect absorption, intent attention, union, bringing into harmony, spiritual absorption

When the object of meditation engulfs the meditator, appearing as the subject, self-awareness is lost. This is samādhi.

When the attentive flow of consciousness merges with the object of meditation, the consciousness of the meditator, the subject, appears to be dissolved in the object. This union of subject and object becomes *samādhi.*

When the object of contemplation shines forth without the intervention of one's own consciousness, *dhyāna* flows into *samādhi.*

When a musician loses himself and is completely engrossed in his music, or an inventor makes his discoveries when devoid of ego, or a painter transcends himself with colour, shade and brush; they glimpse *samādhi.* So it is with the yogi: when his object of contemplation becomes himself, devoid of himself, he experiences *samādhi.*

The difference is that the artist or musician reaches this state by effort, and cannot sustain it; whereas the yogi, remaining devoid of ego, experiences it as natural, continuous and effortless. Consequently it is difficult for an artist to infuse his vision of the sublime, which is associated with the performance and realization of a particular art form, into his ordinary daily existence. For the yogi, however, whose 'art' is formless and whose goal has no physical expression like a painting, a book or a symphony, the fragrance of *samādhi* penetrates every aspect of his 'normal' behaviour, activities and state of being.

Uninterrupted flow of attention dissolves the split between the object seen and the seer who sees it. Consciousness appears to have ceased, and to have reached a state of silence. It is devoid of 'I', and merges into the core of the being in a profound state of serenity. In *samādhi*, awareness of place vanishes and one ceases to experience space and time.

In I.27–28, Patañjali deals with *japa* (prayer), *artha* (meaning and purpose) and *bhāvana* (feeling or experiencing). *Japa* of *mantra* may be associated with *dhāraṇā*; *artha* with *dhyāna*, and *bhāvana* with *samādhi.*

(See also I.41 and 43.)

त्रयमेकत्रसंयमः ।४।

III.4 trayam ekatra saṁyamaḥ

trayam	these three
ekatra	jointly, together
saṁyamaḥ	defining, holding together, integration

These three together – dhāraṇā, dhyāna *and* samādhi – *constitute integration or* saṁyama.

Saṁyama is a technical word defining the integration of concentration (*dhāraṇā*), meditation (*dhyāna*) and absorption (*samādhi*). In *saṁyama* the three are a single thread, evolving from uninterrupted attention to *samādhi*.

Dhāraṇā is single-pointed attention. It modifies into *dhyāna* by being sustained in time whilst dissolving its one-pointed character implicit in the word 'concentration'. When it becomes all-pointed, which is also no-pointed (that is to say equally diffused, but with no drop in attentiveness) it leads to total absorption (*samādhi*). Continuous prolongation of these three subtle aspects of yoga thus forms a single unit, called *saṁyama*. *Saṁyama*, is a state of immobility, and a *saṁyami* is one who subdues his passions and remains motionless.

The following analogy shows the organic relationship between *dhāraṇā*, *dhyāna* and *samādhi*. When one contemplates a diamond, one at first sees with great clarity the gem itself. Gradually one becomes aware of the light glowing from its centre. As awareness of the light grows, awareness of the stone as an object diminishes. Then there is only brightness, no source, no object. When the light is everywhere, that is *samādhi*.

As *dhāraṇā* is external to *dhyāna*, *dhyāna* to *samādhi*, *samādhi* to *saṁyama* and *saṁyama* to *nirbīja samādhi*, so the mind is external to intelligence, intelligence to consciousness and consciousness to the seer.

Dhāraṇā brings stability in mind, *dhyāna* develops maturity in intelligence and *samādhi* acts to diffuse the consciousness.

Dhāraṇā, *dhyāna* and *samādhi* intermingle to become *saṁyama*, or integration. The intermingling of mind, intelligence and consciousness is *saṁyama* of the three. The vision of the seer is equivalent to *nirbīja samādhi*.

तज्जयात् प्रज्ञालोकः ।५।

III.5 tajjayāt prajñālokaḥ

tad	from that
jayāt	by mastery, by attainment, conquest
prajñā	awareness, wisdom, judgement, discrimination
ālokaḥ	light, lustre, insight

From mastery of saṁyama *comes the light of awareness and insight.*

When mastery of integration (*saṁyama*) is achieved, the lustre of wisdom and insight shine brilliantly, reconciling the known with the knowable and revealing the soul.

Awareness and cognition become firmer and sharper through direct spiritual perception.

Ordinarily, our intelligence flits from object to object and from place to place, making it impossible to penetrate fully any one thing. In *saṁyama*, the knower comes closer and closer to the known and, merging in it, loses his separateness.

(See I.47, III.36 and IV.29.)

तस्य भूमिषु विनियोगः ।६।

III.6 tasya bhūmiṣu viniyogaḥ

tasya	its (*saṁyama*)
bhūmiṣu	degree, step, stage
viniyogaḥ	application

Saṁyama *may be applied in various spheres to derive its usefulness.*

Patañjali explains that this insight and wisdom are to be properly distributed in the various spheres of one's life.

Saṁyama can be applied in various spheres. In *samādhi pāda*, concepts such as *pratyaya* and various aspects of *saṁprajñāta samādhi* and *nirbīja samādhi* were explained (I.17–22 and I.51). But one who has not mastered the lower stages cannot attain the higher, nor can he skip the intermediate stages. If each stage is followed in turn, one becomes acquainted with them by degrees and full insight develops.

Full insight may also dawn by the grace of God, won through one's previous virtuous *karmas*. Vāmadeva, Prahlāda, Śukadeva and Rāmakṛṣṇa in the past, and Aurobindo, Rāmaṇa Māharṣi and Mahātma Gāndhi of the present century were such great personalities who had the blessings of God and attained fullness of knowledge.

This sūtra affirms that no-one can expect success or mastery without regular practice, and also warns one not to jump to higher stages of practice without first establishing a firm foundation through the primary steps of yoga.

There are many examples, even in modern literature, of people quite unexpectedly experiencing *saṁyama* even if they have been following no fixed path of yogic discipline. The Japanese refer to this sudden lifting of the curtain of ignorance as a 'flash'. This is undoubtedly a moment of grace, but it is not the same thing as enlightenment. If the recipient of this sudden grace is sensible, he will go back to the beginning, find a suitable path, and follow it assiduously even for many years, to construct consciously and by worthy effort what had once been yielded in a moment of grace.

The modern fancy of '*kuṇḍalini* awakening' has probably arisen through these freakish experiences of 'integration'. Patañjali does not mention *kuṇḍalini* but speaks of the energy of nature flowing abundantly in a yogi (IV.2). *Kuṇḍalini* is a neologism. This energy of nature (*prakṛti shakti*) was originally known as *agni* or fire. Later yogis called this fire *kuṇḍalini* (the coiled one) as its conduit in the body is coiled 3½ times at the base of the spine. It is, however, clear that many who undergo an overwhelming experience of fusion with the universal consciousness reap, through their unpreparedness, more pain than benefit. To the lucky, healthy few such an experience can serve as a spur to begin a true spiritual search, but to many others it can bring severe physical and psychological disorders. The eightfold path, although it may appear mystical to the uninitiated, is ultimately a path of spiritual evolution whose motto might well be 'safety first'. The foundation must be secure, as Patañjali emphasizes when he places *yama* and *niyama* first, and when he marks a definite step up between *āsana* and *prāṇāyāma*.

Vyāsa has elucidated this sūtra thus: 'Yoga is to be known by yoga. Yoga is the teacher of yoga. The power of yoga manifests through yoga alone. He who does not become careless, negligent or inattentive, he alone rests in yoga and enjoys yoga.'

'Yogena yogojñātavya yogo yogātpravartate
yo pramattastu yogena sa yogo ramate ciram.'

(See I.17, 40; II.27.)

त्रयमन्तरङ्गं पूर्वेभ्यः ॥७॥

III.7 trayam antaraṅgaṁ pūrvebhyaḥ

trayam	these three (*dhāraṇā*, *dhyāna* and *samādhi*)
antaraṅgaṁ	interior parts, the mind and the heart
pūrvebhyaḥ	in relation to the preceding ones

These three aspects of yoga are internal, compared to the former five.

Compared to the former five aspects of yoga, it may be seen that *dhāraṇā*, *dhyāna* and *samādhi* are more subtle, internal, intimate and subjective practices. The first five, which deal with the seen or cognizable sheaths, are called the external quest. *Yama* purifies the organs of action; *niyama*, the senses of perception; *āsana* cleanses the physical and organic aspects of the body; *prāṇāyāma* stops wastage of energy and increases stamina; *pratyāhāra* cleanses the mind.

More intimately, *dhāraṇā* develops and sharpens intelligence, *dhyāna* purifies consciousness and *samādhi* leads consciousness towards the soul. These three are directly involved in the subtle sheaths of mind, intelligence and consciousness and are very close to the spiritual heart. They directly affect the spiritual path, and are therefore called the inner quest, or *sabīja samādhi*, because the *sādhaka* now has one-pointed consciousness.

In *samādhi pāda*, Patañjali explained that truth-bearing wisdom (*ṛtaṁbhara prajñā*) is the threshold between *sabīja* and *nirbīja samādhis*. Here he describes *saṁyama* as the penultimate step towards *nirbīja samādhi*.

In the next sūtra Patañjali explains that *saṁyama* is external to *nirbīja samādhi*, and then proceeds, in III.9–16, to penetrate the transformations in the very substance of the consciousness, leading one to experience its finest state, which appears to be subtler than *saṁyama*.

तदपि बहिरङ्गं निर्बीजस्य ।८।

III.8 tadapi bahiraṅgaṁ nirbījasya

tat	that
api	even, too
bahiraṅgaṁ	external part
nirbījasya	to the seedless

Similarly, saṁyama *is external when compared to seedless* (nirbīja) samādhi.

Even this perfection of *dhāraṇā, dhyāna* and *samādhi* appears external to one who has experienced the seedless *samādhi,* the direct vision of the soul.

Vyāsa's commentary on 1.2 divides *citta* into five states:

1 *kṣipta,* a mental force which is scattered, in a state of disarray and neglect
2 *mūḍha,* a foolish and dull state
3 *vikṣipta,* agitated and distracted, neither marshalled nor controlled
4 *ekāgra,* a state of one-pointed attention
5 *niruddha,* where everything is restrained, for the *sādhaka* to reach the threshold of *kaivalya.*

Sūtras III.7–8 describe the distinction between *sabīja* and *nirbīja samādhi.* Sūtra III.7 explains that the conquest of the vehicles of nature and of nature itself is of the foremost importance in opening the gates of *kaivalya.* In III.8 it is said that as *saṁyama* is dependent on a support or a form, it is called 'external' compared to *nirbīja samādhi.* Once the vehicles of nature (body, organs of action, senses of perception, mind, intelligence, reason and consciousness) cease to function, the soul (*ātman*) shines forth, and the *sādhaka* dwells in *kaivalya* and not on its threshold.

Sleep comes naturally when mental activities cease without effort. In the same way, perfection in *sabīja samādhi* takes one towards the seedless state of *samādhi* or *kaivalya,* as effortlessly as falling asleep. The soul surfaces of its own accord.

(See I.16–18, I.41–45 and III.13.)

व्युत्थाननिरोधसंस्कारयोरभिभवप्रादुर्भावौ निरोधक्षणचित्तान्वयो निरोधपरिणामः ।९।

III.9 vyutthāna nirodha saṁskārayoḥ abhibhava prādurbhāvau nirodhakṣaṇa cittānvayaḥ nirodhapariṇāmaḥ

vyutthāna	emergence of thoughts, rising thoughts
nirodha	suppression, obstruction, restraint
saṁskārayoḥ	of the subliminal impressions
abhibhava	disappearing, subjugating
prādurbhāvau	reappearing
nirodha	restraint, suppression
kṣaṇa	moment
citta	consciousness
anvayaḥ	association, permeation, pervasion
nirodha	restraint, suppression
pariṇāmaḥ	transformation, effect

Study of the silent moments between rising and restraining subliminal impressions is the transformation of consciousness towards restraint (nirodhapariṇāmaḥ).

Transformation by restraint of consciousness is achieved by study of the silent moments that occur between the rising of impressions and our impulse to restrain them, and between the restraining impulse and the resurgence of thought.

The central thread of Patañjali's philosophy is the relationship between the Self, *puruṣa*, and nature, *prakṛti*. We are born into nature, and without it nothing would move, nothing would change, nothing could happen. We seek to free ourselves from nature in order to transcend it, to achieve lasting freedom.

Sensory involvement leads to attachment, desire, frustration and anger. These bring disorientation, and the eventual decay of our true intelligence. Through the combined techniques and resources of *yama*, *niyama*, *āsana*, *prāṇāyāma* and *pratyāhāra* we learn control. These are all external means of restraining consciousness, whether we focus on God, or the breath, or in an *āsana* by learning to direct and diffuse consciousness. All this learning develops in the relationship between subject and object. It is comparatively simple because it is a relative, dual process. But how can subject work on subject, consciousness on consciousness? How, in other words, can one's eyes see one's own eyes? In III.9–15 Patañjali shows the way.

One may well ask why one ought to do this. III.13–14 answer this question and enable one to identify, within one's consciousness, the subtle properties of nature, to discriminate between them, and to distinguish between that which undergoes the stresses and changes of time and that which is immutable and permanent. In so doing we gain from the inner quest the same freedom from nature that we have struggled to achieve in the external. The freedom we gain from the tyranny of time, from the illusion that is absolute, is especially significant. Cutting our ties to sense objects within our consciousness carries immensely more weight than any severance from outside objects; if this were not so, a prisoner in solitary confinement would be halfway to being a yogi. Through the inner quest, the inner aspects of desire, attraction and aversion are brought to an end.

In III.4, Patañjali shows *dhāraṇā*, *dhyāna* and *samādhi* as three threads woven into a single, integrated, unfolding strand. Then he introduces three transformations of consciousness related directly to them, and successively ascending to the highest level, at which consciousness reflects the light of the soul. These transformations are *nirodha pariṇāma*, *samādhi pariṇāma* and *ekāgratā pariṇāma*. They are related to the three transformations in nature: *dharma*, *lakṣaṇa* and *avasthā pariṇāma* (III.13), resulting from our heightened perception, our penetration of nature's reality on a higher level. The word transformation suggests to our imagination a series of steps in a static structure, but it is more helpful to conceive of a harmonious flux, such as that offered by modern particle physics.

Nirodha pariṇāma relates to the method used in meditation, when *dhāraṇā* loses its sharpness of attention on the object, and intelligence itself is brought into focus. In *dhāraṇā* and *nirodha pariṇāma*, observation is a dynamic initiative.

Through *nirodha pariṇāma*, transformation by restraint or suppression, the consciousness learns to calm its own fluctuations and distractions, deliberate and non-deliberate. The method consists of noticing then seizing and finally enlarging those subliminal pauses of silence that occur between rising and restraining thoughts and vice versa.

As long as one impression is replaced by a counter-impression, consciousness rises up against it. This state is called *vyutthāna citta*, or *vyutthāna saṁskāra* (rising impressions). Restraining the rising waves of consciousness and overcoming these impressions is *nirodha citta* or *nirodha saṁskāra*. The precious psychological moments of intermission (*nirodhakṣaṇa*) where there is stillness and silence are to be prolonged into extra-chronological moments of consciousness, without beginning or end.

The key to understanding this wheel of mutations in consciousness is to be found in the breath. Between each inbreath and outbreath, we experience the cessation of breath for a split second. Without this gap, we cannot inhale or exhale. This interval between each breath has another advantage: it allows the heart and lungs to rest. I call this rest period '*śavāsana*' of the heart and lungs.

The yogis who discovered *prāṇāyāma* called this natural space *kumbhaka*, and advised us to prolong its duration. So, there are four movements in each breath: inhalation, pause, exhalation and pause. Consciousness, too, has four movements: rising consciousness, a quiet state of consciousness, restraining consciousness and a quiet state of consciousness.

Inhalation actually generates thought-waves, whereas exhalation helps to restrain them (see I.34). The pauses between breaths, which take place after inhalation and exhalation are akin to the intervals between each rising and restraining thought. The mutation of breath and mutation of consciousness are therefore identical, as both are silent periods for the physiological and intellectual body. They are moments of void in which a sense of emptiness is felt. We are advised by Patañjali to transform this sense of emptiness into a dynamic whole, as single-pointed attention to no-pointed attentiveness. This will become the second mode – *samādhi pariṇāma*.

The mind wavers like the waves of the sea, and we must make efforts to direct its attention to a chosen thought or object. In this process we often lose awareness on account of suppression and distraction. Having understood these silent intervals, we have to prolong them, as we prolong breath retention, so that there is no room for generation or restraint of thoughts.

(Lord Kṛṣṇa says in the *Gītā* that 'What is night for other beings, is day for an awakened yogi and what is night for a yogi is day for others' (II.69). This sūtra conveys the same idea. When generating thoughts and their restraint keep the seeker awake, it is day for him, but night for the seer. When the seer is awake in the prolonged spaces between rising and restraining thought, it is day for him, but night for the seeker. To understand this more clearly, think of the body as a lake. The mind floats on its surface, but the seer is hidden at the bottom. This is darkness for the seer. Yoga practice causes the mind to sink and the seer to float. This is day for the seer.)

Just as one feels refreshed after a sound sleep, the seer's consciousness is refreshed as he utilizes this prolonged pause for rejuvenation and recuperation. But at first, it is difficult to educate the consciousness to restrain each rising thought. It is against the thought current (*pratipakṣa*) and hence creates restlessness, whereas the movement from restraint towards rising thought is with the current (*pakṣa*) and brings restfulness. The first method requires force of will and so is tinged with *rajas*. The second is slightly *sāttvic*, but tinged with *tamas*. To transform the consciousness into a pure *sāttvic* state of dynamic silence, we must learn by repeated effort to prolong the intermissions (see I.14). If no impressions are allowed to intervene, the consciousness will remain fresh, and rest in its own abode. This is *ekāgratā pariṇāma*.

Some commentators equate *nirodha pariṇāma* with *asaṁprajñāta samādhi* (or *manolaya*) on the grounds that it implies the suppression of the 'I' consciousness. They maintain that it should come last and that the order of the sūtras should therefore be reversed giving the sequence III.12, III.11 and finally, III.9. They thus place *ekāgratā pariṇāma* first, relating it to the one-pointed focusing of the mind in *dhāraṇā*. There is a similarity since the surface meaning of *ekāgratā* does refer to one-pointed focusing on an object, but its deeper meaning is 'one without a second'. There is the soul and nothing but the soul. When we recognize this profound meaning then the reason for Patañjali's order is clear. Patañjali's discussion of *dharma*, *lakṣaṇa* and *avasthā pariṇāmas* (III.13) further clarifies this point.

Consciousness has three *dhārmic* characteristics; to wander, to be restrained and to remain silent. The silent state must be transformed into a dynamic but single state of awareness. Patañjali warns that in restraint old impressions may re-emerge: the *sādhaka* must train to react instantly to such appearances and cut them off at their source. Each act of restraint re-establishes a state of restfulness. This is *dharma pariṇāma*. When a serene flow of tranquillity is maintained without interruption then *samādhi pariṇāma* and *lakṣaṇa pariṇāma* begin. During this phase the *sādhaka* may become trapped in a spiritual desert (see I.18). At this point he must persevere to reach oneness with the soul and abide in that state (*avasthā pariṇāma*) everlastingly. This final goal is reached through *ekāgratā pariṇāma*. (See I.20.)

Table 12: *The order of transformations of* citta *and* prakṛti

Citta Transformations	*Prakṛti* Transformations
1 *Nirodha Pariṇāma* (Restraining transformation)	1 *Dharma Pariṇāma* (Transformation to exalted state)
2 *Samādhi Pariṇāma* (Transformation to *samādhi*)	2 *Lakṣaṇa Pariṇāma* (Transformation to awareness of perfection)
3 *Ekāgratā Pariṇāma* (Transformation from one-pointed to no-pointed attention)	3 *Avasthā Pariṇāma* (Maintenance of perfected state)

तस्य प्रशान्तवाहिता संस्कारात् ।१०।

III.10 tasya praśāntavāhitā saṁskārāt

tasya	its (*nirodha pariṇāma*)
praśānta	tranquillity, a peaceful state
vāhitā	flow
saṁskārāt	faculty of impressions, polished, refined

The restraint of rising impressions brings about an undisturbed flow of tranquillity.

By maintaining perfect awareness in the intervals between rising and restraining impressions, steadiness becomes effortless and natural. Then the stream of tranquillity flows without any ripples in the consciousness (III.9).

By skilful repeated efforts, consciousness is transformed, cultured, refined and polished. It develops freedom from all forms of fluctuations so that undisturbed peace may flow. As each drop of water helps to form a lake, so one must continue to prolong each tranquil pause between rising and restraining impressions. An adept of *abhyāsa* and *vairāgya* keeps himself steady, so that calmness can flow uninterruptedly. Thus he is freed from all previous impressions of consciousness.

The words used earlier by Patañjali for the state of tranquillity are *citta prasādanam*, *adhyātma prasādanam*, *svarasa vāhinī* and *ananta samāpattiḥ*. When disturbed consciousness is brought to an undisturbed state, it is *citta prasādanam* (favourable disposition of *citta*). When sorrows are conquered, it is *svarasa vāhinī* (flow of the soul's fragrance). When exertion in search of the soul ceases, it is *ananta samāpattiḥ* (assuming the original and eternal form). Proficiency in meditation is *adhyātma prasādanam* (manifestation of the light of the soul). All convey the same meaning – that the seeker and the sought are one; that the seeker is the seer.

(See I.12, 33, 47; II.9, 47. IV.29, 32.)

सर्वार्थतैकाग्रतयोः क्षयोदयौ चित्तस्य समाधिपरिणामः ।११।

III.11 sarvārthatā ekāgratayoḥ kṣaya udayau cittasya samādhipariṇāmaḥ

sarvārthatā	all-pointedness, many-pointedness
ekāgratayoḥ	one-pointedness
kṣaya	decay
udayau	the rise
cittasya	of the consciousness
samādhi	spiritual absorption
pariṇāmaḥ	transformation

The weakening of scattered attention and the rise of one-pointed attention in the citta *is the transformation towards* samādhi.

Consciousness oscillates between multi-faceted and one-pointed attention. When one-pointed attention is established, multi-faceted attention disappears; when one-pointed attention fades, consciousness is scattered. Observing these alternations and learning to hold steadfastly to singlepointed attention is the second phase of the transformation: *samādhi pariṇāma*.

Citta has two properties, dispersiveness (*sarvārthatā citta*) and one-pointedness (*ekāgratā citta*), with which it can direct its attention externally or internally. It can fuse these two powers into one, to move towards spiritual absorption.

Citta takes the form of any object seen, observed or thought of. It can spread itself as much as it desires. When it spreads, it is multi-faceted; when it remains steadily focused, it is one-pointed. When it is scattered, distraction and restlessness set in. This restlessness can be subdued, but nothing which exists can be destroyed; it can only be transformed: made to disappear or fade by thoughtful attention, enabling the stream of conscious restfulness to flow steadily. In this way, consciousness is influenced by its own action. It forms the habit of absorption in a single thought, which prepares one for spiritual absorption. This type of attention, *samādhi pariṇāma*, stabilizes the state of restfulness.

In *nirodha pariṇāma*, the emergence of thought-waves is restrained and stilled. In *samādhi pariṇāma*, the intervals between the emergence and the restraint of thoughts and vice versa are studied. From this study emerges a stillness which leads to silence. One should know that stillness is rigidity and silence is passive and meditative. In the state of silence, the fragrance of the soul emerges as the centre of attention. This is *ekāgratā pariṇāma*, which is dealt with in the next sūtra.

(See I.2, 5, 32, 43, 50.)

ततः पुनः शान्तोदितौ तुल्यप्रत्ययौ चित्तस्यैकाग्रतापरिणामः ।१२।

III.12 tataḥ punaḥśānta uditau tulya pratyayau cittasya ekāgratāpariṇāmaḥ

tataḥ	then
punaḥ	again
śānta	subsiding state, quiescent state
uditau	rising state
tulya	similar
pratyayau	cognitions, means of action, cause
cittasya	of consciousness (mind)
ekāgratā	(*eka* = singular, one, alone, unique, pre-eminent; *agra* = first, a resting place, base, prominent, excellent, best, chief and summit; *ekāgra* = turned towards one point, intent upon one object: here, *ekāgra* means the indivisible (*abhedya*) soul and the foundation of life) one-pointedness
pariṇāmaḥ	transformation

When rising and falling thought processes are in balance, one-pointed consciousness emerges. Maintenance of awareness with keen intensity from one-pointed attention to no-pointed attentiveness is ekāgratā pariṇāma.

Even in this focus on the property of *citta* alone, the sensitivity of attention may be intense or light. To maintain a steady, uninterrupted flow and intensity of attention in *citta* is the third phase of transformation.

At times, consciousness is thoughtfully silent but then it suddenly gushes out into vibrant activity. In a split second, this activity may be controlled and balance regained. This control requires effort, and effort involves time. By skilful practice, the depth of silence which at first appears only in glimpses, is made to permeate and fill the entire *citta*. Then the feeling of time disappears. Past and future are reabsorbed into the timeless.

Mind and time are interdependent. As the moments of the mind come to an end, so does time. *Citta* and the seer (*ātman*) are the two sharp edges of a blade. In one-pointed attention (*ekāgratā saṁskāra*) the energies of the seeker and the seer become one. The seeker does, the seer is. To do plus to be equals to become: a dynamic quality of becoming ensues which has neither subject nor object. The focal point is now on the seer, for the seer, by the seer. This is *ekāgratā pariṇāma*.

When the state of restraint is reached (*nirodha saṁskāra*), glimpses of silence are prolonged and fill the consciousness (*samādhi saṁskāra*). Then the third phase of *ekāgratā saṁskāra* should be practised. Here, the consciousness which was dependent on external objects moves inwards to impregnate the seedless seat of the soul.

In III.9–12 Patañjali explains the three levels of transformation of consciousness in sequential order: *nirodha*, *samādhi* and finally *ekāgratā*. *Ekāgratā*, as explained earlier, has two meanings. One is concentration on a given object: at this external level, it has the same meaning as *dhāranā*. The other is 'one without a second': that is, the soul. This level of transformation of consciousness is the highest. I feel, therefore, that Patañjali's meaning is this: *ekāgratā pariṇāma* is the final phase of the transformation in which consciousness is uplifted to the level of the soul, and is one with it.

(See I.47, 51; II.19–20.)

एतेन भूतेन्द्रियेषु धर्मलक्षणावस्थापरिणामा व्याख्याताः ।१३।

III.13 etena bhūtendriyeṣu dharma lakṣaṇa avasthā pariṇāmāḥ vyākhyātāḥ

etena	by this
bhūtendriyeṣu	the elements, body and sense organs
dharma	propriety, law, duty, right, virtue, religion
lakṣaṇa	character, mark, sign, quality, description
avasthā	condition, state, position
pariṇāmāh	change, effect, transformation
vyākhyātāḥ	visible, described, unfolded, enumerated

Through these three phases, cultured consciousness is transformed from its potential state (dharma) *towards further refinement* (lakṣaṇa) *and the zenith of refinement* (avasthā). *In this way, the transformation of elements, senses and mind takes place.*

The three stages of transformation described in III.9–12 affect the entire being: organs, senses, body and mind, and bring about a stable, steady state of consciousness.

Both *puruṣa* and *prakṛti* are eternal. *Puruṣa* remains eternally changeless. *Prakṛti* goes on eternally changing due to the interaction between its own *guṇas* of *sattva*, *rajas* and *tamas*.

Earth, water, fire, air and ether; their counterparts smell, taste, sight, touch and sound; the senses of perception and organs of action; mind, intelligence, consciousness and ego are all parts of nature. Ego, consciousness and intelligence are sensitive and subtle. They accumulate experiences of objects perceived through the senses of perception, organs of action and mind. These experiences vary according to their relation to circumstances. In this way, consciousness is limited by the qualities of nature. It is also linked with time as it oscillates with thoughts of past, present and future.

By disciplined study and effort, experiences are observed to move qualitatively towards the best.

Through study one realizes that consciousness has four tendencies or attributes. The first, when *avidyā* is predominant, is its wandering nature, *vyutthāna saṁskāra*. The dawning power of discrimination leads to the second tendency: restraint, *nirodha saṁskāra*, *dharma pariṇāma*. The effect of restraint is the flow of tranquillity (*praśānta vāhita saṁskāra*), experienced between *vyutthāna* and *nirodha saṁskāras*. This is the third tendency: *lakṣaṇa pariṇāma*. The effort to prolong this silent intermission brings the *sādhaka* to the zenith of emancipation (*avasthā pariṇāma*), the fourth or final attribute of consciousness.

When consciousness loses all these tendencies and becomes pensive, it rests in the seer. This affects the behavioural patterns in the body, senses and mind, which also remain peaceful. Consciousness becomes pensive. This wholly peaceful state is *ekāgratā pariṇāma*. By thoughtful action, consciousness traces the source of its attributes, moves towards it, and is dissolved therein. At that moment, body, senses and mind are devoid of evolution and dissolution, of birth and death. This is *viveka khyāti* (II.26). The *sādhaka* transforms himself to an exalted state (*dharma pariṇāma*), develops awareness of perfection (*lakṣaṇa pariṇāma*) and maintains himself without losing the acquired perfection (*avasthā pariṇāma*).

The two analogies that follow will help to explain the concepts of property (*dharma*), changes (*lakṣaṇa*) and condition (*avasthā*).

The dust of clay is formed into a lump, to make a pot. The dust of the clay is its property (*dharma*), the lump is the modification (*lakṣaṇa*) and the pot is the final condition (*avasthā*). If the potter wants to change the pot's pattern, he breaks it down to its original state for re-shaping it. It is the same with a gold ring. To remake it, the goldsmith has to melt it down to its original state.

A man may be a son, brother, nephew, brother-in-law, son-in-law, father, uncle, father-in-law, or grandfather, but he is still the same man. The man is the *dharma*, the original substance; his different relationships with others the *lakṣaṇa*; and his culminating state the *avasthā*.

Dharma pariṇāma is the knowledge of *prakṛti* and *puruṣa*; *lakṣaṇa pariṇāma* is the way one makes use of them; and *avasthā pariṇāma* is steadily maintaining them, once they have been cleansed of trial and error, in the established state. In this way the elements, organs of action, senses of perception and mind are transformed: *puruṣa* is recognized and understood. All these transformations are stabilized, and the changing states in body, mind and ego come to an end, enabling the *sādhaka* to rest in the eternal changeless *puruṣa*. The search terminates and the duality between the seeker and the sought ends as the seer realizes that he alone was the seeker, seeking his own form, *svarūpa*. From now on, he drinks the nectar of his own self-generating pure fragrance.

These three phases of conscious transformation culminate in tranquillity. Awareness flows peacefully, and virtue arises as *dharma pariṇāma*. This is the true character of intelligence and consciousness. Now, the *sādhaka* is highly cultured and civilized. This is *lakṣaṇa pariṇāma*. Maintaining this qualitative state of conscious progression towards the zenith is *avasthā pariṇāma* (see I.3; II.15, 18, 19, 20; III.5, 45 and 48.)

शान्तोदिताव्यपदेश्यधर्मानुपाती धर्मी ।१४।

III.14 śānta udita avyapadeśya dharma anupātī dharmī

śānta	appeased, allayed, calmed, quietened, pacified
udita	rise, ascended, manifested
avyapadeśya	not defined, latent, lying in potential form
dharma	propriety, usage, law, duty, religion, virtue
anupātī	closely followed, common to
dharmī	virtuous, just, religious, characterized

The substrata is that which continues to exist and maintain its characteristic quality in all states, whether manifest, latent, or subdued.

Table 13: *The four planes of consciousness*

1 Unconscious plane	1 *Śānti citta* (calm)	1 Profound sleep state	1 *Nidrāvasthā* or *Suṣuptyāvasthā*
2 Subconscious plane	2 *Kṣaya citta* (sleeping)	2 Dream-filled state	2 *Svapnāvasthā*
3 Conscious plane	3 *Udaya citta* (rising)	3 Waking state	3 *Jāgratāvasthā*
4 Superconscious plane	4 Transcendence of 1, 2, and 3	4 *Kaivalya*, or eternal emancipation	4 *Turyāvasthā*

The inherent characteristic quality of nature (*mūla-prakṛti*) has three properties: pacified or calmed (*śānta*), manifested (*udita*) or latent (*avyapadeśya*). They appear indistinctly or clearly according to one's intellectual development.

The substratum of nature remains the same for all time, though transformations take place. The moulding of consciousness takes place owing to the changes in the *guṇas* of nature.

In III.9 Patañjali explains the three phases of consciousness as rising, being restrained and the pauses between the two. In III.10, he describes these pauses as tranquil consciousness. If these pauses are prolonged, all pointedness and one-pointedness meet, and there is no room for rising or subsiding of thoughts (III.11). Sūtra III.12 explains that maintaining these quiet moments brings about a balanced state of consciousness, which is described in III.13 as a cultured and harmonious state. Rising and restraining thoughts are the tendencies (*dharma*) of the *citta*, and the tranquil state is its characteristic quality (*dharmī*).

The rising *citta* is felt in the sensory body. Citta then appears at the external level as *bahiraṅga citta*. Watching the movement of rising thoughts is an external or *bahiraṅga sādhana*. The delicate restraint of rising thoughts moves *citta* inwards from the peripheral body: this is inner or *antaraṅga sādhana*. Stabilizing the tranquillity that takes place in the intervals is innermost or *antarātmā sādhana*: that state is considered to be an auspicious moment of consciousness. It is like re-discovering the dust which existed before the pot.

From III.9 to III.14, we learned that consciousness has three phases, external, internal and innermost. As we trace and retrace these, we see their relevance to our practices of *āsana*, *prāṇāyāma* and meditation, in which consciousness moves from the skin inwards, and each cell and fibre is infused with the tranquillity of the seer.

Today, everyone is aware of constant 'stress and strain' in life. These aspects of consciousness which complicate life are by no means new to mankind. Patañjali's word *vyutthāna*, used to designate the 'emergence of rising thought', is equivalent to the appearance of 'stress'. *Nirodha*, 'restraint of rising thought' is equivalent to the 'strain' of trying to control that stress. Striking the balance between the two is called 'relaxation' (*śānti citta*). Restraining of rising thought is against the current (*pratipakṣa*). Hence restraint is strain.

A person who has undergone childhood is *śānta*, because that childhood stage has passed and is over. As one stands at the threshold of youth, he is in the present or *udita* state. In course of time, one moves towards old age, which has yet to come: this is *avyapadeśya*, old age which is still in an unmanifested form and indistinct. But the person remains the same through all these changes. That unchanging person is *dharmī*. Similarly, milk is the property which separates into curds and whey, or changes into butter. It is the same with dust, which is formed into clay to make a jar. The dust stands for the past, the clay for the present, the jar for the future. Thus all changes from the source move in time as past, present and future.

In II.18, the properties of nature are explained as luminosity (*prākāśa*), vibrancy (*kriyā*) and inertia (*sthithi*). By the use of these qualities, one may be enmeshed in a mixture of pleasure and pain, or go beyond them to unalloyed bliss.

The properties of nature exist for the purpose of one's evolution and involution. Consciousness, being a part of nature, is bound by the spokes of the wheel of time.

If an aspirant sows the right seed through knowledge and discrimination (*viveka*) and develops consciousness, he reaps the fruit of self-realization through *ekāgratā*. He becomes the force which distinguishes between the hidden properties and the transformations of nature. He recognizes his true, pure state of existence which is changeless and virtuous. This is the fruit earned through the judicious effort of *sādhana*.

The import of this sūtra can be used to practical advantage while practising *āsana*, *prāṇāyāma* or meditation. If we observe the various scattered dust cells lying latent in the body, and charge them so that they cohere (lump of clay), we can feel the inner unity and transform body, breath and consciousness into designs in the form of different *āsanas* and *prāṇāyāmas*, as the potter forms his clay into a variety of shapes.

In *āsana*, if the energy of the body is harmonized to a 'point zero' whilst in a state of tension, we reach precision. The same can be applied to the intake of breath, its distribution or discharge in *prāṇāyāma*, and in meditation. The combining of single-pointed attention with all-pointed attention at the core of one's being is the essence of this sūtra.

'Point zero' indicates the point of balance and harmony at which we can unlock and liberate the knotty confusion of matter and emotion. It also conveys the importance of finding the exact centre of the meeting points of vertical extension and horizontal expansion in body, breath and consciousness.

क्रमान्यत्वं परिणामान्यत्वे हेतुः ।१५।

III.15 krama anyatvaṁ pariṇāma anyatve hetuḥ

krama	going, proceeding, advancing, regular course, method, order of sequence, succession
anyatvaṁ	different, distinct
pariṇāma	change, transformation, effect
anyatve	different, distinct, variant
hetuḥ	cause, reason

Successive sequential changes cause the distinctive changes in the consciousness.

Differences in changes in consciousness are caused by the changing order of sequence in the method of practice.

According to the sequence of practice, distinct transformations take place.

Krama means regular sequence. Let us return to our earthenware pot, and look at the clay dust as the first principle of evolution, which has a property (*dharma*), the lump of malleable clay which embodies the qualitative mark (*lakṣaṇa*), and the jar which culminates the process and which represents the evolved state (*avasthā*). Only by following a certain sequence of actions can we turn earth into pottery. This is harmonious and organic growth.

In yoga practice a regular sequence must also be followed. The *sādhaka* first acquires restraint in consciousness (*nirodha pariṇāma*) in order to experience tranquillity (*samādhi pariṇāma*). Then he proceeds towards the 'one without a second', the seer (*ekāgratā pariṇāma*). Only then does he become a fulfilled yogi (*kṛtārthan*) (see I.18, 19, and IV.32).

Although consciousness may be considered partly to exist outside time, the work needed to transform that consciousness definitely exists inside the framework of time. It may well be that there is an evolutionary 'tilt' to the cosmos by which all things tend to evolve for the better in the long run. But we cannot count on that, and so some individual effort is necessary, especially as the world itself, the only known theatre of action for this evolutionary drama, is now in danger from man's excesses of pollution, greed and war. Such was not the case in Patañjali's day, yet he saw fit to furnish us with an exact evolutionary map so that our advance might be orderly and expeditious.

There is a logic to the involutionary spiritual journey, just as there is in the growth of a plant from seed, to stem, to bud, to flower, to fruit. The original, pure consciousness which we trace through Patañjali's method is the seed of transformation in oneself. Our own self is the maker of our own spiritual destiny.

The importance of structure and sequence can be shown in the example of language-learning.

If we set out to learn a language without structured tuition, we may learn it or we may not. It is a 'hit or miss' process. But if we seek to learn in a structured way, there is a definite order of procedure. We start with the present tense of the verbs 'to be' and 'to have' and certain basic nouns and prepositions. To start with complex grammatical forms would be ludicrous and self-defeating. The structure of evolution and progress in all things has its own inner logic and harmony. This is sequence, or *krama*.

परिणामत्रयसंयमादतीतानागतज्ञानम् ।१६।

III.16 pariṇāmatraya saṁyamāt atīta anāgatajñānam

pariṇāma	change, transformation, effect
traya	threefold
saṁyamāt	integration, control
atīta	past
anāgata	future
jñānam	knowledge

By mastery of the three transformations of nature (dharma), *quality* (lakṣaṇa) *and condition* (avasthā), *through* saṁyama *on the* nirodha, samādhi, *and* ekāgratā *states of consciousness, the yogi acquires knowledge of the past and the future.*

Now Patañjali explains the properties of yoga, commonly known as supernatural powers, which accrue by transformations of consciousness.

In III.14, the words *śānta* (appeasement), *udita* (generation) and *avyapadeśya* (non-manifestation) were used for the past, present and future. III.15 speaks of the order of sequence from the source (*dharmī*), involving time and effort for transformation. By following this order, the *sādhaka* observes the natural flow of the present moving into the past, to manifest later as the future, and thereby gains mastery over time.

In this sūtra, Patañjali begins to identify the accomplishments which come to the aspirant who has advanced in yogic discipline. The first is the awareness of time. The yogi's consciousness has crossed the frontier of time: he sees time as ever flowing. Hence he has knowledge of past and future. (Present time is deliberately not mentioned, because its presence is felt.) He perceives the orderly sequence of the present slipping into the past, and rolling towards the future; he knows time, its meaning and its impact.

The so-called supernatural powers, discussed from III.16 to III.50, are evidence that the *sādhaka*'s yoga practices are correct. He is advised to intensify them with sustained faith and enthusiasm and to be indifferent to his achievements, so as to avoid deteriorating into affliction, fluctuation and self-gratification.

(see IV.1 and 28.)

शब्दार्थप्रत्ययानामितरेतराध्यासात् संकरस्तत्प्रविभागसंयमात्
सर्वभूतरुतज्ञानम् ।१७।

III.17 śabda artha pratyayānām itaretarādhyāsāt saṅkaraḥ tatpravibhāga saṁyamāt sarvabhūta rutajñānam

śabda	word, sound
artha	object, purpose, meaning
pratyayānām	feelings, emotions, ideas, contents
itaretara	one for the other
adhyāsāt	superimposing, coinciding
saṅkaraḥ	mixing together, intermixture, becoming one
tat	their
pravibhāga	distinction, differentiation, resolution
saṁyamāt	restraint, check, control, subdue, govern
sarva	all
bhūta	living beings
ruta	sounds, speech
jñānam	knowledge

Words, objects and ideas are superimposed, creating confusion; by saṁyama, *one gains knowledge of the language of all beings.*

Conventional usage of a word, its fundamental meaning, content and feeling may all coincide, or may be confused due to intermixture or superimposition. The same word may convey altogether different meanings in another language. A perfect yogi acquires accurate knowledge of the meaning and feeling of any sound or word, in any language produced by any being.

For example, Jesus's disciples are said to have received the gift of speaking in all languages.

We do not ordinarily differentiate between a word, its original purpose and meaning, and its contemporary usage; they are considered by those of average intellect to coincide. A cultured intellect, however, may penetrate deeply to understand just what is conveyed by the sound, meaning and sense of a word. An accomplished yogi intuitively perceives and precisely distinguishes the meaning and feeling of each word or sound uttered by any living being, according to how they express themselves.

संस्कारसाक्षात्करणात् पूर्वजातिज्ञानम् ।१८।

III.18 saṁskāra sākṣātkaraṇāt pūrvajātijñānam

saṁskāra	subliminal impressions, instinct, realization of past perception
sākṣātkaraṇāt	to see in reality, by direct observation, by direct perception, by bringing to the surface of consciousness
pūrva	earlier, previous
jāti	descent, status in life, lineage, condition, rank, birth
jñānam	knowledge

Through direct perception of his subliminal impressions, the yogi gains knowledge of his previous lives.

The yogi is able to recollect the impressions of past incarnations which have moulded his present life. In the continuity of life, instinct, memory and desire play important roles. Memory belongs to the subconscious mind, and the fruits of desires (pains and pleasures experienced in the present life as a result of good and bad actions in past lives) to the unconscious.

When a yogi is free from all instincts and desires, he sees directly, independent of memory, and of feelings of joy or sorrow. Through intuition, in the orderly sequence of time, he *actually sees* his past lineage and future status, and also the lives of others.

(See II.12, 13, 39, and IV.33.)

प्रत्ययस्य परचित्तज्ञानम् ।१९।

III.19 pratyayasya paracittajñānam

pratyayasya	conception, idea, perception
para	of others, another's
citta	mind, consciousness
jñānam	knowledge

He acquires the ability to understand the minds of others.

Through his purity of consciousness, the yogi realizes directly the nature of his own mind and consciousness, and also that of others.

The word *sākṣātkaraṇāt*, used in III.18, means seeing reality. The word *pratyaya* means perceiving the content of the mind. Both convey the same meaning. By mastery over his own mind and consciousness, the yogi develops clairvoyance and can read the minds of others.

न च तत्सालम्बनं तस्याविषयीभूतत्वात् ।२०।

III.20 na ca tat sālambanaṁ tasya aviṣayī bhūtatvāt

na	not
ca	and
tat	that (knowledge)
sālambanaṁ	support, use
tasya	that

aviṣayī	unperceived, beyond the reach of mind, not within the reach of
bhūtatvāt	in life

A yogi who is able to read the minds of others in general, can also, if necessary, precisely identify specific contents which are beyond the reach of the mind.

This sūtra is sometimes omitted on the grounds that it is a later addition, the argument being that if, as the previous sūtra says, the yogi is able to read minds in general then the contents of particular minds must be equally transparent. Some combine sūtras 19 and 20 or omit sūtra 20, interpreting it to mean that the yogi's concentration is only on the idea in another's mind and not on its supporting object. It is really immaterial. A true yogi, though he possesses the general and specific gifts of mental insight, is unlikely to waste his time looking into other people's minds and risk losing the grace of yoga, except when he needs an exact knowledge of another's motives to know how best to act towards that person. The *sādhaka* prefers to incline his attention towards those who are free of desire: his master's mind, for example, so that his consciousness, by sympathetic attraction, may take on a more graceful disposition.

To gauge the mind of an individual requires more sensitivity than to sense the contents of mass consciousness. Successful politicians are said to be adept at the latter, but the former may be compared to a gallery visitor looking at an abstract painting, who attributes to the artist his own feelings as he tries to interpret it. A yogi would be able to penetrate the artist's state of mind, and his exact thoughts and feelings while at work on the canvas.

कायरूपसंयमात् तद्ग्राह्यशक्तिस्तम्भे चक्षुष्प्रकाशासंप्रयोगेऽन्तर्धानम् ।२१।

III.21 kāya rūpa saṁyamāt tadgrāhyaśakti stambhe cakṣuḥ prakāśa asaṁprayoge antardhānam

kāya	body
rūpa	form
saṁyamāt	constraint, control
tad	from that form
grāhya	to be seized, taken, received, perceivable

śakti	power, capacity, emanation
stambhe	suspension
cakṣuḥ	eye
prakāśa	light
asaṁprayoge	there being no contact
antardhānam	disappearance, invisibility

By control over the subtle body, the yogi can suspend at will the rays of light emanating from himself so that he becomes invisible to onlookers. He may again make himself visible by bringing back the power of perceptibility.

एतेन शब्दाद्यन्तर्धानमुक्तम् ।२२।

III.22 etena śabdādi antardhānam uktam

etena	by this
śabdādi	sound and others
antardhānam	disappearance
uktam	said, described

In the same way as described above, he is able to arrest sound, smell, taste, form and touch.

Some texts omit this sūtra, on the grounds that if a yogi can manipulate appearance and disappearance of form, his ability to manipulate the other senses can be inferred.

सोपक्रमं निरुपक्रमं च कर्म तत्संयमादपरान्तज्ञानमरिष्टेभ्यो वा ।२३।

III.23 sopakramaṁ nirupakramaṁ ca karma tatsaṁyamāt aparāntajñānam ariṣṭebhyaḥ vā

sopakramaṁ	immediate effect, intensively operative, active
nirupakramaṁ	slow in fruition, non-operative, dormant
ca	and, or
karma	action
tat	those, these, them
saṁyamāt	by restraint, control, mastery
aparānta	death
jñānam	knowledge
ariṣṭebhyaḥ	by portents, omens
vā	or

The effects of action are immediate or delayed. By saṁyama *on his actions, a yogi will gain foreknowledge of their final fruits. He will know the exact time of his death by omens.*

The fruits of action (*karmaphala*) are linked to time (*kāla phala*). If a piece of wet cloth is fully spread out, it dries quickly; if folded or rolled up it takes a long time to dry. Similarly, the fruits of action may be felt immediately or at a later time.

Omens or premonitions of death are of three types. They may strike one directly by intuition, by elemental disturbances, and through the voice of the divine. For example, if one no longer hears the vibrations of the body, or cannot see a finger held before the eyes, it is an omen of approaching death.

Those who know something of Indian philosophy will probably be aware of *sañcita karma*, *prārabdha karma* and *kriyamāṇa karma*, the three types of actions which bear fruit. The first is the merit or demerit accumulated from former lives. The second refers specifically to the good or bad actions which have formed our present life. The third we generate by our actions in this life. The effects of *kriyamāṇa karma* are to come later: we can therefore assume that Patañjali has included *kriyamāṇa karma* and *sañcita karma* in the category of *nirupakrama*, and *prārabdha karma* in *sopakrama*.

(See II.12, 14; III.15, 18; IV.7.)

मैत्र्यादिषु बलानि ।२४।

III.24 maitryādiṣu balāni

maitrī	friendliness
ādiṣu	so forth
balāni	strength, power (moral and emotional)

He gains moral and emotional strength by perfecting friendliness and other virtues towards one and all.

The yogi who perfects friendliness, compassion and benevolence, and who regards things impartially without becoming involved, keeps his consciousness free of desire, anger, greed, lust, pride and envy. With his mind cleansed of such weaknesses, an amiability evolves which spreads happiness to all. His equipoise of mind creates a graceful disposition of heart.

(See I.33.)

बलेषु हस्तिबलादीनि ।२५।

III.25 baleṣu hasti balādīni

baleṣu	by *saṁyama* on strength
hasti	elephant
bala	strength (physical and intellectual)
ādīni	the others

By saṁyama *on strength, the yogi will develop the physical strength, grace, and endurance of an elephant.*

By *saṁyama* (integration), the yogi may acquire the strength and grace of an elephant, or if he wishes, develop his powers so as to become the strongest of the strong, the most graceful of the graceful, the swiftest of the swift.

प्रवृत्त्यालोकन्यासात् सूक्ष्मव्यवहितविप्रकृष्टज्ञानम् ।२६।

III.26 pravṛtti āloka nyāsāt sūkṣma vyavahita viprakṛṣṭajñānam

pravṛttyaḥ	the super-sensory activity, super-sense perception
āloka	light
nyāsāt	directing, projecting, extending
sūkṣma	small, fine, subtle
vyavahita	hidden, veiled, concealed
viprakṛṣṭa	remote, distant
jñānam	knowledge

Concealed things, near or far, are revealed to a yogi.

By integration of the inner light, that is, the insight of the soul, a yogi develops super-sensitive powers of perception. Such insight brings the power of seeing things which are subtle and fine, concealed or at a distance.

(See III.34.)

भुवनज्ञानं सूर्ये संयमात् ।२७।

III.27 bhuvanajñānaṁ sūrye saṁyamāt

bhuvanajñānaṁ	knowledge of the worlds
sūrye	on the sun
saṁyamāt	by constraint, by integration

By saṁyama *on the sun the yogi will have knowledge of the seven worlds, and of the seven cosmic centres in the body.*

As the sun illumines the world with its rays, so the light of the soul reaches the *sahasrāra*, the thousand-petalled *cakra*, also known as *brahmakapāla*. The yogi knows the functions of both the outer and the inner worlds.

According to Indian philosophy, there are fourteen worlds or divisions of the universe: seven above and seven below. Those above are called the aerial region. They are *bhūloka*, *bhuvarloka*, *suvarloka*, *mahāloka*, *janoloka*, *tapoloka* and *satyaloka*. Those below are the nether region. They are *atala*, *vitala*, *sutala*, *rasātala*, *talātala*, *mahātala* and *pātala*. All these worlds are interdependent and interconnected.

As the microcosm represents the macrocosm, man's body epitomizes the entire structure of the great universe. The fourteen worlds are represented in the various regions of the body from the crown of the head to the soles of the feet. Taking the bottom portion of the torso as the central point, the aerial regions are situated above, and the nether regions below it. The several aerial regions correspond as follows: pelvic region to *bhūloka*, navel to *bhuvarloka*, diaphragmatic to *suvarloka*, heart to *mahāloka*, neck to *janoloka*, eyebrow centre to *tapoloka* and crown of the head to *satyaloka*. The seven nether worlds are represented as follows: hips to *atala*, thighs to *vitala*, knees to *sutala*, calves to *rasātala*, ankles to *talātala*, metatarsals to *mahātala* and soles of the feet to *pātala*.

According to yogis, within the aerial regions are the seven major *cakras*. They are *mūlādhāra* (seat of the anus), *svādhiṣṭāna* (sacral area), *maṇipūraka* (navel), *anāhata* (heart), *viśuddhi* (throat), *ājñā* (eyebrow centre) and *sahasrāra* (crown of the head). There are other *cakras*, such as *sūrya* (corresponding to the sympathetic nervous system), *candra* (parasympathetic nervous system) and *manas* (seat of the mind). All these are interconnected, like the solar system. The light that shines from the seat of the soul is the sun of life. It passes through *sūrya nāḍī* at the gates of *sūrya cakra* and illumines the seven states of awareness in the yogi's consciousness (II.27).

Patañjali speaks not only of external, but of internal, achievements. He instructs the aspirant to direct his mind towards the inner body, to study and gain knowledge of the soul.

चन्द्रे ताराव्यूहज्ञानम् ।२८।

III.28 candre tārāvyūhajñānam

candre	on moon
tārā	stars
vyūha	galaxy, system, orderly arrangement, disposition
jñānam	knowledge

By saṁyama *on the moon, the yogi will know the position and system of the stars.*

In the last sūtra, the sun, *sūrya*, refers to the core of one's being. The moon, *candra*, refers to the mind and consciousness. The solar plexus is situated in the region of the trunk; the lunar plexus has its seat in the cerebrum. By *saṁyama* on that region, the yogi gains further knowledge.

The brain is equated with the moon which cools the solar system; the lunar plexus maintains a steady, constant temperature in the body even though the seasonal temperature varies. It also controls and directs the parasympathetic system and regulates the functioning of the central nervous system.

The galaxies of stars stand for galaxies of thought-waves which, like stars, twinkle, disappear, reappear and shine forth once again.

ध्रुवे तद्गतिज्ञानम् ।२९।

III.29 dhruve tadgatijñānam

dhruve	fixed, firm, permanent, the Pole Star, era, tip of the nose
tat	from that, of their
gati	movement, course of events, fortune
jñānam	knowledge

By saṁyama *on the Pole Star, the yogi knows the course of destiny.*

By *saṁyama* on the Pole Star (*dhruva nakṣatra*), a yogi knows the movements of stars and their effect on the events of the world. *Dhruva* also stands for the roof (*ājñā cakra*) as well as the tip of the nose (*nāsāgra*). The yogi will know beforehand his own destiny as well as that of others.

King Uttānapāda had two wives, Sunīti and Suruchi. Though Sunīti was the queen, the king was very fond of his second wife Suruchi. Each of them had a son. The elder one was Dhruva and the younger one was Uttama. One day Prince Uttama was playing sitting on his father's lap. Dhruva too came to sit on his father's lap; but Suruchi, the mother of Uttama pulled him away, scolding him that he had to do *tapas* to take birth in her in order to have the privilege. Dhruva went to his own mother, narrated the incident and begged her to permit him to go to the forest to do *tapas* and to gain the kingdom. It so happened that the *saptarṣis*, the seven stars of the constellation Ursa Major, gave him a *mantra* and with that *mantra*, he steadfastly prayed to Lord Viṣṇu to bless him with the kingdom. Lord Viṣṇu was pleased by his steadfast *tapas* at such a youthful age; He granted his wish and named a star after him, Dhruva Nakṣatra, known to all of us as the Pole Star.

नाभिचक्रे कायव्यूहज्ञानम् ॥३०॥

III.30 nābhicakre kāyavyūhajñānam

nābhi	the navel
cakre	mystical centres, 'wheels', energy centres
kāya	the body
vyūha	system, disposition, orderly arrangement
jñānam	knowledge

By saṁyama *on the navel, the yogi acquires perfect knowledge of the disposition of the human body.*

By *saṁyama* on the navel area or *nābhi cakra*, also called *maṇipūraka cakra*, a yogi can gain perfect knowledge of the constitution of the human body. He knows the activities of his each and every cell and therefore becomes a master of his own body.

According to yoga texts, the navel is known as *kandasthāna* (*kanda* = egg or bulb; *sthāna* = region). The root of all the nerves is in the navel. From the navel, 72,000 root nerves (in *haṭha yoga* terminology, *nāḍīs*) branch out. Each root nerve is connected with another 72,000 nerves. These 72,000 multiplied by another 72,000 branch off into various directions, supplying energy to the entire system. The navel is considered to be the pivot of the sympathetic, and the brain of the parasympathetic nervous system.

Let us recall the five *kośas*, or sheaths of the body.

The anatomical sheath consists of seven substances: skin, blood, flesh, sinew, bone, marrow and semen. They function in combination with the three humours: wind (*vāta*), bile (*pitta*) and phlegm (*śleṣma* or *kapha*).

The physiological sheath consists of the circulatory, respiratory, digestive, excretory, endocrine, lymphatic, nervous, and reproductive systems. The psychological sheath is the seat of motivation; the intellectual sheath reasons and judges. The spiritual sheath, body of bliss, is also called the causal body.

Only the yogi can know the fine dividing line between body and mind, mind and soul, and become master of himself.

कण्ठकूपे क्षुत्पिपासानिवृत्तिः ।३१।

III.31 kaṇṭhakūpe kṣutpipāsā nivṛttiḥ

kaṇṭha	throat
kūpe	the pit, the well
kṣut	hunger
pipāsā	thirst
nivṛttiḥ	subdued, conquered

By saṁyama *on the pit of the throat, the yogi overcomes hunger and thirst.*

By *saṁyama* on the pit of the throat (*khecarī mudrā*), a yogi can arrest pangs of hunger and thirst and conquer them.

Kaṇṭha kūpa stands for the *viṣuddhi cakra* of later yoga texts, which is said to be situated in the region of the pit of the throat. (Certain *mudrās*, for example *kāka mudrā* and *khecarī mudrā*, help to overcome hunger and thirst.)

कूर्मनाड्यां स्थैर्यम् ।३२।

III.32 kūrmanāḍyāṁ sthairyam

kūrma	tortoise, name of a nerve
nāḍyāṁ	nerve, a vessel
sthairyam	steadiness, immovability

By saṁyama *on* kūrmanāḍī, *at the pit of the throat, the yogi can make his body and mind firm and immobile like a tortoise.*

By mastery over *kūrma nāḍī*, the yogi not only keeps his physical body immobile like a tortoise, alligator or snake, but also has the power to hibernate mentally by completely immobilizing the functions of the body and intellect. *Kūrma nāḍī* corresponds to the epigastric region.

Kūrma nāḍī is rather hard to locate in the human system. The teachers who knew about the nervous system may have recorded their knowledge, but their teachings have been lost over the centuries. Also, in those days, instructions were imparted orally, and in the communication gap between teacher and pupil the location of such nāḍis may have been forgotten.

The functions of the body are performed by five types of vital energy, *prāṇa vāyus*: *prāṇa*, *apāna*, *samāna*, *udāna* and *vyāna*. *Prāṇa* moves in the thoracic region and controls breathing. *Apāna* moves in the lower abdomen and controls elimination of urine, semen and faeces. *Samāna* stokes the gastric fire, aiding digestion and maintaining the harmonious functioning of the abdominal organs. *Udāna*, working in the throat, controls the vocal chords and the intake of air and food. *Vyāna* pervades the entire body, distributing the energy from the breath and food through the arteries, veins and nerves.

There are also five *upavāyus* known as *upa-prāṇas*. They are *nāga*, *kṛkara*, *devadatta*, *dhanaṁjaya* and *kūrma*. *Nāga* relieves pressures of the abdomen by belching; *kṛkara* prevents substances from passing up the nasal passages and down the throat by making one sneeze or cough. *Devadatta* causes yawning and induces sleep. *Dhanaṁjaya* produces phlegm, nourishes the body, remains in it even after death and sometimes inflates a corpse. *Kūrma* controls the movements of the eyelids and regulates the intensity of light for seeing by controlling the size of the iris. The eyes are the index of the brain. Any movement in the brain is reflected in the eyes. By stilling the eyes, i.e., by the control of *kūrma vāyu*, one can still one's thoughts and make one's brain immobile (see I.18–19).

(For details, see *Light on Prāṇāyāma*.)

In yoga texts one can read of the main *nāḍīs* such as *iḍā*, *piṅgalā*, *suṣumnā*, *citrā*, *gāndhārī*, *hastijihvā*, *pūṣā*, *yaśasvinī*, *ālumbusā*, *kuhū*, *śarasvatī*, *vāruṇī*, *viśodharī*, *payasvinī*, *śaṅkhiṇī*, *śubhā*, *kauśikī*, *śūrā*, *rākā*, *vijñāna*, *kūrma* and many others. The beginning and end of some of the *nāḍis* are described; for others, only the end points are recorded. The functions of some are dealt with, others are not. *Kūrma nāḍī*'s functions are explained but not its source or its terminus. This *nāḍī* may represent the epigastric region, and may directly affect emotional upheavals and their control.

One's mental functions revolve mainly around lust, anger, greed, infatuation, pride and envy, considered the enemies of the soul. They are represented by the four legs, mouth and tail of the tortoise. The tortoise draws its head and limbs into the shell and does not come out, come what may.

By mastery over the *kūrma nāḍī*, the yogi stops the movements of these six spokes of the mind which are influenced by the qualities of *sattva*, *rajas* and *tamas*. He brings these enemies of the soul to a state of steadiness, and through the dominance of *sattva guṇa* transforms them into friends. He remains like a tortoise in his shell, his emotional centre undisturbed, under all circumstances. He has developed emotional stability, the prerequisite of spiritual realization.

मूर्धज्योतिषि सिद्धदर्शनम् ।३३।

III.33 mūrdhajyotiṣi siddhadarśanam

mūrdha	the head
jyotiṣi	on the light
siddha	the perfected beings
darśanam	vision

By performing saṁyama *on the light of the crown of the head* (ājñā cakra), *the yogi has visions of perfected beings.*

Siddhas are those who have perfected themselves in the field of enlightenment. *Mūrdhajyoti* represents the *ājñā cakra* of the yoga texts.

A yogi can develop a balanced head and a poised heart, and from his visions of *siddhas*, yogis and *ācāryas* (great teachers) he may obtain guidance and inspiration to further his *sādhana*.

प्रातिभाद्वा सर्वम् ।३४।

III.34 prātibhāt vā sarvam

prātibhāt	the effulgent light, brilliant conception, intuitive knowledge, faculty of spiritual perception
vā	or
sarvam	all, everything

Through the faculty of spiritual perception the yogi becomes the knower of all knowledge.

A yogi can intuitively perceive anything and everything. By *saṁyama* on the effulgent light, he becomes the knower of all knowledge. All knowledge is mirrored in a yogi.

In short, as day follows the dawn, impulsive nature is transformed into intuitive thought through which the yogi possesses universal knowledge. It is the conquest of nature.

हृदये चित्तसंवित् ।३५।

III.35 hṛdaye cittasaṁvit

hṛdaye on the heart
citta consciousness
saṁvit knowledge, awareness

By saṁyama *on the region of the heart, the yogi acquires a thorough knowledge of the contents and tendencies of consciousness.*

The citadel of *puruṣa* is the heart. It is *anāhata cakra*, the seat of pure knowledge as well as of consciousness. By *saṁyama*, a yogi can become aware of consciousness and of true, pure knowledge. He learns to unfold and tap the source of his being, and identify himself with the Supreme.

सत्त्वपुरुषयोरत्यन्तासंकीर्णयोः प्रत्ययाविशेषो भोगः परार्थत्त्वात् स्वार्थसंयमात् पुरुषज्ञानम् ।३६।

III.36 sattva puruṣayoḥ atyantāsaṁkīrṇayoḥ pratyaya aviśeṣaḥ bhogaḥ parārthatvāt svārthasaṁyamāt puruṣajñānam

sattva	intelligence, one of the three *guṇas*, certain, real, true
puruṣayoḥ	of the soul
atyanta	absolute, extreme
asaṁkīrṇayoḥ	distinct from each other, unmingled
pratyayaḥ	awareness
aviśeṣaḥ	not distinct
bhogaḥ	experience
parārthatvāt	apart from another
svārtha	one's own, self-interest
saṁyamāt	by constraint, control
puruṣajñānam	knowledge of the soul

By saṁyama, *the yogi easily differentiates between the intelligence and the soul which is real and true.*

Since it serves the purposes of the Self and nature, pure intelligence and the seer appear to be one, but they are quite distinct from each other. By *saṁyama* on that which exists for itself, comes knowledge of the soul.

The refined illuminative intelligence (*sattva buddhi*) is free from egoism. It is quite distinct from the light of the soul. *Saṁyama* on one's own self brings to light the difference between intelligence and self and crowns the yogi with the knowledge of the soul. This sūtra, by the use of the word *svārtha* for the seer and *parārtha* for the intelligence, clearly shows the difference between the two. Failure to discriminate between them leads to entanglement in worldly pleasures. Knowing the distinction enables one to enter the gates of the soul.

Though the refined illuminative intelligence is the pinnacle of nature, it is subject to varied experiences. The soul being immutable, its light is constant, steady and unalterable. To the *sādhaka*, the intellect appears to be *puruṣa*. By *saṁyama*, the yogi has to disentangle the knot that binds the intellect and the self, and isolate the refined intelligence. From this comes isolation of the senses, mind and ego, and finally the release of the light of the soul.

We rightly admire such men as Albert Einstein, Rāmānuja, Arnold Toynbee, Śakuntalā Devi and C. G. Jung. Their towering intellects, directed to the service of humanity, inspire us all. Nevertheless, their spirituality was that of the refined illuminative intelligence belonging to human nature, and not that of the luminescent immutable *puruṣa*.

(See I.3; II.18, 20; III.35 and IV.34.)

ततः प्रातिभश्रावणवेदनादर्शास्वादवार्ता जायन्ते ।३७।

III.37 tataḥ prātibha śrāvaṇa vedana ādarśa āsvāda vārtāḥ jāyante

tataḥ	therefrom, thence
prātibha	light, faculty of spiritual perception
śrāvaṇa	faculty of hearing, auditory sense
vedana	faculty of touch
ādarśa	faculty of vision
āsvāda	faculty of taste
vārtāḥ	faculty of smell
jāyante	produced

Through that spiritual perception, the yogi acquires the divine faculties of hearing, touch, vision, taste and smell. He can even generate these divine emanations by his own will.

Through the dawn of the self-luminous light of intuitive understanding, divine perceptions in hearing, feeling, seeing, tasting and smelling, beyond the range of ordinary perceptions, arise of their own accord.

As the mind is the centre of the functions of the senses of perception, it limits their powers of hearing, feeling, seeing, tasting and smelling. When the limitations of the mind are removed, the yogi contacts the very core of his being, and has direct, divine perceptions independent of the sense organs. He is able to hear, feel, see, taste and smell through unlimited space.

(See III.26 and 34.)

ते समाधावुपसर्गा व्युत्थाने सिद्धयः ।३८।

III.38 te samādhau upasargāḥ vyutthāne siddhayaḥ

te	they (divine perceptions)
samādhau	in *samādhi*
upasargāḥ	hindrances, obstacles
vyutthāne	rising up, following one's own inclination, outgoing mind
siddhayaḥ	powers

These attainments are impediments to samādhi, *although they are powers in active life.*

Divine perceptions are hindrances to a yogi whose wisdom is supreme and whose goal is spiritual absorption. They are great accomplishments, but he should know that they fall within the range of the *guṇas* of nature, and in acquiring them he might forget his main aim in life and luxuriate in them. If they are shunned, however, they become aids to *samādhi*.

The yogi may mistake these accomplishments and rewards for the end and aim of yogic practices. He may imagine that he has attained great spiritual heights, and that whatever is attainable through yoga has been achieved. In this way he may forget the goal of Self-Realization.

Patañjali warns yogis to treat these powers as obstacles in their *sādhana*. One should control them as whole-heartedly as one fought earlier to conquer the afflictions of the body and the fluctuations of the mind. Then one can move forwards towards *kaivalya*, emancipation.

बन्धकारणशैथिल्यात् प्रचारसंवेदनाच्च चित्तस्य परशरीरावेशः ।३९।

III.39 bandhakāraṇa śaithilyāt pracāra saṁvedanāt ca cittasya paraśarīrāveśaḥ

bandha	bondage
kāraṇa	cause
śaithilyāt	laxity, relaxation

pracāra	movement, passage, channel, flow
saṁvedanāt	from knowing, from sensitivity
ca	and
cittasya	of the consciousness
para	another's, other's
śarīra	body
āveśaḥ	entrance, occupation

Through relaxation of the causes of bondage, and the free flow of consciousness, the yogi enters another's body at will.

A perfect yogi can enter the body of another individual or, in order to free himself from the bondage of *karmas*, he can leave his own body at will.

The yogi's consciousness can enter the body of another when the cause of bondage (*karmāśaya*) ceases and the knowledge of moving from one body into another is acquired. This is the conquest of the element of earth.

This is *saṁyama* on the causes of bondage: ignorance, egoism, desire, malice and fear of death.

It is said that Śrī Śaṅkarācārya did *parakāya praveṣa* (*para* = other; *kāya* = body, and *praveṣa* = entry), i.e., entered into another's body.

There was a philosopher by the name of Maṇḍana Miśra in Śrī Śaṅkarācārya's time. He was a follower of *pūrva mīmāṁsā*. He was very conscious of his duties and performed the sacred rituals regularly. He was a householder and his wife's name was Bhāratī. She too was a learned lady, who had full knowledge of the sacred texts. People who heard Śrī Śaṅkara's philosophy of monism (*advaita*) maintained that if he could persuade Miśra, a believer in rituals with many followers, to accept his philosophy and become a *sannyāsin* (monk), it would assist Śrī Śaṅkara to establish his teachings. He was also told that he could easily recognize Miśra's house as he would hear parrots chanting the *Vedas* at his doorstep.

Śrī Śaṅkara wandered from place to place in search of Miśra's house. Hearing parrots chanting the *Vedas*, he realized he had arrived at the right place. Miśra was performing rituals for his parents' death anniversary. Śrī Śaṅkara was made to wait till the ritual was over. Then they agreed to hold a debate on the respective merits of *pūrva mīmāṁsā* and *advaita*. The stipulation was that if one of them was defeated in argument, he would embrace the other's philosophy. They chose Śrīmatī Bhāratī, Miśra's wife to be the judge. She said that as she was busy with household affairs, she would garland both and whichever garland withered first, its wearer would be declared the loser. The arguments lasted for days. Slowly Miśra's garland began to fade, and Bhāratī declared that he had lost the debate. He accepted defeat and agreed to become Śrī Śaṅkara's pupil.

Then Bhāratī challenged Śrī Śaṅkara: as the other half of her husband, he must debate with and defeat her, too, before they could become his pupils. She chose the subject and asked Śrī Śaṅkara to debate on the experiences of the life of a householder. Being a monk, he was in a quandary. Though he was baffled at first, he accepted the challenge and asked for time. She consented to wait for a stipulated period. Through his insight he came to know that a king by the name of Amarakā was dying. Śrī Śaṅkara told his pupils to hide his body in a safe place and to guard it until his return. Then, by his power of *saṁyama* on *citrā nāḍī* (see *Light on Prāṇāyāma*), he left his body and entered the dead body of the king. The king was revived and Śrī Śaṅkara in the form of King Amarakā ruled the country. However, Amarakā's queen became suspicious of the king's behaviour as it was not the same as that of her husband. So the queen sent messengers to search for corpses and to bring them to the court at once. Coming to know of the queen's plans, Śrī Śaṅkara feared that the queen might destroy his original body. He at once left the king's body which fell to the ground, and returned to his original body.

Then Śrī Śaṅkara appeared before Bhāratī. She saw through her yogic powers that he now possessed the experiences of a householder, and accepted defeat.

After returning to the South from his triumphant tour of North India, Śrī Śaṅkara built a Śāradā temple at Śṛṅgeri in honour of Bhāratī, the great scholar. It is now one of the famous cloisters known as Śṛṅgeri Śaṅkarācārya maṭha, a place for religious learning according to the teachings of Śrī Śaṅkarācārya.

उदानजयाज्जलपङ्ककण्टकादिष्वसङ्ग उत्क्रान्तिश्च ।४०।

III.40 udānajayāt jala paṅka kaṇṭakādiṣu asaṅgaḥ utkrāntiḥ ca

udāna	one of the five *prāṇas* or vital airs
jayāt	by conquest, mastery
jala	water
paṅka	mud
kaṇṭaka	thorns

ādiṣu	and so forth, and the rest
asaṅgaḥ	non-contact
utkrāntiḥ	ascension, levitation, going up and beyond
ca	and

By mastery of udāna vāyu, *the yogi can walk over water, swamps and thorns without touching them. He can also levitate.*

By *saṁyama* on *udāna vāyu*, the yogi can make his body so light that he is able to walk over water, mud and thorns without coming in contact with them. He can make *prāṇa* ascend through *brahmarandhra* and so die at will.

It is said in III.37 that the yogi has the power of knowing the *tanmātras*, sound, touch, sight, taste and smell, which are the counterparts of the elements, while III.40–43 speak of the conquest of the elements water, fire, air and ether.

Prāṇa is usually translated as 'breath', yet this is only one of its manifestations in the human body. If breathing stops, so does life. Ancient Indian sages knew that all functions of the body were performed by five types of vital energy (*prāṇa vāyus*): *prāṇa*, *apāna*, *samāna*, *udāna* and *vyāna*. They are specific aspects of the one vital cosmic force, the primeval principle of existence in all beings. The functions of the five *prāṇa vāyus* were described in III.32.

In *prāṇāyāma, prāṇa vāyu* is activated by the inbreath and *apāna vāyu* by the outbreath. *Vyāna* is essential for the functioning of *prāṇa* and *apāna*, as it is the medium for transferring energies from one to the other. *Udāna* raises the energy from the lower spine to the brain.

This sūtra explains the powers gained by the yogi who masters *udāna vāyu*: he raises the energy, and is then able to walk over water.

(See *Light on Yoga* and *Light on Prāṇāyāma.*)

The following are some stories illustrating the powers gained by various yogis.

In the 8th century, a saint by the name of Tirumangai Ālwār was on a pilgrimage, visiting various famous temples in South India. Accompanying him were four disciples, each of whom was gifted with a miraculous power. One was able to fascinate with his power of speech. His name was Tolarvalla Vān. The second, Taludhavān, could open any lock by the power of his breath. The third, Nilalai Pidippan, could stop people from moving by tapping on their shadows, while the fourth, Nīrmel Nadappan by name, could walk over water.

Tirumangai Ālwār and his disciples arrived at the most holy shrine of Śrī Raṅganātha at Śrīraṅgam on the bank of the river Kāveri. It was in a deplorable condition and the saint wanted to rebuild it. He asked a number of wealthy people for financial help, but no one responded to his appeal. He therefore made up his mind to become a leader of a band of robbers and asked his four pupils to use their powers to raise money for the temple. They obeyed the orders of their guru and collected money, materials and men for construction. It took years to complete the temple which is known as the seven walls of Śrīraṅgam temple near Tiruchināpally (Trichy). When it was completed he gave up robbery, but the workers started pestering him for money. As he did not respond to their demands, they wanted to murder him. He asked them to go to the opposite bank of the river, where he had hidden some money, and to distribute it equally among themselves. Then he whispered to his pupil who could walk over water that he should take them in a boat and sink the boat in the middle of the river. Due to the rains, the river was in spate. The disciple obeyed the orders of his guru, took them all aboard the boat, sank it and rejoined his guru.

Sadānandācārya, a pupil of Śrī Śaṅkarācārya, walked over water at the call of his guru, who was on the other side of the river Gaṅgā at Vārāṇasi, modern-day Benares. People saw the imprints of his feet bearing a lotus flower, hence Sadānandācārya was known as Padmapādācārya (*padma* = lotus; *pāda* = foot).

It is said that Brahmendra Svāmi, the guru of Bājirao I of Mahārāṣṭra used to sit on a palm leaf and cross the sea. It is also related of Jesus Christ that he walked over a lake to meet his disciples who were waiting for him on the other side.

समानजयाज्ज्वलनम् ।४१।

III.41 samānajayāt jvalanam

samāna	one of the five *prāṇa vāyus*
jayāt	conquest, mastery
jvalanam	shining, burning, blazing, fire

By saṁyama *on* samāna vāyu, *a yogi glows like fire and his aura shines.*

By the conquest of *samāna vāyu*, the yogi gains control over the element of fire (*tejastattva*).

The middle of the torso is the region of *samāna* which stokes the gastric fire, aiding digestion and maintaining harmonious functioning of the abdominal organs. It controls the functioning of the heart, and through it the life force.

Kapilā, the founder of *sāṁkhya* philosophy, seems to have had the power of emitting fire from his eyes, which burnt the sons of King Sagara. The Mahārāṣṭrian saint Jñāneśvar, who wrote a translation and commentary on the *Bhagavad Gītā*, also had this power. Nearer our time, it is said that a pupil of Śrī Rāmakṛṣṇa used to light the path for his master on a dark night.

श्रोत्राकाशयोः संबन्धसंयमाद्दिव्यं श्रोत्रम् ।४२।

III.42 śrotra ākāśayoḥ saṁbandha saṁyamāt divyaṁ śrotram

śrotra	of hearing
ākāśayoḥ	in space, ether
saṁbandha	relation
saṁyamāt	by performing constraint
divyaṁ	divine
śrotram	power of hearing

By saṁyama *on the relation between space and sound, the yogi acquires the power of hearing distant and divine sounds. The organ of hearing, the ear, grasps sound in space. This is the conquest of air.*

कायाकाशयोः संबन्धसंयमाल्लघुतूलसमापत्तेश्चाकाशगमनम् ।४३।

III.43 kāya ākāśayoḥ saṁbandha saṁyamāt laghutūlasamāpatteḥ ca ākāśagamanam

kāya	body
ākāśayoḥ	ether
saṁbandha	relation
saṁyamāt	constraint

laghu	light
tūla	cotton fibre
samāpatteḥ	coalescence, becoming one
ca	and
ākāśa	space, levitation
gamanam	passage, going, movement, motion

By knowing the relationship between the body and ether, the yogi transforms his body and mind so that they become as light as cotton fibre. He can then levitate in space. This is the conquest of ether.

This is one of the supernatural powers called *laghimā*, or becoming as light as cotton.

In the *purāṇas*, it is said that Lord Hanumān (son of the Wind God) jumped up to the sky to fetch the sun, which he thought was an apple. There is also the story from the Rāmāyaṇa that he leaped to the Himālayās to fetch the elixir of life, called *sañjīvanī*, to save the life of Lord Rāma's brother who was wounded in a fight with Rāvaṇa's son. Nārada, who composed the *Bhakti Sūtras*, is said to wander in the three worlds from time immemorial to this day.

बहिरकल्पिता वृत्तिर्महाविदेहा ततः प्रकाशावरणक्षयः ।४४।

III.44 bahiḥ akalpitā vṛttiḥ mahāvidehā tataḥ prakāśa āvaraṇakṣayaḥ

bahiḥ	external, outside
akalpitā	unimaginable, actual, inconceivable
vṛttiḥ	fluctuations, modifications
mahā	great
videhā	without a body
tataḥ	then
prakāśa	light, illumination
āvaraṇa	covering
kṣayaḥ	destruction, dissolution

By saṁyama on mahāvideha (*the disembodied state*), *where consciousness acts outside the body, the veil covering the light of illumination is destroyed.*

By *saṁyama* on the consciousness, the yogi lives without a body; this is something that is unimaginable, yet it is a fact. It is a *siddhi*, called *mahāvideha siddhi* or great discarnation. It removes the veil covering the light of illumination. The yogi in this state has true and pure intelligence.

If consciousness moves outside the body but abides in the body, it is called an imaginable state. When the same consciousness moves outside the body, independent of and without abiding in it, it is an unimaginable state. In *mahāvideha*, the yogi disconnects his body from consciousness, so that afflictions do not influence him. He is beyond the *guṇas*. In this non-attached state, *citta* becomes divine and universal and can absorb anything in space without the use of the body, senses, or ego.

From his biography, we know that Śrī Aurobindo was in that state while imprisoned during the freedom movement.

(See I.19.)

स्थूलस्वरूपसूक्ष्मान्वयार्थवत्वसंयमात् भूतजयः ।४५।

III.45 sthūla svarūpa sūkṣma anvaya arthavatva saṁyamāt bhūtajayaḥ

sthūla	gross
svarūpa	form, attributes
sūkṣma	subtle
anvaya	all-pervasiveness, interpenetration, conjunction
arthavatva	purpose, fullness
saṁyamāt	by restraint
bhūtajayaḥ	mastery over the elements

By saṁyama *on the elements – their mass, forms, subtlety, conjunction and purposes, the yogi becomes Lord over them all.*

By restraint, the yogi gains control over the gross and subtle elements of nature, their forms and *guṇas*, as well as their purpose.

The Universe is made from the constituents of the basic elements of nature, earth (*pṛthvi*), water (*āp*), fire (*tejas*), air (*vāyu*) and ether (*ākāśa*). Each element possesses five attributes, mass (*sthūla*), subtlety (*sūkṣma*), form (*svarūpa*), all-pervasiveness or interpenetration (*anvaya*), and purpose or fruition (*arthavatva*).

The characteristic of the gross forms of elements are solidity, fluidity, heat, mobility and volume. Their subtle counterparts are smell, taste, sight, touch and sound. Their all-pervasiveness or interpentration are the three *guṇas*, and their purpose is either worldly enjoyment or freedom and beatitude.

The earth element has five properties of sound, touch, sight, taste and smell. Water has four: sound, touch, sight and taste. Fire has three: sound, touch and sight. Air has sound and touch. Ether has only the one quality of sound (see '*praṇavaḥ*', 1.27).

(See II.18–19.)

Table 14: *The elements and their properties*

ELEMENT			PROPERTY		
	(Sound	Touch	Sight	Taste	Smell)
Earth	+	+	+	+	+
Water	+	+	+	+	
Fire	+	+	+		
Air	+	+			
Ether	+				

ततोऽणिमादिप्रादुर्भावः कायसंपत् तद्धर्मानभिघातश्च ।४६।

III.46 tataḥ aṇimādi prādurbhāvaḥ kāyasaṁpat taddharma anabhighātaḥ ca

tataḥ	from it, thence
aṇimādi	powers such as minuteness and so forth
prādurbhāvaḥ	manifestation, appearance
kāya	of the body
saṁpat	perfection, wealth
tad	their, of them

dharma	attributes, functions
anabhighātaḥ	non-resistance, non-obstruction, indestructibility
ca	and

From that arises perfection of the body, the ability to resist the play of the elements, and powers such as minuteness.

The yogi can reduce himself to the size of an atom, or expand. He can become light or heavy. He can pierce rocks, have access to everything and master everything.

From *saṁyama* on the elements, their counterparts, forms, conjunctions and fruits, the yogi develops the eight supernatural powers and gains perfect wealth of the body without falling victim to the obstacles posed by the elements. This is said to be the best wealth of the body: perfection and freedom from all hindrances.

This sūtra indicates that by the conquest of the elements a yogi gains mastery in three fields. The first is the acquirement of the eight supernatural powers. The second is perfection of the body, which means that earth does not soil him, water dampen him, or fire burn him. Wind cannot move him and space can conceal his body anywhere at any time. The third is immunity from the play of the elements and their characteristics, and from the obstructions and disturbances which they create.

(See I.30, 31, 40; II.55.)

रूपलावण्यबलवज्रसंहननत्वानि कायसंपत् ।४७।

III.47 rūpa lāvaṇya bala vajra saṁhananatvāni kāyasaṁpat

rūpa	graceful forms, appearance
lāvaṇya	grace, beauty, charm, loveliness, ability to attract
bala	strength, force
vajra	a thunderbolt, adamantine, hard, diamond, impenetrable
saṁhananatvāni	firmness, compactness
kāya	body
saṁpat	perfection, wealth

Perfection of the body consists of beauty of form, grace, strength, compactness, and the hardness and brilliance of a diamond.

(For details, see *Art of Yoga*.)

ग्रहणस्वरूपास्मितान्वयार्थवत्त्वसंयमादिन्द्रियजयः ।४८।

III.48 grahaṇa svarūpa asmitā anvaya
arthavattva saṁyamāt indriyajayaḥ

grahaṇa	power of cognition
svarūpa	real appearance, natural state, one's form, one's visage
asmitā	egoism, the individual self
anvaya	conjunction
arthavattva	purposefulness, reason for being
saṁyamāt	by constraint
indriya	senses
jayaḥ	conquest

Through saṁyama *upon the purpose of the conjunction of the process of knowing, the ego, and nature, there is mastery over the senses.*

By *saṁyama* upon the natural states of the senses of perception, their function and receptivity with or without their conjunction with nature and the perception of the individual self (*asmitā*), the yogi recognizes the purpose of the conjunction of nature, senses and self and acquires mastery over them all.

Having in III.47 discussed the excellence of the body, Patañjali now speaks of the wealth of the senses.

This sūtra is both complementary and supplementary to III.45, in which the five qualities of the natural elements were objectively categorized. Here Patañjali describes the five specific qualities, particularly in relation to the senses of perception and the ego. The properties of the senses of perception are: knowing their own natural state; cognition or recognition of external objects; the reason for this contact; and the involvement of the individual self in these states, which change it from objective to subjective.

Everything we experience in the universe is transmitted through the medium of the senses to the 'I' consciousness. The senses by their nature are attracted to worldly objects conducive to pleasure, and their yearning for more and more entangles them. At some stage, when the senses are appeased, they and the organs of action become passive, and a state of quietness is experienced. An ordinary individual will go on following the senses when they are again aroused to their pursuit of pleasure, but the cultured intelligence will reflect, and consider that it is possible to turn inwards. This reflection on the receptivity of the senses and mind can now be diverted and directed by the intelligence toward exploring the realm of the seer so that senses, mind and ego are brought to rest permanently in the abode of the soul.

(See II.6, 21, 22; IV.4.)

ततो मनोजवित्वं विकरणभावः प्रधानजयश्च ।४९।

III.49 tataḥ manojavitvaṁ vikaraṇabhāvaḥ pradhānajayaḥ ca

tataḥ	thence, from it, therefrom
manojavitvaṁ	quickness of mind, speed of mind
vikaraṇabhāvaḥ	feeling of change, modification, without the help of the senses, freedom from the senses of perception
pradhāna	first cause, chief, main, pre-eminent, most excellent, best, first cause, primary or original matter
jayaḥ	mastery, conquest
ca	and

By mastery over the senses of perception, the yogi's speed of body, senses and mind matches that of the soul, independent of the primary causes of nature. Unaided by consciousness, he subdues the first principle of nature (mahat).

When the properties of nature have been conquered, and both body and consciousness purified, the self perceives directly and quickly, independent of nature. Body, senses, mind and consciousness stand equal to the seer in their movements, and the soul drinks its own sweetness. Sage Vyāsa, commenting on this state, calls it *madhu pratīka* (*madhu* = sweetness, honey; *pratīka* = turned towards). The taste of honey is the same from whichever side of the comb it is drawn. Similarly, the organs of action and senses of perception, body and mind are made as pure as the soul when they are transformed to the level of the soul. In this spiritual elation, they lose interest in sensual gratification and pleasure. Each cell reflects the light of the pure Self and each cell drinks the nectar of the soul. This is *madhu pratīka*.

(See I.41, 48; III.26, 37.)

सत्त्वपुरुषान्यताख्यातिमात्रस्य सर्वभावाधिष्ठातृत्वं सर्वज्ञातृत्वं च ।५०।

III.50 sattva puruṣa anyatā khyātimātrasya sarvabhāva adhiṣṭhātṛtvaṁ sarvajñātṛtvaṁ ca

sattva	pure, illuminative
puruṣa	soul
anyatā	distinction, discrimination, difference
khyāti	awareness, understanding knowledge
mātrasya	only, of that
sarva	all
bhāva	manifestations, states
adhiṣṭhātṛtvaṁ	supremacy, overlordship
sarvajñātṛtvaṁ	all knowingness, omniscience
ca	and

Only one who knows the difference between the illuminative intelligence and the seer attains supreme knowledge of all that exists and all that manifests.

The yogi distinguishes between intelligence, consciousness, ego and the soul. Through knowledge of the soul, he gains mastery over all states of manifestations and becomes master of all knowledge. He is omnipresent, omnipotent and omniscient.

He alone is the observer, perceiving everything directly, and he alone is the actor, independent of mind, senses of perception and organs of action.

(See I.36, 47; II.18, 20; III.36 and IV.25.)

तद्वैराग्यादपि दोषबीजक्षये कैवल्यम् ।५१।

III.51 tadvairāgyāt api doṣabījakṣaye kaivalyam

tadvairāgyāt	from non-attachment to them, indifferent towards them, desirelessness towards them
api	even
doṣa	defect, bondage, imperfection
bīja	seed
kṣaye	on destruction
kaivalyam	pure, simple, unmingled, perfect in one's self, perfect aloneness, eternal emancipation, absorption in the supreme soul

By destruction of the seeds of bondage and the renunciation of even these powers, comes eternal emancipation.

By renouncing the supernormal powers, the yogi reaches eternal emancipation. Indifference to all supernatural experiences destroys the seed of sorrows and leads the yogi to live in his own self. If he does not spurn them he will be caught in the web of subtle afflictions, and may find it very difficult to come out of them.

In II.16, Patañjali spoke of afflictions and pains which may affect the *sādhaka* at a later time through pride or want of understanding. Now that the *sādhaka* has developed intellectual sensitivity, he is ready to hear that afflictions will instantly engulf one (see IV.28) who succumbs to the temptation of the *siddhis*. If he fails to see their hidden dangers, he ends up in sorrow. If he cultivates non-attachment to, and detachment from them, the seeds of sorrow, weakness or bondage that spring from *siddha vidyā* are destroyed. From renunciation springs eternal emancipation, unalloyed purity. This is *kaivalya*. The self, now, has achieved absolute independence and abides in its own nature.

(See I.3; II.25; IV.27, 30.)

स्थान्युपनिमन्त्रणे सङ्गस्मयाकरणं पुनरनिष्टप्रसङ्गात् ।५२।

III.52 sthānyupanimantraṇe saṅgasmayākaraṇaṁ punaraniṣṭa prasaṅgāt

sthāni	a place or position, rank, dignity, presiding deities
upanimantraṇe	on invitation, on being invited
saṅga	coming together, union, contact, association
smaya	wonder, surprise, smile
akaraṇaṁ	non-performance
punaḥ	again
aniṣṭa	undesirable, unfavourable
prasaṅgāt	connection, event

When approached by celestial beings, there should be neither attachment nor surprise, for undesirable connections can occur again.

Celestial beings try to seduce the yogi from the grace of yoga. The yogi must maintain his hard-won freedom, and must not fall victim to temptations that can pull him down from the height of spirituality.

Like sirens, celestial beings try to lure the successful yogi to his doom. If he submits to their blandishments, he is again caught in sensory pleasures and afflictions, and falls from the grace of yoga.

There are four types of yogis. They are known as *prathama kalpika, madhubhūmika, prajñājyotī* and *atikrāntabhāvanīya. Prathama kalpika* yogis have worked hard in their yogic practices, and the power of progress has just begun to dawn. *Madhubhūmika* yogis have learned to differentiate between *citta* and the seer and try to gain further mastery. (They are also called *ṛtambharā prajñās.*) The *prajñājyotis* have succeeded in subjugating the elements of nature, the qualities of the senses of perception, mind and desires and have realized the seer, while the *atikrāntabhāvanīyas* have attained the highest knowledge of the seer and have the power of *paravairāgya* (highest dispassion).

Patañjali warns all classes of yogis not to let themselves be enticed into angelic 'traps', but to distance themselves from these divine temptations so that their hearts have no room to harbour undesirable feelings and urges.

(See I.16, 21, 48; II.27.)

क्षणतत्क्रमयोः संयमाद्विवेकजं ज्ञानम् ।५३।

III.53 kṣaṇa tatkramayoḥ saṁyamāt vivekajaṁ jñānam

kṣaṇa	an instant, a moment, an infinitesimal unit in time
tat	that, its
kramayoḥ	order, sequence, succession
saṁyamāt	by constraint
vivekajaṁ	exalted intelligence, total awareness
jñānam	knowledge, sacred knowledge, cognizance

By saṁyama *on moment and on the continuous flow of moments, the yogi gains exalted knowledge, free from the limitations of time and space.*

Patañjali now shows an altogether different method of reaching *samādhi*: by *saṁyama* on the continuous flow of moments which move in a succession known as time, the yogi gets direct understanding of time and relativity. From this, he recognizes that a moment in time is timeless, and that this timelessness is real and eternal, while its movement is confined to the past and the future. Movement is timebound, transient and ever-changing. The moment is everlasting, changeless, sacred: it is, in fact, the secret of *samādhi*. The moment is unconditioned reality, while the sequence of moments is conditioned reality; it is relative to the absolute and illusory. This realization is termed exalted intelligence.

In moment, neither psychological nor chronological time is felt. Moment comes between rising impressions and their restraints and vice-versa: it is a quiet intervening state, auspicious and pure, and is to be stabilized, prolonged and expanded so that consciousness becomes absolute.

This is *vivekaja jñāna*, the gateway to *kaivalya*. The yogi has learned the orderly sequence of practice and of time, and now cannot be trapped by the temptations of celestial beings. (But, should this happen, he is reminded to pursue his *sādhana*, and to keep Self-Realization as his goal.)

As the atom is the minutest particle of matter, the moment is the minutest particle of time. The moment is singularly alone. Moments succeed one another in sequence, and these sequences put together constitute time. Thus the spokes of moments move into the wheel of time. The movement of mind in a continuum is psychological time. The movement of moments in present, past and future is chronological time.

The yogi keeps aware of the moment and thus conquers psychological and chronological time. He remains attentive to the moment, and does not allow his attention to slip into the movement of moments. He remains undisturbed, and with the loss of the time factor, his consciousness, too, loses its significance. Then, he catches sight of the soul. This is *vivekaja jñāna*, exalted intelligence, the secret and sacred knowledge. (Read and re-read II.9–15).

This sounds extremely complicated, and certainly its absolute realization is unbelievably difficult, like trying to thread a needle when the thread is thicker than the needle's eye. Yet there is a seed lesson here from which everyone can learn, and improve the quality of their lives.

Poets and wise men since the beginning of the written word have enjoined us in all cultures to live in the present moment because it is all we really have. Have you ever wondered, while watching nature films on television in which herds of beautiful gazelles are constantly surrounded by marauding predators, why their life is not a living hell of fear and insecurity? How can they live their family lives of courtship, procreation, joy in their own physical perfection, knowing that the inevitable end will be in the lion's maw? You cannot say it is dull fatalism, or lack of imagination. If they lacked imagination why would they run away so fast? The answer must be that they have the capacity to live in the present moment *as it is* and not as it might be. Those who live in reality, which can only be the present, will assuredly die, but will have lived before they die. Many people die without having lived. This is true cellularly as well as psychologically. By perfect positioning in *āsana*, we flood our cells with life, which is nothing but present awareness. The cells too will die – but first they will have lived.

One of the reasons why, as a teacher of *āsana*, I am so intense, and was in the past even harsh, is that I want to give the students one and a half hours of present life in a lesson. As I shout at them to straighten their legs in *Sīrṣāsana* (headstand), they cannot be wondering what is for dinner or whether they will be promoted or demoted at work. For those who habitually flee the present, one hour's experience of 'now' can be daunting, even exhausting, and I wonder if the fatigue felt by some students after lessons is due more to that than to the work of performing *āsanas*. Our perpetual mental absences are like tranquillizing drugs, and the habit dies hard. For the keen student, the effect of *āsana* is exhilarating.

The 'elsewhere' or 'otherwise' mentality to which we are bound by psychological time, causes us to emasculate our present reality with our illusory unreality. It is as if we were staying in a town with only one hotel, not a very nice one, and all night we are miserable because we are thinking of the lovely hotel we stayed in the night before. But as the town has only one hotel, we are destroying our night's sleep for the sake of fantasy. Now the atom of the moment, the minutest particle of time, is like the town with only one hotel. If we can live with that, such as it is, good, bad or indifferent, without a forwards, backwards or sideways glance, then we are free. If I seem to have over-simplified the subject, it is in an effort to demystify a topic which has become a plaything for intellectuals.

(See IV.12 and 13.)

जातिलक्षणदेशैरन्यतानवच्छेदात् तुल्ययोस्ततः प्रतिपत्तिः ।५४।

III.54 jāti lakṣaṇa deśaiḥ anyatā anavacchedāt tulyayoḥ tataḥ pratipattiḥ

jāti	class, descent, rank, race, lineage
lakṣaṇa	distinctive mark, a sign, quality
deśaiḥ	place, position in space
anyatā	otherwise, in a different manner
anavacchedāt	not bounded, not separated, undefined
tulyayoḥ	of the same kind or class, similar, equal
tataḥ	thereby, from it
pratipattiḥ	understanding, knowledge

By this knowledge the yogi is able to distinguish unerringly the differences in similar objects which cannot be distinguished by rank, qualitative signs or position in space.

With this exalted intelligence the yogi is capable of distinguishing, faultlessly and instantaneously, the minutest differences between two similar kinds of things or objects, irrespective of rank, creed, quality, place or space.

A yogi who has attained spiritual realization has clarity and sensitivity even in the subtlest of things. He sees all things distinctly and expresses himself faultlessly.

This quality of intelligence cannot be possessed even by evolved souls unless they are anchored in the sacred divine spiritual knowledge, *vivekaja jñānam*.

तारकं सर्वविषयं सर्वथाविषयमक्रमं चेति विवेकजं ज्ञानम् ।५५।

III.55 tārakaṁ sarvaviṣayaṁ sarvathāviṣayaṁ akramaṁ ca iti vivekajaṁ jñānam

tārakaṁ	shining, radiant, clear, clean, excellent
sarva	all
viṣayaṁ	objects, pursuits, affairs, aims
sarvathā	in all ways, by all means, wholly, completely, at all times
viṣayaṁ	objects, pursuits, affairs, aims
akramaṁ	without succession, without method or order, without sequence
ca	and
iti	this
vivekajaṁ jñānam	exalted knowledge, sacred spiritual knowledge

The essential characteristic of the yogi's exalted knowledge is that he grasps instantly, clearly and wholly, the aims of all objects without going into the sequence of time or change.

Exalted in understanding, clear in action, he dominates and transcends nature and reaches, through yogic practices, the light of the soul.

(See I.36; II.52; III.34 and 36.)

सत्त्वपुरुषयोः शुद्धिसाम्ये कैवल्यमिति ।५६।

III.56 sattva puruṣayoḥ śuddhi sāmye kaivalyam iti

sattva	pure illuminative consciousness
puruṣayoḥ	soul
śuddhi	of purity
sāmye	becoming equal
kaivalyam	perfect aloneness, unmingled freedom, pure, simple, perfect in one's self
iti	this

When the purity of intelligence equals the purity of the soul, the yogi has reached kaivalya, *perfection in yoga.*

When the vestures of the soul are equal in purity to that of the soul, there is harmony between them. There comes freedom, *kaivalya*, of the seer, uncontaminated by the qualities of nature.

By yogic discipline, the veil of ignorance is lifted from the intelligence. This is the real and true light: *vivekaja jñānam*, illuminative consciousness. It becomes equal to that of the light of the soul, *puruṣa*. The distinction between intelligence and consciousness comes to an end. Both dissolve in the beacon light of the soul. They are isolated from contact with nature's objects. The seeds of affliction are burnt up. The vestures either become isolated and functionless or are lifted to the level of their wearer. This is freedom. Now the Soul shines in its pristine form, in its pure effulgence: it reigns supreme. This is *kaivalya*, the indivisible state of existence.

(See II.23; III.49 and IV.26.)

Here ends the exposition on *vibhūti*, the third *pāda* of Patañjali's *Yoga Sūtras*.

part four

कैवल्य पादः।

Kaivalya Pāda

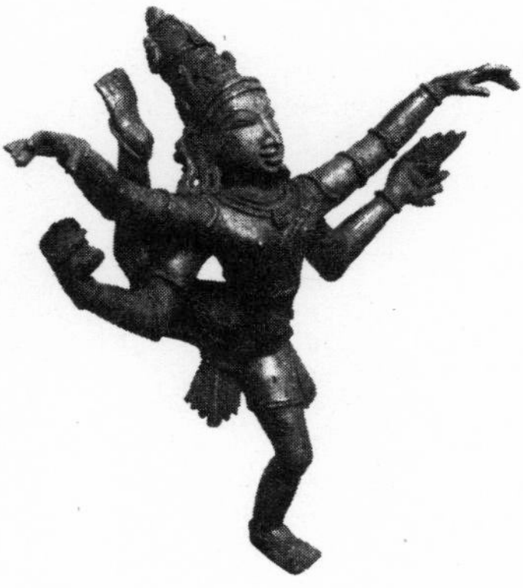

Kaivalya pāda is the fourth and final chapter of Patañjali's exposition of yoga.

In his individual way, Patañjali set out the three cornerstones of Indian philosophy: the path of devotion, *bhakti mārga*, in *samādhi pāda*; the path of action, *karma mārga*, in *sādhana pāda*; the path of knowledge, *jñāna mārga*, in *vibhūti pāda*. In *kaivalya pāda*, he describes the path of renunciation, *vairāgya mārga* or *virakti mārga*, the path of detachment from worldly objects and of freedom from worldly desires. In so doing, he brings out the whole essence of the Indian outlook on life.

This *pāda* is complex and difficult to comprehend at first glance, as it appears to be more theoretical than practical, but hidden practical aspects are present in each sūtra.

Here, Patañjali explains how consciousness can become pure, intelligent and ripe, and free itself from the clutches of nature, enabling the yogi to reach the goal of Absolute Freedom, auspicious bliss and beatitude. These, according to Patañjali, are the qualities of a perfect yogi. He then deals with the course of action which the exalted yogi should follow after enlightenment.

Patañjali says that when the intelligence is cultivated to the point of ripeness, ego, *ahaṁkāra*, loses its potency naturally and consciousness reaches a state of divine purity. The rivers of intelligence and consciousness lose their identities and merge in the river of the soul. This is the crowning glory of the yoga *sādhana*, the attainment of *kaivalya* or *Brahma jñāna*.

Let us briefly summarize our journey so far. By now, the reader is familiar with the fact that *samādhi pāda* is an internal quest in which the art and meaning of yoga are described, the functions of mind, intelligence and consciousness explained, and methods of developing and sustaining a permanently balanced, stable consciousness shown.

Sādhana pāda deals with the body, senses and mind, and connects them to the intelligence and consciousness. The external sheaths – body, senses and mind – are perceptible and distinguishable; intelligence and consciousness are not easily perceptible. *Sādhana pāda* thus describes the external quest, beginning with the distinguishable sheaths and proceeding to the penetration of the core of being through intelligence and consciousness.

Samādhi pāda begins with the fluctuations of consciousness and ends with a state in which the mind does not function. *Sādhana pāda* begins with the afflictions of the body and their emotional implications and sets out means to overcome them through the various disciplines of yoga.

The first two *pādas* thus emphasize the art, theory and practice of yoga.

Vibhūti pāda describes the properties of yoga. Here, having guided the *sādhaka* through the external quest, Patañjali takes him through the internal quest and then deeper into integration, *saṁyama*.

Saṁyama is the art of contemplating wholly, so that the yogi becomes one with the object of contemplation. Patañjali calls this communion of subject and object the innermost quest. In it, he says, sparks of superconsciousness and extraordinary powers accrue, which might affect the yogi's divinity and hinder his progress towards self-awareness and universal consciousness. He advises yogis who have acquired such powers to move away from them by screening out their 'I' centre from them, and to further filter and purify consciousness for attainment of exalted intelligence, *vivekaja jñānam*. Then the seer reigns supreme.

These three *pādas* of the *Yoga Sūtras* speak of the growth of man from an unfulfilled state of mind, to the glory of illumined intelligence and consciousness.

In *kaivalya pāda*, without forgetting the internal and external sheaths, Patañjali draws the yogi towards the subtlest, the soul. *Kaivalya pāda* can therefore be called the quest of the soul, *antarātma sādhana*. Here Patañjali speaks of the ways in which such exalted yogis should live and serve humanity with their supreme wisdom, maintaining the radiance of their souls with untainted intelligence and unalloyed peace.

Interestingly, Patañjali begins this chapter with the rebirth of such adepts. Having attained refined states of intelligence through yoga, they may have become proud or arrogant, or indifferent or negligent in their practices, and fallen from the grace of yoga. Patañjali uses the phrase '*jātyantara pariṇāma*' for such fallen yogis (*jātyantara* = change of birth, birth into another class, another state of life; *pariṇāma* = transformation).

Adepts are born according to the standard of their previous *sādhana*. The potentialities of nature flow in them abundantly so that they may continue their *sādhana* with renewed vigour and intensity (see I.21).

Patañjali explains four types of actions (*karma*). He first describes three actions common to all, white, grey and black. Then he speaks of the fourth type, which has no reaction and is meant for the attainment of untainted purity. He cautions that these must be maintained, sustained and upheld throughout one's *sādhana*. Then consciousness will realize that it has no light of its own, that it exists only by the borrowed light of the soul (*ātman*). At this stage, consciousness gravitates towards and merges in its Lord, the soul (*ātman*).

The yogi is now free from the fourfold aims of life: religious duty (*dharma*), purpose of life and duty of earning a livelihood (*artha*), joy of life (*kāma*) and liberation (*mokṣa*). He is free from the gravitational pull of the *guṇas*, *sattva*, *rajas* and *tamas*. He is a *guṇātītan*, free from the *guṇas*. This is the summit of yoga.

In the *Bhagavad Gītā*, Lord Kṛṣṇa beautifully describes to Arjuṅa the characteristics of a perfect yogi (II.55–59, 61, 64–72).

He who is free from desire in thought, word, deed and content in his soul, is clean and clear in his intelligence. 55

He who remains unperturbed amidst sorrows; who does not long for pleasures and lives free from passion, fear and anger, has steadfast wisdom. 56

He who has no attachment on any side and remains indifferent to good or evil, is firmly established in his intelligence. 57

He who draws away his senses effortlessly from their pastures as a tortoise draws in its limbs, his wisdom is firmly set. 58

He who abstains from feeding the desires of the senses and mind and allows the tastes of desires to fade out on their own, is one with the soul. 59

He whose senses and mind are under control, he who is firmly set in his wisdom remains firm in yoga intent on Me. 61

He who has disciplined his *citta* remains unresponsive to likes and dislikes, and is filled with purity and tranquillity. 64

He, in that tranquil state, extinguishes all miseries and is established in his exalted intelligence. 65

He who is not able to restrain fluctuations of his consciousness, cannot concentrate, and without concentration cannot attain salvation. With efforts of practice and renunciation, he has to gain control over the mind. 66

If one's *citta* is mingled with the senses that rove among objects, one loses the power of discriminative discernment and will be carried away from the path of evolution like the wind carrying away a ship in waters. 67

Therefore, Lord Kṛṣṇa says, he whose senses are completely restrained from their objects, his intelligence is under control. 68

What is night for all beings is day for a disciplined yogi, as he is one with the vision of the soul (*apavarga*); when all beings are active with worldly pleasures (*bhoga*), the yogi considers this as night by keeping himself aloof from worldly thoughts. 69

Just as waters flow into the ocean, yet the level of the ocean neither changes nor becomes ruffled, similarly he who is steadfast in intelligence, pleasures do not haunt him, he attains liberation. 70

He who renounces all desires and keeps away from attachment, attains freedom and beatitude (*kaivalya*). 71

He who is free from delusion and keeps himself in contact with the divine consciousness, even at the moment of death, reaches *kaivalya* and the Supreme Lord. 72

जन्मौषधिमन्त्रतपःसमाधिजाः सिद्धयः ॥१॥

IV.1 janma auṣadhi mantra tapaḥ samādhijāḥ siddhayaḥ

janma	birth
auṣadhi	medicinal plant, herb, drug, incense, elixir
mantra	incantation, charm, spell
tapaḥ	heat, burning, shining, an ascetic devotional practice, burning desire to reach perfection, that which burns all impurities
samādhi	profound meditation, total absorption
jāḥ	born
siddhayaḥ	perfections, accomplishments, fulfilments, attainments

Accomplishments may be attained through birth, the use of herbs, incantations, self-discipline or samādhi.

There are five types of accomplished yogis (*siddhayaḥ*):

1 by birth with aspiration to become perfect (*janma*)
2 by spiritual experience gained through herbs, drugs or elixir (*auṣadha*)
3 by incantation of the name of one's desired deity (*mantra*)
4 by ascetic devotional practice (*tapas*)
5 by profound meditation (*samādhi*)

There is an important distinction between these means of spiritual accomplishment. Followers of the first three may fall from the grace of yoga through pride or negligence. The others, whose spiritual gains are through *tapas* and *samādhi*, do not. They become masters, standing alone as divine, liberated souls, shining examples to mankind.

Nandi, Rāmakṛṣṇa Paramahaṁsa, Sai Bābā of Śirḍi and Rāmaṇa Māharṣi were accomplished yogis by birth.

Sage Māṇḍavya and King Yayāti developed supernatural powers through an elixir of life. Today many drug users employ mescalin, LSD, hashish, heroin, etc. to experience the so-called spiritual visions investigated by Aldous Huxley and others. Artists and poets in the past have also relied on drugs to bring about supernormal states to enhance their art.

Māṇḍavya was a sage and a yogi. In his childhood days his only game was to kill flies. When he grew up, he reached *samādhi* by *tapas*. Local thieves were stealthily using his *āśrama* as a resting place after pillaging and bringing back their booty. People went to the king and told him of their agony and fear for their lives. The king, at once, ordered his attendants to find the thieves and put them to the gallows. The party traced the thieves to the yogi's *āśrama* and brought all of them, including the sage, and hanged them. All died except the sage. Seeing this wonder, the king came and apologized and released him from the gallows. But the sage kicked and broke the gallows and died of his own will.

Attendants of Yama (Lord of Death) carried the sage to hell. He was shocked to find himself there and asked the God of death the reason for bringing him to hell. The Lord replied that, having killed flies in his childhood, he had come to hell. The sage was enraged and thundered that the crimes of childhood days belong to the parents, and not to the children. The sage said to the Lord: 'You do not know *dharma* (science of duty), hence I curse you to be born on earth as the son of a *śūdra* for having failed in your duty as an impartial judge of man's sins', and then the sage returned to his old hermitage as young as ever. Due to this curse, the Lord of Death took birth as Vidura and acted as adviser to King Dhṛtarāṣṭra of *Mahābhārata* fame.

King Yayāti was the son of Nahūṣa. He had two wives. One was Devayāni (daughter of Śukrācārya, preceptor of the demons and inventor of the elixir of life – *sanjīvani*), and the other was Śarmiṣṭhā. As the king's worldly power grew, his lust for sensual joy increased, and he committed adultery. Devayāni, incensed by her husband's infidelity, returned to her father and complained of her husband. Śukrācārya cursed the king with premature old age. Then her affection for Yayāti sprang out and she pleaded with her father that the curse was too strong. Listening to his daughter's pleas, he consented to transfer the curse to any one of the king's sons if they would accept it. None of his sons came forward except his youngest son, Purū. Purū accepted his father's old age and the father kept his youth. Later in life, Yayāti realized that lust (*kāma*) cannot be quenched at all. He returned his youth to his son along with his kingdom. He took back his old age and returned to the forest to devote the rest of his life to meditation.

Many *sādhakas* initiated through ṃantras did penance and became spiritual masters, poets and scholars. The dacoit Ratnākar became the author of the famous epic Rāmāyaṇa; Dhruva, the son of King Uttānapāda, reached God-hood; while young Prahlāda, the son of the demon King Hiraṇyakaśipu, made God come out of a pillar.

जात्यन्तरपरिणामः प्रकृत्यापूरात् ।२।

IV.2 jātyantara pariṇāmaḥ prakṛtyāpūrāt

jātyantara	in another class, change of birth, another state of life
pariṇāmaḥ	change, transformation
prakṛti	nature, creative cause, nature's energy
āpūrāt	becoming full, being full, abundant flow

The abundant flow of nature's energy brings about a transformation in one's birth, aiding the process of evolution.

Just as water can be transformed into vapour or ice, and gold into ornaments, so afflictions and fluctuations can be brought under control and transformed by vanquishing *avidyā*.

In IV.I, Patañjali explained that nature's energy flows in such abundance in certain adepts that their consciousness is transformed, enabling them to live in a pure dynamic state in this present life. (If a *sādhaka* fails to reach perfection during this life, nature may abundantly penetrate and perfect his *sādhana* in the next, so that he may then experience freedom.)

Due to the power of his practices, nature's energy flows in such a *sādhaka* with such force as to transform him into an immortal. This accords with the theory of evolution. It is interesting to note also that nature itself is the power-house for spiritual evolution.

Buddha, Ādi Śaṅkara, Śrī Rāmānūjācārya, Jñāneśvar, Tukārām and Nandanār attained *kaivalya* during their lives here on earth without yogic *sādhana* because of the fruits of yogic practices in their previous lives (*jātyantara pariṇāma*).

Similarly, *ācāryāṇīs* Maitreyī, Gārgī, Arundhatī, Lilāvatī, Sulabhā, Śāradā Devi, yoginī Lallā of Kashmir and yoginī Motibai of Jaipur, all attained liberation through *jātyantara pariṇāma*. See *Great Women of India*, Advaita Āśrama, Almora, Himālayas; also see *Yoga, A Gem for Women*, by Geeta S. Iyengar, Allied Publishers, Delhi.)

निमित्तमप्रयोजकं प्रकृतीनां वरणभेदस्तु ततः क्षेत्रिकवत् ।३।

IV.3 nimittaṁ aprayojakaṁ prakṛtīnāṁ varaṇabhedaḥ tu tataḥ kṣetrikavat

nimittaṁ	incidental, instrumental, efficient cause, a pretext
aprayojakaṁ	not useful, of no use, those which do not move into action
prakṛtīnāṁ	of natural tendencies or potentialities
varaṇam	covers, veils, obstacles
bhedaḥ	split, division, separation
tu	but, on the contrary, on the other hand, nevertheless
tataḥ	from that
kṣetrikavat	like a farmer, like a peasant, like a husbandman

Nature's efficient cause does not impel its potentialities into action, but helps to remove the obstacles to evolution, just as a farmer builds banks to irrigate his fields.

Culture of the sprouted consciousness is of paramount importance in yoga. As a farmer builds dykes between fields to regulate the flow of water, evolved yogis channel the abundant flow of nature's energy to free themselves from the bondage of their actions and develop spiritual insight. Even if *sādhana* fails to bring about complete transformation in the life of a *sādhaka*, it certainly serves to remove obstacles in the path of his evolution.

Past good actions (*karmāśaya*) indirectly become instrumental in accelerating the flow of natural tendencies for the good of the consciousness. A farmer heaps up banks of earth to collect water and soak part of a field. When one area is soaked, he opens the bank to enable the water to flow into the adjoining area, continuing until the entire field is thoroughly irrigated. Then he sows the best seeds to get the best of harvests, and enjoys the fruits. Through yogic discipline, the yogi removes all obstacles to his evolution, and enjoys emancipation.

Thus disciplined, the yogi's enhanced energy spontaneously removes all fluctuations and afflictions which hinder his spiritual growth, enabling him to gain insight into his very being, his soul.

This sūtra is a beauty in itself. Nature's energy now flows abundantly in the *sādhaka*. This energy is built up and concentrated through practice of *āsana, prāṇāyāma* and *bandha*, which can be thought of as 'dykes' in the system to regulate and channel energy, so that mind and intelligence may diffuse evenly throughout one's being.

Judicious use of energy builds courage, strength, wisdom and freedom. This is cultivation of talent, which may transform itself to the level of genius.

(See I.2, 18, 29–39; II.2, 12, 13, 18; II.29–III.15.)

निर्माणचित्तान्यस्मितामात्रात् ।४।

IV.4 nirmāṇacittāni asmitāmātrāt

nirmāṇa	measuring, forming, making, fabricating, creating, creation
cittāni	spheres of consciousness, the stuff of the mind
asmitā	sense of individuality
mātrāt	from that alone

Constructed or created mind springs from the sense of individuality (asmitā).

From a sense of self-awareness, numerous activities become associated in one's consciousness, thereby giving rise to mental states called moods, which form themselves into *nirmita*, or cultivated, *citta*. They taint, distort and disturb the intelligence, creating various afflictions and fluctuations. If this distorted consciousness is re-channelled in the right direction, it develops refinement and sensitivity. Then *nirmita citta* changes into *nirmāṇa*, or *sās-mita, citta*, or a sense of *sāttvic* individuality, and nature makes the intelligence wise, which in turn keeps the consciousness pure.

This sūtra explains the quality of constructive and creative mind through *asmitā*. The seat of the mind-matter is the brain. It creates fluctuations, bias and prejudices which cause pain and distress, and need to be restrained.

The mind at its source is single and pure. It is known as the core of the being (*ātman*) or the seat of the spiritual heart. When it sprouts into a seedling, it becomes the self-conscious centre (*antaḥkaraṇa*), and forms *sāsmitā* or a sense of *sāttvic* individuality. This develops into consciousness (*citta*), which branches out into ego (*ahaṁkāra*), intelligence (*buddhi*) and mind (*manas*). These manifest themselves as multiple thought-waves, which, if allowed free play, give rise to afflictions and fluctuations (*vyutthāna citta*).

By regular practice, the fire of yoga develops the *sādhaka*'s ability to discriminate between the original mind and its off-shoots, single mind and multifaceted, complex mind. He does this by careful observation of his behaviour, channelling his energies to retrace the source of these thought-waves (*citta vṛttis*) and eradicate them at this very source. This is *śānta citta* or *samāhita citta*, which takes the *sādhaka* to the verge of the single state of consciousness, and converts the sprouted or created consciousness into a cultured consciousness, *nirmāṇa citta*. This, in turn, traces the core of his individual existence. This becomes meditation, *dhyāna*, at which point the distortions of the multiple mind disappear. The conscious awareness of head and heart unite, and the consciousness becomes mature and pure (*divya citta*). This pure *citta* is the root consciousness, *mūla citta*.

For example, one can compare the single state of consciousness to the trunk of a tree and the multiple mind to the branches of the tree. Though the branches shoot out from the main trunk, they remain in contact with it. Similarly, the *sādhaka* has to draw back the branches of consciousness, i.e., the 'I' consciousness, from the head towards its base, so as to lose its identity.

(See I.2; II.6 and III.12–13.)

प्रवृत्तिभेदे प्रयोजकं चित्तमेकमनेकेषाम् ॥५॥

IV.5 pravṛtti bhede prayojakaṁ cittam ekam anekeṣām

pravṛtti	moving forward, proceeding, progressing
bhede	difference
prayojakaṁ	effect, usefulness, benefit
cittam	consciousness
ekam	one
anekeṣām	numberless, numerous

Consciousness is one, but it branches into many different types of activities and innumerable thought-waves.

Consciousness, though single, directs multiple thoughts, sometimes creating disparities between words and deeds. It is indirectly responsible for numerous activities, and becomes the source of desires and their fulfilment. If it stops directing thoughts, the need to culture the consciousness towards transformation (*nirmāṇa citta*) does not arise.

Patañjali wants us to channel the energies of the multiple mind in the right direction, so that no disparities or distortions arise between words, thoughts and deeds.

It has already been said that from the sense of 'I' consciousness in the sphere of activity, multiple thoughts arise. Owing to lack of understanding, *avidyā*, their fluctuations create doubts, confusion, desires and greed, bringing afflictions that disturb the mind. These are 'weeds' of the mind (*vyutthāna* or *nirmita citta*). By using the discriminative faculty (*nirodha citta*) gained through yoga, and analysing the fluctuating changes, the weeds are uprooted and a state of silence (*praśānta citta*), is created: an intermediate state between the original, universal mind and the individual mind. In that state of silence, comes a refining and purifying spark from within (*divya citta*). When this occurs, nature becomes a real friend to consciousness, culturing and transforming it, with its abundant energies, and purifying the intelligence of the heart. Intelligence and consciousness then realize that they are one, not separate and different, and all sorrows and joys come to an end.

The intelligence of the heart is nothing but the seer, in whom both intelligence and consciousness rest and remain forever, with purity and divinity.

(See I.2, 17; II.6; III.13, 14; IV.1, 3.)

तत्र ध्यानजमनाशयम् ।६।

IV.6 tatra dhyānajam anāśayam

tatra	of them, of these
dhyānajam	born of meditation
anāśayam	free from impressions or influences

Of these activities of consciousness of perfected beings, only those which proceed from meditation are free from latent impressions and influences.

Having explained the creation by the single mind of multiple thoughts which disturb the poise of the original mind, Patañjali says here that this 'sprouted' mind should be cultured, stilled and silenced through profound meditation. This puts an end to the influence of impressions, and frees the consciousness from entanglements with objects seen, heard or known.

Meditation not only frees consciousness from past impressions but also removes the obstacles to the progressive evolution of the mind. Impressions of attachment and affliction continue to torment others.

These obstacles, lust, anger, greed, infatuation, pride and jealousy, are the spokes of the emotional wheel. Meditation helps to subdue them so that the emotional centre (the consciousness of the heart) can expand in a new dimension of spiritual growth. Then consciousness will have neither merits nor demerits, virtue nor vice, fluctuations nor afflictions. It becomes 'cultured' (*samāhita citta*), and is conducive to experiencing *kaivalya*.

(See I.23, 29, 32; II.11, 12; III.51.)

कर्माशुक्लाकृष्णं योगिनस्त्रिविधमितरेषाम् ॥७॥

IV.7 karma aśukla akṛṣṇaṁ yoginaḥ trividham itareṣām

karma	action
aśukla	non-white
akṛṣṇaṁ	non-black
yoginaḥ	of a yogi
trividham	threefold (black, white and mixed, or grey)
itareṣām	for others

A yogi's actions are neither white nor black. The actions of others are of three kinds, white, black or grey.

This sūtra speaks of three types of actions and their effects on an average individual, but there are in fact four. The fourth is free, uncoloured and pure. The yogi follows this kind of action to be free from its fruits.

White, black and mixed or grey actions produce fruits and chain reactions. Black actions produce *tāmasic*, grey actions *rājasic*, and white *sāttvic* effects. White actions result in virtue, black in vice. Grey actions result in a mixture of effects, and of positive and negative emotions.

The unmixed actions of the yogi are beyond *sattva, rajas* and *tamas*. They produce no positive or negative reactions in consciousness and hence are free from duality. This fourth type of action is propitious and auspicious. This is the real 'skill in action' of the yogi (see *Bhagavad Gītā*, II.50).

An average person is full of ambition. He desires rewards for his deeds, but forgets that they carry the seeds of pain. If his ambition is transformed into spiritual aspiration, he loses interest in rewards and comes to understand *sādhana* for the sake of *sādhana*, or action for the sake of action. He becomes refined; his mind and consciousness become clear and his actions clean. He collects no impressions. He takes future births only to cleanse himself of past accumulated impressions. He anchors his mind and consciousness unreservedly to the will of the divine. All his actions are free from the seeds of reactions.

There is a tendency to associate the renunciate of Patañjali's eightfold path with the recluse who conquers the temptations of the flesh simply by rejecting the civilized world and dwelling in places where no temptations exist. Of all discussions on how to belong to the world, act in it and yet remain unsullied, pride of place is often given to the debate between Lord Kṛṣṇa and Arjuṅa on the eve of battle. There, Kṛṣṇa makes it plain that action cannot be avoided; because inaction is also action; and that selfish actions, and attachment to their fruits, lead to ensnarement.

With respect to this triumph of world literature and philosophy, the *Bhagavad Gītā*, we must acknowledge that in this sūtra, Patañjali, in his usual terse style, has said exactly the same thing. Not even the superbly expressive style of the *Gītā* can eclipse Patañjali's genius in going straight to the heart of the matter.

How does a free man act, and yet remain free? This is the main thrust of the *kaivalya pāda*. Here Patañjali clearly states that free action, beyond causality, is his who acts without motive or desire – as if a kite were released in the sky, without a string to bring it back to earth.

(See II.12–15 and IV.4.)

ततस्तद्विपाकानुगुणानामेवाभिव्यक्तिर्वासनानाम् ।८।

IV.8 tataḥ tadvipāka anuguṇānām eva abhivyaktiḥ vāsanānām

tataḥ	thence
tad	those impressions, their tendencies, potentialities
vipāka	ripening, fruition
anuguṇānām	correspondingly, accordingly
eva	only

abhivyaktiḥ manifestation
vāsanānām of desires, of tendencies

These three types of actions leave impressions which become manifest when conditions are favourable and ripe.

Of the four kinds of action, the first three leave behind potential residues which are accumulated as impressions in the memory. Memories create desires, and the results of desires in turn become memories. They move together and form latent impressions, which, according to their maturity, either manifest immediately or remain dormant, to appear unexpectedly later in this life or in future lives.

Desire is the motivating force which stimulates the body and mind and strives for fulfilment. Desires and their fulfilment bind consciousness to the threefold actions. Desire and memory compel the mind to act for their gratification, determining one's future class of birth, span of life, and the kinds of experiences to be undergone. If the impressions are good, they create situations favourable to spiritual life. Unfavourable impressions bind one to lust, anger, greed, infatuation, pride and envy, creating disturbances in the consciousness. But even then, if one turns one's consciousness towards the seer by sincerely and reverentially following the eightfold path of yogic discipline, one's actions will no longer be of the threefold type, but of the fourth, which do not give rise to desire for fruits or rewards. This is the literal meaning of *Yogaḥ karmasu kauśalam*, 'skill of yogic action'.

(See I.12, 43; II.12, 13, 28; III.18, 23 and 38.)

जातिदेशकालव्यवहितानामप्यानन्तर्यं स्मृतिसंस्कारयोरेकरूपत्वात् ।९।

IV.9 jāti deśa kāla vyavahitānām api ānantaryaṁ smṛti saṁskārayoḥ ekarūpatvāt

jāti class, lineage, descent, race, rank
deśa place, locality
kāla time, effect, point
vyavahitānām placed in between, separated, impeded, laid aside, surpassed, done well
api even

ānantaryaṁ	uninterrupted sequences, immediate succession
smṛti	memory
saṁskārayoḥ	potential, impressions
ekarūpatvāt	one in form, same in appearance, of common identity

Life is a continuous process, even though it is demarcated by race, place and time. Due to the uninterrupted close relationship between memory and subliminal impressions, the fruits of actions remain intact from one life to the next, as if there were no separation between births.

According to Indian philosophy, the law of *karma* functions uninterruptedly throughout successive lifetimes, though each life is separated by rank, place and time. Desires and impressions are stored in the memory and connect the behavioural patterns of previous lives with present and future lives.

The theory of *karma*, or the law of cause and effect, is explained to inspire the *sādhaka* to pursue non-white and non-black *karmas*, which will free him from the desires and results which are simply the accumulated actions of his previous lives. Such desireless actions culture and refine the consciousness and enable it to explore the kingdom of the soul. This is another aspect of *nirmāṇa citta*.

In the previous sūtra, the common identity of latent habitual impressions and memories is pointed out. Memories and impressions are interrelated, interconnected, interwoven. They act as stimuli in the present life. Even if previous lives are divided by social condition, status, time and place, the oneness of memory and impression flashes consciously, subconsciously or unconsciously and moulds the pattern of the present life. For example, if a man's life has taken shape after undergoing many lives in the form of other species, memory and impressions at once connect the past to the present life even though the interval between them may be a long one. We may therefore conclude that the seed of future lives is planted in the present life. 'As you sow, so shall you reap': we are responsible in this life for moulding our future lives.

The theory of *karma*, far from being a fatalistic theory of 'predestination', as many people misunderstand it to be, serves to make us aware of our responsibility and our power to affect the future course of our lives. It acts as a guide, inspiring us to perform virtuous actions which will gradually lead us towards the skill of performing desireless actions.

तासामनादित्वं चाशिषो नित्यत्वात् ।१०।

IV.10 tāsām anāditvaṁ ca āśiṣaḥ nityatvāt

tāsām	those memories and impressions
anāditvaṁ	without beginning, existing since eternity
ca	and
āśiṣaḥ	desires
nityatvāt	permanent, eternal

These impressions, memories and desires have existed eternally, as the desire to live is eternal.

Just as the universe is eternal, so are impressions and desires. They have existed from time immemorial. For one whose seeds of defects are eradicated, and whose desires have come to an end, the upheavals of the universe appear to have come to an end.

Nobody knows the timeless, primeval, absolute One, or when the world came into being. Both *puruṣa* and *prakṛti*, spirit and nature, existed before man appeared. When creation took place, man was endowed with consciousness, intelligence, mind, senses of perception, organs of action and body. At the same time the characteristics or qualities (*guṇas*) of nature, illumination (*sattva*), action (*rajas*) and inertia (*tamas*) entered man's body. Set on the wheel of time with the spokes of the *guṇas* of nature, man began to function in accordance with these three fundamental, intermingling qualities. Though born with a pure heart, he gradually became caught in the web of nature and fell prey to the polarities of pleasure and pain, good and evil, love and hatred, the permanent and transient. That is how desires (*vāsanā*) and imprints (*saṁskāra*) rooted themselves in man's life, and why this sūtra says that desires have existed from time immemorial.

Caught in these opposites, man felt the need of a personal divinity, unaffected by afflictions, untouched by actions and reactions, and free from the experience of joy and sorrow. This led to a search for the highest ideal embodied in *puruṣa*, or God. Through this search came culture, and then civilization. Man learned to distinguish between good and evil, virtue and vice, and what is moral and immoral. That is how yoga was discovered.

Through yoga *sādhana*, the desires that have existed since the beginning of time are eradicated so that *kaivalya* can be experienced.

In II.12, Patañjali explained that the causes of actions are hidden accumulated impressions of our past deeds. In this chapter he speaks of pure actions, which collect and store no imprints.

The essential nature of *citta* is tranquillity, *śānta citta*. When the *sādhaka* does not allow thought-waves to arise (*vyutthāna citta*), naturally there is no need for their restraint, *nirodha citta*. As both are filtered by *śānta citta*, the *sādhaka* dwells in this quiet state and does his duties. His actions are pure, and their outcome too will be pure (see IV.7).

Due to ignorance, joy and sorrow arise and intensify according to one's surroundings. If allowed free rein, they disturb the serene state of consciousness and the gates of *kaivalya* may remain closed forever. But one can sever the links of desires by developing the mind through the grace of yoga. As long as one practices yoga, one is free from desire. Devoted, life-long practice of yoga stops the wheel of desires, so that one lives in the state of poise and peace.

(See I.35; II.1, 9; III.51.)

हेतुफलाश्रयालम्बनैः संगृहीतत्वादेषामभावे तदभावः ।११।

IV.11 hetu phala āśraya ālambanaiḥ saṅgṛhītatvāt eṣām abhāve tad abhāvaḥ

hetu	cause, motive, impulse
phala	effect, fruit
āśraya	support, shelter, refuge, anything closely connected
ālambanaiḥ	dependent upon, resting upon, assistance, help
saṅgṛhītatvāt	held together
eṣām	of these
abhāve	in the absence of
tad	of them, of these
abhāvaḥ	disappearance

Impressions and desires are bound together by their dependence upon cause and effect. In the absence of the latter, the former too ceases to function.

Lack of understanding, *avidyā*, creates afflictions, which in turn create desires. This causes the cycle of rebirths. The accumulated impressions of memory are without beginning, but have a definite end provided the individual becomes cultured and discerning. When the formation of desire is kept in abeyance, the cycle of rebirths comes to an end.

The sight of an object creates motivation, which acts as a springboard for desire. Desire sustains motive, and motive ignites action aimed at fulfilment of the desire. This nourishes further desires which then lodge permanently in the seat of the consciousness, binding the soul forever.

Through regular, reverential practice of yoga, and the use of discriminative intelligence, this web of object, motivation, desire and reward is made to wither away. Then the pairs of opposites – vice and virtue, pain and pleasure, aversion and attachment – gradually fade and then disappear.

This brings sensitivity and refinement to the consciousness, which now avoids desires and thoughts of reward, and directs its attention towards the exploration of the seer.

(See I.4; II.3–9, 12–14, 18.)

अतीतानागतं स्वरूपतोऽस्त्यध्वभेदाद्धर्माणाम् ।१२।

IV.12 atīta anāgataṁ svarūpataḥ asti adhvabhedāt dharmāṇām

atīta	the past
anāgataṁ	the future
svarūpataḥ	in its true form, essential form, real nature
asti	exists
adhvabhedāt	condition being different
dharmāṇām	characteristics, inherent properties

The existence of the past and the future is as real as that of the present. As moments roll into movements which have yet to appear as the future, the quality of knowledge in one's intellect and consciousness is affected.

The understanding of time releases one from bondage. Time is a system revealing the sequential relation that one event has to another and another and so on, as past, present, or future. Time is regarded as an indefinite continuous duration in which events succeed one another.

The past and future are as real as the present. The orderly rhythmic procession of moments (*kṣaṇa cakra*) into movements is the wheel of time (*kāla cakra*). Its existence is real and eternal.

The present may fade into the past, or manifest clearly at a future time.

Due to the play of the *guṇas* of nature, conditions change, producing the illusion that time has changed.

Past and future are woven into the present, though they appear different due to the movement of moments.

Desire nourishes action aimed at its gratification. The intermission between desire, action and fulfilment involves time, which manifests as past, present and future. True understanding of motivation and the movement of moments releases a yogi from the knot of bondage.

Moment is changeless and eternal. Moments flow into movements eternally and are measurable as past, present and future. This measurable time is finite, when contrasted with eternity.

The negative effects of time are intellectual (lack of spiritual knowledge, *avidyā*, and pride, *asmitā*); emotional (attachment to pleasure, *rāga*, and aversion to pain, *dveṣa*); and instinctive (the desire to cling to life, *abhiniveśa*). Time's positive effect is the acquisition of knowledge. The experience of the past supports the present, and progress in the present builds a sound foundation for the future. One uses the past as a guide to develop discriminative power, alertness and awareness which smooth the path for Self-Realization. The yogi who studies in depth this unique rotation of time keeps aloof from the movement of moments; he rests in the present, at which crucial point desires are kept in abeyance. Thus he becomes clear of head, clean of heart, and free from time, which binds consciousness. When the conjunction between the movement of moments and consciousness terminates, freedom and beatitude, *kaivalya*, are experienced.

(See III.14, 16; IV.33.)

ते व्यक्तसूक्ष्मा गुणात्मानः ।१३।

IV.13 te vyakta sūkṣmāḥ guṇātmānaḥ

te	they (past, present and future)
vyakta	manifest
sūkṣmāḥ	subtle
guṇātmānaḥ	the nature of qualities

The three phases of time intermingle rhythmically and interweave with the qualities of nature. They change the composition of nature's properties into gross and subtle.

Desires, actions and rewards are not only entwined with the cycle of time but are composed and hidden according to the rhythmic movement of *sattva*, *rajas* and *tamas*. They may manifest and be brought to the surface, or remain hidden and emerge later.

Bound to the wheel of time by the *guṇas*, man started to form ideas fuelled by desires in the fire of consciousness. Then, through past actions and experiences, he began to mould his life in order to gain freedom from dualities. This involved time, which has no beginning or end, but is simply a succession of moments. Though each moment is eternal and real in its continuous flow, it changes into movement. To be free from the cycles of cause and effect, man has to mould his behaviour from moment to moment. The cause is subtle but the effect is felt. The effects of our actions of yesterday are the cause of today's; and the experience of our actions today becomes the seed of our actions tomorrow. All actions revolve around time and the qualities of nature.

A yogi has learned to weaken ignorance and increase the light of knowledge. He has moved from ignorance to knowledge, and darkness to light, from death to immortality. He alone knows how to live freely, unaffected by the onslaughts of nature. This is *kaivalya*.

(See II.18–19.)

परिणामैकत्वाद्वस्तुतत्त्वम् ।१४।

IV.14 pariṇāma ekatvāt vastutattvam

pariṇāma	change, alteration, modification, transformation, expansion
ekatvāt	due to oneness, on account of unity
vastu	object, thing, nature
tattvam	essence, real, abiding substance, essential property

Unity in the mutation of time caused by the abiding qualities of nature, sattva, rajas *and* tamas, *causes modifications in objects, but their unique essence, or reality, does not change.*

As there is a harmonious mutation between *sattva*, *rajas* and *tamas* (*prakāśa*, *kriyā* and *sthiti*), both in nature and in the individual self, so there are differences in the way we see objects. According to the predominating *guṇas* in one's intelligence, an object is perceived differently although its essence remains the same.

The yogi penetrates the harmonious combination of nature with its *guṇas*, understands clearly their mutations, and keeps aloof from them. This study helps him to remain in the essence of his object of contemplation which is not bound by time or by the qualities of nature. This object is the unchangeable seer, or the soul. The seer is not bound by time, whereas mind is.

This sūtra is a good guide for us. In our practice of *āsana* and *prāṇāyāma*, we are the subjects, the performers. The different *āsanas* and *prāṇāyāmas* are the objects which we try to perceive and conceive clearly, so as to understand their principles and essence. Due to our accumulated desires and impressions, our ways of thinking, seeing and feeling change. If we learn to observe carefully, and memorize the basic principles of every posture and every breathing practice, we will be able to grasp their true essence.

Truth is One, and we must experience it in its real essence, without distinctions. If it seems to vary, that is because our intelligence and perception vary, and this prevents us from seeing the essential truth. If intelligence and consciousness are filtered and refined, both subject and object retain and reflect their real essence.

When Patañjali says that dualities disappear when *āsanas* are performed perfectly (II.48), he is telling us that the essence of an object does not vary: subject and object merge into one, so distinctions between them do not arise. Similarly in *prāṇāyāma*, the veil that covers the intelligence is lifted, and subject and object reveal their true essence. This conclusion applies equally to the essence of all other objects.

(See II.18–19.)

वस्तुसाम्ये चित्तभेदात् तयोर्विभक्तः पन्थाः ।१५।

IV.15 vastusāmye cittabhedāt tayoḥ vibhaktaḥ panthāḥ

vastu	object
sāmye	being the same
citta	consciousness
bhedāt	being different
tayoḥ	theirs, of these two

vibhaktaḥ	different, divided, partitioned, separated, parted
panthāḥ	paths, ways of being

Due to the variance in the quality of mind-content, each person may view the same object differently, according to his own way of thinking.

The object (nature or *prakṛti*) is as real as the subject (*puruṣa*), but though the substance of nature or object remains the same, the perceptions of it vary according to the difference in the development of each person's consciousness.

Here, consciousness is the perceiver and the object perceived becomes the object to be known. On account of the wheel of time, substance and qualities of nature, and consciousness as perceiver develop differently in each individual. Though different perceivers see an object in different ways, it remains the same. For example, the same man or woman is a pleasure to a beloved or a lover and a pain to a rival. He or she may be an object of indifference to an ascetic and of no interest to a renunciate. Thus, the object is the same, the perceiver sees in the light of the interplay of the various guṇas.

In *āsana* and *prāṇāyāma*, owing to differences in one's constitution and frame of mind, techniques and sequences change, but not their essence. As soon as the consciousness is purified by removal of the impurity, *āsana* and *prāṇāyāma* disclose their essence. When an even balance is achieved, the essence of subject and object are revealed in their purest and truest forms.

When the yogi realizes that the perceiver in the form of consciousness is not the real perceiver but an instrument of its lord – the seer or *puruṣa* – it begins to discard its fluctuations and also its outer form, ego, so as to blend into a single unvacillating mind. This allows the single mind to merge in the seer, and the seer to shine forth in the light of the soul. This is *ātma jñāna*, leading to *Brahma jñāna*. (See I.41–43.)

न चैकचित्ततन्त्रं चेद्वस्तु तदप्रमाणकं तदा किं स्यात् ।१६।

IV.16 na ca ekacitta tantraṁ ced vastu tat apramāṇakaṁ tadā kiṁ syāt

na	not
ca	and
eka citta	one consciousness

tantraṁ	dependent
ced	it
vastu	object
tat	that
apramāṇakam	unobserved, unapproved, unrecognized
tadā	then
kiṁ	what
syāt	would happen

An object exists independent of its cognizance by any one consciousness. What happens to it when that consciousness is not there to perceive it?

The essence of an object is not dependent upon one's mind or consciousness. If the mind or consciousness does not recognize the object, it means that mind or consciousness does not see, or that the seer is not stimulated by, the object. But this does not mean that the object does not exist.

As *prakṛti* is as real and eternal as *puruṣa*, so are object and subject. Due to unripe intelligence and differences in the development of consciousness, each individual perceives objects according to his own intellectual 'wavelength', though their essence does not change. When a yogi reaches perfection in his *sādhana*, intelligence and consciousness touch the supreme knowledge: he becomes a fulfilled yogi, and remains merely an uninvolved witness of objects.

Man is a trinity of body, mind and soul. I have already shown that according to Indian philosophy, mind is treated as the eleventh sense. The five organs of action, five senses of perception and the mind are considered to be the eleven senses. Body, senses, mind, intelligence and self are interdependent: they are part of the cosmic consciousness (*mahat*), and susceptible to mutation and change, unlike the soul, which is changeless. The mind ignites stimuli in the senses of perception, or vice versa, and the organs of action participate so that the mind can experience objects. These experiences are imprinted according to the development of the mind, and in turn create impressions on the consciousness.

If an object does not stimulate the mind, it remains unperceived by the mind or the mind fails to grasp it. When the mind is freed from the play of the *guṇas*, it sees objects in their true reality, and remains free from impressions. Its contact with perceived objects is severed. Then mind and soul become one, and are one with the essence of all objects.

(See I.43; II.22; IV.22, 31, 32.)

तदुपरागापेक्षित्वाच्चित्तस्य वस्तु ज्ञाताज्ञातम् ॥१७॥

IV.17 taduparāga apekṣitvāt cittasya vastu jñāta ajñātam

tad	thereby
uparāga	conditioning, colouring
apekṣitvāt	expectation, hope, desire, want, need
cittasya	by the consciousness, for the consciousness
vastu	object
jñāta	known
ajñātam	unknown

An object remains known or unknown according to the conditioning or expectation of the consciousness.

Consciousness is not the seer, but an instrument of the seer. A conditioned mind can never perceive an object correctly. If the mind sees the object without expectation, it remains free.

An object is understood and known according to the expectation of the mind, or remains unrecognized owing to the absence of reflection. When the object attracts the mind, contact and reflection begin. This gives rise to knowledge. If the mind fails to come in contact with the object, it does not perceive it and the object remains unknown.

If consciousness is conditioned or coloured (see *vṛttis* and *kleśas* – I.6 and II.6), knowledge of the object also becomes coloured. When the consciousness reflects on the object without condition, taint or expectation, its real essence is known. Similarly, if the consciousness reflects on the essence of the seer without conditioning, bias, or prejudice, the mind becomes enlightened. It knows that it is not itself the seer, but only an instrument of the seer. The unenlightened mistake mind and consciousness for the seer.

(See I.2–4, 41; II.3, 12–14, 20.)

सदा ज्ञाताश्चित्तवृत्तयस्तत्प्रभोः पुरुषस्यापरिणामित्वात् ।१८।

IV.18 sadā jñātāḥ cittavṛttayaḥ tatprabhoḥ puruṣasya apariṇāmitvāt

sadā	always
jñātāḥ	known
citta vṛttayaḥ	fluctuations of the consciousness
tatprabhoḥ	of its lord
puruṣasya	of the soul
apariṇāmitvāt	an account of changelessness

Puruṣa *is ever illuminative and changeless. Being constant and master of the mind, he always knows the moods and modes of consciousness.*

The Lord of consciousness is the seer. He is changeless, constant, and never alters or falters.

In deep sleep, consciousness forgets itself. It is *puruṣa*, as a witness which reminds the mind of sleep after waking. This indicates that *puruṣa* is ever alert and aware (*sadā jñātā*). *Puruṣa*'s alertness will be known to the *sādhaka* only when consciousness is purified and freed from rising thoughts and their restraints. Then the *sādhaka*, the seeker, becomes the seer.

The seer knows his consciousness and its ramifications. He is the seed and root, and consciousness is the seedling. Its stem is the 'I' consciousness (*asmitā*), which branches forth as ego, intelligence and mind. The seer, being the seed and root of consciousness, observes the changes and transformations taking place in it.

(See II.17, 20, 22–24; IV.30.)

न तत् स्वाभासं दृश्यत्वात् ।१९।

IV.19 na tat svābhāsaṁ dṛśyatvāt

na	not
tat	that
svābhāsaṁ	self-illuminative
dṛśyatvāt	because of its knowability or perceptibility

Consciousness cannot illumine itself as it is a knowable object.

Consciousness can be seen as an object. It is knowable and perceptible. It is not self-illuminative like the seer.

Consciousness being the seedling of the seer, its growth and luminosity depend upon the seed, the light of the seer. Its own light is as that of the moon, which is reflected light from the sun. The seer represents the sun, and consciousness the moon. As a child feels strong and secure in the presence of its parents, consciousness, the child of the seer, draws its strength from the seer.

Consciousness, like the senses of perception, can normally see an object but not its own form. For an average person, the eyes pose as the seer when apprehending worldly objects. For an intellectual person, the eyes become the seen, and the mind the seer. For an enlightened person, mind and intelligence become objects for the consciousness. But for the wise seer, consciousness itself becomes the object perceived.

The seer can be subject and object at the same time; consciousness cannot. It may therefore be inferred that consciousness has no light of its own. When the borrowed light of consciousness is drawn back to its source, the seer, or soul, glows brilliantly.

(See II.19–20.)

एकसमये चोभयानवधारणम् ।२०।

IV.20 ekasamaye ca ubhaya anavadhāraṇam

ekasamaye	at the same time
ca	and
ubhaya	of both
anavadhāraṇam	cannot comprehend, cannot be held with affirmation or assurance

Consciousness cannot comprehend both the seer and itself at the same time.

It cannot comprehend subject–object, observer–observed, or actor–witness at the same time, whereas the seer can.

Day and night cannot exist simultaneously. Similarly, restlessness and restfulness cannot co-exist in absolute juxtaposition. In between night and day there is dawn. In the same way, there is space between the flow of restlessness, *cittavṛtti* or *cittavāhinī*, and restfulness, *praśānta vṛtti* or *praśānta vāhinī*. In between these two rivers of restlessness and restfulness, and underneath them, flows the concealed invisible secret river, the river of the soul. This is dawn, or the sudden arrival of enlightenment.

For a yogi, restlessness is the night and restfulness is the day. In between, there is a third state which is neither day nor night but dawn. It is the diffusion of consciousness, in which the rivers of restlessness and restfulness unite in the seat of absolute consciousness.

When the water of a lake is unruffled, the reflection of the moon on its surface is very clear. Similarly, when the lake of consciousness is serene, consciousness disseminates itself. This is known as a glimpse, or a reflection, of the soul.

The seer, being constant and unchangeable, can perceive the fluctuations as well as the serenity of his consciousness. If consciousness itself were self-luminous, it too could be the knower and the knowable. As it has not the power to be both, a wise yogi disciplines it, so that he may be alive to the light of the soul.

It is said in the *Bhagavad Gītā* (II.69) 'One who is self-controlled is awake when it appears night to all other beings, and what appears to him as night keeps others awake'. A yogic *sādhaka* thus realizes that when consciousness is active, the seer is asleep and when the seer is awake, it is night to the consciousness.

Similarly, in the *Haṭha Yoga Pradīpikā*, the word *ha* is used to signify the seer as the 'sun', which never fades; while *ṭha* represents consciousness as the 'moon', which eternally waxes and wanes.

(See I.2, 33, 38, 47; III.10.)

चित्तान्तरदृश्ये बुद्धिबुद्धेरतिप्रसङ्गः स्मृतिसंकरश्च ।२१।

IV.21 cittāntaradṛśye buddhibuddheḥ atiprasaṅgaḥ smṛtisaṅkaraḥ ca

citta	consciousness
antaradṛśye	being knowable by another
buddhibuddheḥ	cognition of cognitions
atiprasaṅgaḥ	impertinence, rudeness, abundance, too many, superfluity
smṛti	memory
saṅkaraḥ	confusion, commingling
ca	and

If consciousness were manifold in one's being, each cognizing the other, the intelligence too would be manifold, so the projections of mind would be many, each having its own memory.

Plurality of consciousness would result in lack of understanding between one mind and another, leading to utter confusion and madness. Patañjali therefore concludes that consciousness is one and cannot be many.

As a tree has many branches, all connected to the trunk, the various wavelengths of thoughts are connected to a single consciousness. This consciousness remains pure and divine at its source in the spiritual heart. When it branches from the source towards the head, it is called created consciousness, *nirmita citta*, which, being fresh, is untrained and uncultured. The moment it comes into contact with objects, it becomes tainted, creating moods in the thought-waves. These moods are the five fluctuations (*vṛttis*) and five afflictions (*kleśas*) (see I.6 and II.3).

The early commentators on Patañjali's *Yoga Sūtras* borrowed terms for the various modes of consciousness from Buddhist philosophy. They are discerning knowledge (*vijñāna*), perceptive knowledge of joys and sorrows (*vedana*), resolution (*saṁjñā*), likeness and semblance (*rūpa*) and impression (*saṁskāra*). All these are monitored by *nirmita citta*.

These moods should not be mistaken for a plurality of minds. The mind remains the same, but moods create an illusion of several minds. If the minds were really many, then each would have its own memory and intelligence. This becomes preposterous. Just as a room fitted with mirrors puzzles the onlooker, the idea of many minds causes confusion and absurdity.

The practice of yoga disciplines and cultures the consciousness of the head, by which it perfects the art of analysis (*savitarka*), judges precisely (*savicāra*), experiences unalloyed bliss (*ānanda*), becomes auspicious (*sāsmitā*) and moves towards mature intelligence (consciousness of the heart) and unalloyed wisdom (*ṛtambharā prajñā*).

The two facets of consciousness have been beautifully and poetically explained in the *Muṇḍakopaniṣad* (section 3, canto 1 and 2). Two birds sit together on a fig tree. One hops restlessly from branch to branch, pecking at different fruits which are variously sour, bitter, salty, and sweet. Not finding the taste it wants, it becomes more and more agitated, flying to ever more far-flung branches. The other remains impassive, steady, silent and blissful. Gradually the taster of fruits draws nearer to his quiet companion and, wearying of his frantic search, also becomes calm, unconsciously losing the desire for fruit, and experiencing non-attachment, silence, rest and bliss.

The yogi can learn from this. The tree represents the body, the two birds are the seer and consciousness, fruits are sprouted or secondary consciousness, and the different tastes of fruits are the five senses of perception which form the fluctuations and afflictions in the wavelengths of the mind.

The steady bird is the eternal, pure, divine, omniscient seer. The other is the sprouted or secondary consciousness absorbed in desire and fulfilment, and exhibiting different moods and modes of thought. After experiencing a variety of pain and pleasure, the secondary consciousness changes its mood and modes, identifies its true nature, reconsiders and returns to rest on its source mind. This return of the consciousness from the seat of the head towards the seat of the spiritual heart is purity of consciousness, *divya citta*. This is yoga.

(See I.4–6, 17, 48; II.3–4.)

चितेरप्रतिसंक्रमायास्तदाकारापत्तौ स्वबुद्धिसंवेदनम् ।२२।

IV.22 citeḥ apratisaṁkramāyāḥ tadākārāpattau svabuddhisaṁvedanam

citeḥ	the seer
apratisaṁkramāyāḥ	changeless, non-moving
tad	its
ākāra	form
āpattau	having accomplished, identified, assumed
sva	one's own
buddhi	intelligence
saṁvedanam	knows, assumes, identifies

Consciousness distinguishes its own awareness and intelligence when it reflects and identifies its source – the changeless seer – and assumes his form.

Through the accomplishment of pure consciousness comes knowledge of the unchangeable seer who rests on his own intelligence and nowhere else.

When consciousness no longer fluctuates, then its pure nature surfaces to comprehend itself. As stated in the commentary on IV.21, consciousness has two facets, one pure, divine and immutable, the other changeable, transient and exhibitive. It has no light of its own but acts as a medium or agent between the seer and the objects seen. Due to ignorance, it does not realize that it is impersonating the seer. But the seer knows the movements of the consciousness.

When one facet of consciousness ceases to operate, it ends its contact with the external world and stops collecting impressions. The other facet is drawn to the seer, and the two unite. Intelligence and consciousness merge in their abode – the *ātman*, and the soul comes face to face with itself.

A dirty mirror obscures reflection, a clean mirror reflects objects clearly. The illumined consciousness becomes purified and reflects objects exactly as they are. The reflector is called *biṁba-pratibiṁba vāda*, or the exposition of double reflection. There is no difference between the source object and the reflected image. The soul reflects the soul. It is the fulfilment of yoga. *Citta* is identified with the seer. This is *svabuddhi saṁvedanam* or intuitive understanding of the inner voice.

An everyday example of our consciousness taking on the absolute quality and form of the object we observe, is when we gaze into the dancing flames of a fire, or at the waves of the sea, or the wind in the tree-tops. We feel totally immersed in watching, without thought or impatience, as though we ourselves were the unending waves or the flickering flames, or the wind-swept trees.

द्रष्टृदृश्योपरक्तं चित्तं सर्वार्थम् ।२३।

IV.23 draṣṭṛ dṛśya uparaktaṁ cittaṁ sarvārtham

draṣṭṛ	the knower, the seer
dṛśya	the knowable, the seen
uparaktaṁ	coloured, reflected, tainted, afflicted
cittaṁ	consciousness
sarvārtham	all-pervading, cognizing, comprehending, apprehending

Consciousness, reflected by the seer as well as by the seen, appears to be all-comprehending.

Consciousness, being in conjunction both with the seer and the seen, appears to an average individual to be all-pervading, omniscient and real. When one is cultured and purified, one realizes that consciousness has no existence of its own but is dependent on the seer.

As the physical frame is the body of consciousness, so consciousness is the body of the seer. Consciousness is the bridge between nature and soul, and its conjunction is either illumined by the seer or tainted by the seen. The wise yogi frees consciousness from the qualities of nature; he keeps it clean so that it is reflected without distortion both by the seer and the seen.

When the waves of the sea subside, they lose their identities and become the sea. Similarly, when the waves of the seer – the senses of perception, mind, intelligence and consciousness – subside, they lose their identities and merge in the ocean of the seer, for the seer to blaze forth independently. This is the sight of the soul.

For a clearer understanding of consciousness, we should read sūtras IV.22–25 as a group.

In IV.22, Patañjali explains that consciousness is no longer a subject but an object. It is not a knower but the known. As it is trained by *sādhana* towards maturity (*paripakva citta*), it gains purity (*śuddha citta*) through pure intelligence (*śuddha buddhi*).

Until now, consciousness was under the impression that it was the reflector (*bimba*) and all other images were its reflected reflections (*pratibimba*). This sūtra explains that consciousness in its immature state takes itself to be all-powerful and all-pervading, but the truth is that the seer is actually the reflector. Patañjali shows that the impersonating consciousness is transformed to the level of the seen, so that both the reflector and its reflection, *citta*, are identical.

It is said in the *Bhagavad Gītā* (VI.19) that as a lamp in a windless place does not flicker, so the sheaths of a cultured yogi do not shake. They remain untouched by the wind of desires for the seer to reflect his own glorious light, *ātmajyoti*, and to dwell in that light, *puruṣa jñāna*.

(See I.41; II.18, 23; IV.4.)

तदसंख्येयवासनाभिश्चित्रमपि परार्थं संहत्यकारित्वात् ।२४।

IV.24 tat asaṅkhyeya vāsanābhiḥ citram api parārthaṁ saṁhatyakāritvāt

tat	that
asaṅkhyeya	innumerable
vāsanābhiḥ	knowledge derived from memory, impressions, desires, trust
citram	variegated, filled with, equipped
api	although
parārthaṁ	for the sake of another
saṁhatya	well knitted, firmly united, closely allied
kāritvāt	on account of it, because of it

Though the fabric of consciousness is interwoven with innumerable desires and subconscious impressions, it exists for the seer on account of its proximity to the seer as well as to the objective world.

Though consciousness has been clouded with impressions (*saṁskāras*) throughout eternity, its aim is not only to satisfy the desires of the senses (*bhoga*) but also to further the emancipation (*apavarga*) of the soul.

Consciousness is tied by a hidden force both to the seer and to nature. It is well equipped to reach the seer, though it has no ambition of its own except to serve its Lord.

Consciousness has innumerable tendencies and impressions derived from memory, among which longing for pleasures and freedom from pleasures stand out. They are desired impressions. From this, it becomes clear that consciousness, being close to nature and spirit, feels that it does not exist for its own sake but for the sake of *puruṣa* and *prakṛti*. In the same way that a lover of God offers food, clothes and comforts as if they were essential to God, consciousness wants to satisfy its Lord with the pleasures of the world. Once consciousness is cultured through yogic discipline, it becomes ripe and illumined. It realizes that the seer is not interested in objects of pleasure and opts to serve with detachment. Now that it understands its inner value, it realizes the triviality of nature's pleasures and turns towards the path of Self-Realization. Thus transformed, it begins its journey towards emancipation.

If one's *karmas* are good, they awaken curiosity and guide it towards the path of *kaivalya*; they reward one's effort with the vision of the soul. Yogic practices speed up this process, beginning with the conquest of the body and ending in the vision of the soul. This is salvation.

(See I.41; II.18–19; 22–23; IV.18, 27.)

विशेषदर्शिन आत्मभावभावनानिवृत्तिः ।२५।

IV.25 viśeṣadarśinaḥ ātmabhāva bhāvanānivṛttiḥ

viśeṣa	distinction, specific quality, peculiarity
darśinaḥ	to whom, who sees, the seer
ātmabhāva	the ideas of the seer, the thought of the seer
bhāvanā	feeling, reflection
nivṛttiḥ	return, disappearance, emancipation

For one who realizes the distinction between citta *and* ātmā, *the sense of separation between the two disappears.*

When the difference between consciousness (*citta*) and the projector of the consciousness (*citi*) is recognized, the search for Self-Realization ends.

From IV.15 to IV.25, Patañjali takes the *sādhaka* progressively to the realization that consciousness is not the all-knower, but simply an instrument of the soul.

For one who is not sure of the difference between consciousness and soul (*citta* and *citi*), an analogy is given; the blades of grass which shoot up during the rainy season prove the existence of the hidden seeds.

In this sūtra Patañjali explains that the seed of the soul (*ātma bīja*) is sown at the right time for the knowledge of the soul (*ātma jñāna*) to be firmly established. As we mistake a rope for a snake at first glance, but realize that upon examination that it is a rope, consciousness at this stage realizes that it is not all-knowing but an instrument of the soul. *Avidyā* is vanquished and the practitioner thoroughly understands objective as well as subjective knowledge, without colourization. Here all moods and modes cease to flow, and consciousness is elevated to the optimum degree to behold the exalted state of the seer. The yogi is no longer drawn towards the temptations of the world. His search for the self ends. He becomes a master of yoga and a master of himself. He is *yogeśvara*. This is the substance (*svarūpa*) of yoga and a distinct attribute of the seer (*viśeṣa darśinaḥ*).

(See I.47; II.10, 12; III.56.)

तदा विवेकनिम्नं कैवल्यप्राग्भारं चित्तम् ।२६।

IV.26 tadā vivekanimnaṁ kaivalya prāgbhāraṁ cittam

tadā	then
vivekanimnaṁ	flow of exalted intelligence in consciousness
kaivalya	indivisible state of existence, emancipation
prāg	towards
bhāraṁ	gravitation, influence, importance
cittam	consciousness

Then consciousness is drawn strongly towards the seer or the soul due to the gravitational force of its exalted intelligence.

When the exalted intelligence is ablaze, consciousness is illumined; it becomes free and tinged with the divine (*citta śuddhi*). Due to this divine light, *citta*, with its exalted intelligence, is drawn as if by a magnet towards its source: the indivisible seer who is alone, free and full.

Before reaching the state of exalted intelligence, consciousness is attracted more towards the pleasures of the world. When intelligence is free from doubts and prejudices, it gravitates towards the absolute seer.

As a farmer builds dykes between his fields to regulate the flow of water, exalted intelligence builds a dyke for the consciousness, so that it does not move again towards the world, but turns and flows towards union with the divine seer. This is *kaivalya*, an existence filled with freedom and beatitude. Such a yogi becomes a king amongst men.

Here, I should like to draw the reader's attention to Patañjali's use of the word 'gravitation', showing that in his day science was not behind modern western scientific thought; indeed, it may have been its precursor.

(See I.49; II.25–26; III.55 and IV.29.)

तच्छिद्रेषु प्रत्ययान्तराणि संस्कारेभ्यः ।२७।

IV.27 tat cchidreṣu pratyayāntarāṇi saṁskārebhyaḥ

tat	that
cchidreṣu	a hole, slit, pore, fissure, defect, rent, flaw, fault, opening
pratyaya	going towards, belief, firm conviction, trust, reliance, confidence, content, notion
antarāṇi	interval, space, intermission
saṁskārebhyaḥ	from impression

Notwithstanding this progress, if one is careless during the interval, a fissure arises due to past hidden impressions, creating division between the consciousness and the seer.

The force of past impressions may create loopholes in the form of intellectual pride or other varying moods or modes of thought, which breach the consciousness and disturb the harmony and serenity of oneness with the pure Self (*ātmabhāva*).

This sūtra shows a way to combat old impressions which may influence the consciousness and fissure it.

Patañjali cautions that even for the supreme intelligence, the subconscious *samskāras* may surface in this intermediate stage and sway the consciousness.

Patañjali advises yogis who wish to be free from worldly life to be constantly vigilant in order to overcome these old habits, lest their consciousness waver between the desire for perfection and actual perfection. The uninterrupted practice of yoga unconditionally vanquishes these fissures in consciousness, and eradicates doubts and prejudices, so that pure wisdom may shine.

(Consciousness in evolved souls is dealt with in I.18, wherein the yogi is on the threshold of *sabīja* and *nirbīja samādhis*.)

In the *Bhagavad Gītā* II.59, Lord Kṛṣṇa says that inherent desire persists as a fissure even in the most austere renunciate. Only the vision of the Supreme resolves these latent faults forever. From that moment no worldly desire or temptation can endanger the equanimity and virtue of the yogi.

(See I.50; III.55–56.)

हानमेषां क्लेशवदुक्तम् ।२८।

IV.28 hānam eṣāṁ kleśavat uktam

hānam	abandonment, extinction, harm, deficiency, damage
eṣāṁ	of these
kleśavat	afflictions
uktam	uttered, spoken, said

In the same way as the sādhaka strives to be free from afflictions, the yogi must handle these latent impressions judiciously to extinguish them.

The gap between consciousness and the seer can breed disharmony and disturbance in one's self. As fire is deprived of fuel, the yogi has to remove the latent impressions from the consciousness and extinguish them, for it to be in harmony with the seer.

Patañjali advises the yogi to eradicate disturbances by reintroducing yogic disciplines with faith, vigour and vitality. As the *sādhaka* earlier strove to rid himself of the afflictions of *avidyā*, *asmitā*, *rāga*, *dveṣa* and *abhiniveśa*, the exalted yogi must, through practice, press, dry out and close the perforations in the consciousness.

IV.27 stated that subconscious impressions surface in the form of intellectual pride, which hinders progress towards the goal of union with the divine seer. As roasted seeds do not germinate, so the fire of wisdom must burn out impressions and ambitions, ending their power to generate disturbing thoughts so that the consciousness maintains its union with the seer forever.

प्रसंख्यानेऽप्यकुसीदस्य सर्वथा विवेकख्यातेर्धर्ममेघः समाधिः ।२९।

IV.29 prasaṁkhyāne api akusīdasya sarvathā vivekakhyāteḥ dharmameghaḥ samādhiḥ

prasaṁkhyāne	highest form of intelligence, evolution, enumeration, reflection, deep meditation
api	even
akusīdasya	free from desires and aversions, one who has no selfish interest or motivation
sarvathā	constant, wholly, entirely, at all times
vivekakhyāteḥ	with awareness, discrimination and attentive intelligence
dharmameghaḥ	rain cloud of virtue, delightful fragrant virtue, rain cloud of justice, showering of *dharma*
samādhiḥ	supreme spirit, union putting together

The yogi who has no interest even in this highest state of evolution, and maintains supreme attentive, discriminative awareness, attains dharmameghaḥ samādhi: *he contemplates the fragrance of virtue and justice.*

When the stream of virtue pours in torrents and the consciousness is washed clean of bias, prejudice and ambition, the light of the soul dawns. This is *dharma megha samādhi*: the fruit of the practice of yoga.

If the yogi, knowing that the highest form of intelligence is also a hindrance, remains uninterested even in this enlightened wisdom as well as in spiritual attainments, virtuousness descends upon him like torrential rain, washing away his individual personality. His only ambition now is to sustain spiritual health. He has purity and clarity. His personality has been transformed. He becomes humane, universal and divine. He lives forever in *dharma megha samādhi**, unsurpassed bliss.

He has renounced everything, and is a *viveki* (one who distinguishes the invisible soul from the visible world), a *jñānin* (sage), a *vairāgin* (renunciate), and a *bhaktan* (divine devotee). Now he has attained *nirbīja samādhi.*

(See I.16, 49–50; III.50, 55–56.)

* A cloud has two facets. It may cover the sky without bringing rain. This makes the atmosphere gloomy and people become inactive and dull. But if the cloud bursts into rain, the atmosphere is cleared, the sun shines, and people go out to work joyfully.

Similarly, the yogi should not make the consciousness quiet in a *tāmasic* way, but in an alert, *sāttvic* way to shine forth brilliantly to live in the delightful, fragrant rain-cloud of virtue.

ततः क्लेशकर्मनिवृत्तिः ।३०।

IV.30 tataḥ kleśa karma nivṛttiḥ

tataḥ	thereafter, thence
kleśa	afflictions
karma	action
nivṛttiḥ	return, disappear, abstaining from action, cessation from worldly concerns and being engaged in the field of emancipation, bliss and beatitude

Then comes the end of afflictions and of karma.

The effect of *dharma megha samādhi* is freedom, freedom from the five afflictions and fluctuations. It is the highest form of intelligence and evolution.

From this rain-cloud of virtue, afflictions cease of their own accord and in their place, divine actions with no reactions flow forth like a river from the yogi. This is freedom.

Avidyā, the mother of afflictions, is eradicated, root and branch, along with residual subliminal impressions. The *sādhaka* will not now deviate from the path of divinity nor perform an act that binds, hinders or preconditions his consciousness. He is free from the bondage of *karma*.

In the *Bhagavad Gītā* (VI.5), Lord Kṛṣṇa says that each individual has to cultivate himself to become enlightened, and to learn not to degrade himself, for the Self alone is the friend of the individual self, and the Self alone is the enemy of the egotistical self.

As the light of a lamp fades as the oil runs out, so the lamp of the mind is extinguished as its fuel, the actions producing joys and sorrows, is exhausted.

As *nirmāṇa citta* is extinguished of its own accord, its root motivation is burnt out leaving no opportunity for the production of effects. The cycle of cause and effect is at an end, and the yogi is freed from the grip of nature. Even in this liberated state, he will not forego his practices. He will continue to maintain them as a divine command, so that the freedom earned may not be lost by neglect*.

(See I.3–5, 47; II.12, 20–21, 24, 52; III.55–56; IV.3, 4 and 25.)

* In II.16, Patañjali spoke of avoidable future pains. There, he urged the *sādhaka* to train his intelligence through right understanding and cultivation of right action from the moment he begins yoga. In this sūtra, as the consciousness has been fully ripened, he cautions the yogi that if fissures are formed in the *citta*, afflictions will affect him instantaneously and not at a future time.

तदा सर्वावरणमलापेतस्य ज्ञानस्यानन्त्याज्ज्ञेयमल्पम् ।३१।

IV.31 tadā sarva āvaraṇa malāpetasya jñānasya ānantyāt jñeyam alpam

tadā	then
sarva	all
āvaraṇa	veil, covering, concealing, surrounding, enclosing, interrupting
mala	impurities
āpetasya	devoid of, bereft of, deprived of, removed
jñānasya	of knowledge
ānantyāt	because of infinity
jñeyam	the knowable
alpam	small, little, trivial

Then, when the veils of impurities are removed, the highest, subjective, pure, infinite knowledge is attained, and the knowable, the finite, appears as trivial.

The stream of virtue eradicates all the veils of impurities. The yogi is devoid of doubts, preconceptions and prejudices. The infinite light of the soul illumines him continuously, and his consciousness and the seer become one. For him, knowledge gained through the organs of cognition and through consciousness are insignificant compared with the infinite wisdom emanating from the soul.

This sūtra describes the characteristics of the yogi who is devoid of afflicting actions. His head becomes clear and his heart clean and pure as crystal.

When the clouds disperse, the sky becomes clear. When the sun is bright, no other light is required. When the light of the soul blazes, the yogi does not need mind or intelligence to develop knowledge.

His knowledge springs eternally from the seed of all knowledge (*ātman*) as *jñāna gaṅgā* (perennial river of wisdom), and he perceives directly. He has reached the state of fulfilment.

(See I.3, 47; II.22, 52; III.49, 56.)

ततः कृतार्थानां परिणामक्रमसमाप्तिर्गुणानाम् ।३२।

IV.32 tataḥ kṛtārthānāṁ pariṇāmakrama samāptiḥ guṇānām

tataḥ	thence, by that
kṛtārthānāṁ	having fulfilled their duties
pariṇāmȧ	change, alteration, transformation, expansion
krama	regular process, course, order, service, succession
samāptiḥ	the end
guṇānām	qualities of nature, *sattva*, *rajas* and *tamas*

When dharmameghaḥ samādhi *is attained, qualities of nature* (guṇas) *come to rest. Having fulfilled their purpose, their sequence of successive mutations is at an end.*

Having transformed the yogi's consciousness by the radiation of the rays of the soul, the orderly mutations and rhythmic sequences of the qualities of nature, *sattva*, *rajas* and *tamas* come to an end. Their tasks are fulfilled, and they return to nature.

The essence of intelligence and the essence of consciousness both now retire to rest in the abode of the soul. The master, the seer or the soul, is independent. He keeps the *guṇas* in abeyance, or uses them when necessary. They willingly serve him as devoted servants, without influencing him as before, and without interfering in his true glory.

(See II.18, 22–24.)

क्षणप्रतियोगी परिणामापरान्तनिर्ग्राह्यः क्रमः ।३३।

IV.33 kṣaṇa pratiyogī pariṇāma aparānta nirgrāhyaḥ kramaḥ

kṣaṇa	moments
pratiyogī	uninterrupted sequences, corresponding to, related to, co-operating with, equally matched, counteracting
pariṇāma	change, transformation, alteration, expansion

aparānta	at the end
nirgrāhyaḥ	distinctly recognizable, entirely apprehensible, entirely comprehensible
kramaḥ	regular process, course, order, series, succession

As the mutations of the guṇas *cease to function, time, the uninterrupted movement of moments, stops. This deconstruction of the flow of time is comprehensible only at this final stage of emancipation.*

The sequence of time is related to the order of movements of the *guṇas* of nature. Only the yogi recognizes this inter-relationship and is free from *guṇas*.

The uninterrupted succession of moments is called time. These movements of moments and the uninterrupted mutation of the *guṇas* of nature are distinctly recognizable at the culminating point of transformation.

The average person is not aware of moments: he understands their movement as past, present and future. When moments slip away from one's awareness, one lives in movements. Memory begins to exert its influence, and consciousness is felt at this juncture in the movements of time.

The perfect yogi lives in the moment without getting involved in movements: the movements of moments are arrested, and psychological and chronological time come to an end. Living in the moment, the yogi sees the seer. This is evolution. Nature eternally helps the intelligence and consciousness towards evolution (*pariṇāma nityan*), while the seer remains eternally changeless (*kūṭastha nityan*). (See IV.21 with reference to the *Muṇḍakopaniṣad*. The first bird, as seer, was called *kūṭastha nityan* as it remained steady and still; the other, as consciousness (*pariṇāma nityan*) was constantly moving in the effort to reach the first one.)

Evolution takes place in a moment. Moment implies instant while movement implies time. When change comes, it arrives at once in a moment, only after a series of efforts involving movements of time. Transformation does not come without effort. As change is noticeable to an average individual, so the end transformation is distinguishable to a yogi by virtue of his pure wisdom: *dharma megha samādhi*. He is free from time, place and space while others remain trapped in this net. He is neither attracted towards nature nor disturbed by it. He is now a divine yogi.

(See II.18; III.13, 15, 53.)

पुरुषार्थशून्यानां गुणानां प्रतिप्रसवः कैवल्यं स्वरूपप्रतिष्ठा वा चितिशक्तिरिति ।३४।

IV.34 puruṣārtha śūnyānāṁ guṇānāṁ pratiprasavaḥ kaivalyaṁ svarūpapratiṣṭhā vā citiśaktiḥ iti

puruṣārtha	fourfold aims of man; discharging one's duties and obligations to oneself, one's family, society and country (*dharma*); pursuit of vocation or profession, following one's means of livelihood and acquisition of wealth (*artha*); cultured and artistic pursuits, love and gratification of desires (*kāma*); emancipation or liberation from worldly life (*mokṣa*)
śūnyānām	devoid of
guṇānāṁ	of the three fundamental qualities
pratiprasavaḥ	involution, re-absorption, going back into the original form
kaivalyaṁ	liberation, emancipation, beatitude
svarūpa	in one's own nature
pratiṣṭhā	establishment, installation, consecration, completion
vā	or
citiśaktih	the power of pure consciousness
iti	that is all

Kaivalya, *liberation, comes when the yogi has fulfilled the* puruṣārthas, *the fourfold aims of life, and has transcended the* guṇas. *Aims and* guṇas *return to their source, and consciousness is established in its own natural purity.*

The yogi with the stream of virtuous knowledge is devoid of all aims of life as he is free from the qualities of nature. *Puruṣārthas* are man's four aims in life: *dharma* (science of duty), *artha* (purpose and means of life), *kāma* (enjoyments of life) and *mokṣa* (freedom from worldly pleasures). They leave the fulfilled seer and merge in nature.

Patañjali speaks of the *purusārthas* only in the very last sūtra. This may puzzle the aspirant. Patañjali is an immortal being who accepted human incarnation with its joys and sorrows, attachments and aversions, in order to live through emotional upheavals and intellectual weaknesses to help us to overcome these obstacles and guide us to freedom. Awareness of the aims of life may have been unconsciously hidden in his heart, to surface only at the end of his work. But his thoughts on the *puruṣārthas* are implicitly contained in the earlier chapters, and expressed clearly at the end. So I feel that the four *pādas* are, consciously or unconsciously, founded on these four aims and stages of activity.

The first *pāda* deals with *dharma*, the science of disciplining the fluctuations of the consciousness. For this reason, it begins with the code of conduct, *Yogānuśāsanam*. The second *pāda* gives detailed information regarding this practice and the purpose (*artha*) behind this discipline. Here, the purpose of yoga is physical health and contentment so that one may enjoy the pleasures of the world or seek emancipation (see II.18). The third *pāda* explains the hidden wealth in the form of extraordinary powers which come through yogic practices, tempting one to make use of them for worldly joys (*kāma*) rather than for spiritual purposes. The fourth *pāda* speaks of cultivating actions which cannot produce reactions, and of renouncing the attractions of yogic powers, so that consciousness may dissolve in the light of the soul (*mokṣa*) for the very Being to shine forth.

As Patañjali ends his work with *mokṣa*, the culmination of the four aims, it is perhaps worth considering the social, cultural and civic conditions of his time which still apply to our lives today. The yogis and sages of India formulated ways and means for creating a harmonious and peaceful life by classifying men's minds according to their avocations (*varṇas*), their stages of life (*āśramas*) and their aims in life (*puruṣārthas*).

Lord Kṛṣṇa says in the *Bhagavad Gītā* (IV.13) that men are born according to their acquired moral, mental, intellectual and spiritual growth. These are known as duties of communities (*varṇa dharma*). Varṇa is the psychological characteristic of man according to his words, thoughts and deeds. The word means colour, cover, abode, sort, kind and quality. The four orders are divided according to man's different stages of evolution; they are *brāhmaṇa* (priestly class), *kṣatriya* (warrior class), *vaiśya* (merchant class), and *śūdra* (working class). In the civic sense, they are divisions of labour and not a rigid caste system as they are often held to be.

Again, according to the *Bhagavad Gītā* (XVIII.40–44), 'serenity, faith, self-restraint, austerity, purity, forbearance, uprightness and knowledge to lead a pure and divine life' are said to be the characteristics of a *brāhmaṇa*. A *brāhmaṇa* is one who knows about the Self (*puruṣa*), and has understood and realized the divinity in himself.

'Heroism, vigour, firmness, resourcefulness, generosity, fighting for the right and upholding justice to maintain truth' are the allotted functions of a *kṣatriya*.

'One who cultivates, tends and looks after the needs of society, conserves, is thrifty and frugal, but struggles to earn wisdom and virtue according to his mental capacity' is a *vaiśya*; while one 'who is servile, a sycophant, submissive and labours hard', is a *śūdra*.

These mental characteristics consciously or unconsciously exist even today in all types of vocation. Here is an example of this, applied to yogic discipline. In the beginning of practice, it is a great struggle and effort and one has to sweat profusely in body and brain to get a grasp of it. It is almost like manual labour. This is *śūdra dharma.*

The second stage of evolution in yogic practice begins when one consciously sets out to accumulate experience in order to teach, so as to earn a living. This is *vaiśya dharma.*

When one builds up courage and becomes firm in striving further to develop skill and mastery over the subject, then one gains the authority to share one's knowledge and experience and to maintain and uphold the subtle refinements of the art. Then one's *sādhana* is that of the *kṣatriya.*

If one further proceeds in his practices in order to experience the indivisible, exalted and absolute state of Being (*jīvātman*) which is the body of the Universal Spirit (Paramātman), and surrenders to Him in word, thought and deed, one is a *brāhmaṇa* in yogic *sādhana.* This is the religious fervour of yoga – the aim of each practitioner.

Man's life is similarly divided into four stages of development. They are that of the student (*brahmacaryāśrama*), the ordinary householder (*gṛhastāśrama*), the householder who begins to learn non-attachment (*vānaprasthāśrama*), and finally that of the man detached from worldly thoughts and attached to God (*sannyāsāśrama*). The hundred-year span of man's life is divided into four parts, each of 25 years, so that one may adjust one's life to evolve through these fourfold stages and fourfold objectives of life towards the experience of True Being.

The aims (*puruṣārthas*) are *dharma*, *artha*, *kāma* and *mokṣa.*

Dharma is the careful observation of one's ethical, social, intellectual and religious duties in daily life. Strictly speaking this is taught at the level of studentship, but it must be followed throughout life; without this religious quality in daily life, spiritual attainment is not possible.

Artha is acquisition of wealth in order to progress towards higher pursuits of life including understanding the main purpose of life. If one does not earn one's own way, dependence on another will lead to a parasitic life. One is not meant to be greedy while accumulating wealth, but only to meet one's needs, so that one's body is kept nourished so that one may be free from worries and anxieties. In this stage one also finds a partner with whom to lead a householder's life. One comes to understand human love through individual friendship and compassion, so that one may later develop a universal fellowship leading to the realization of divine love. The householder is expected to fulfil his responsibilities of bringing up his children and helping his fellow men. Therefore, married life has never been considered a hindrance to happiness, to divine love or to the union with the Supreme Soul.

Kāma means enjoyment of the pleasures of life provided one does not lose physical health, or harmony and balance of mind. The Self cannot be experienced by a weakling, and the body, the temple of the soul, has to be treated with care and respect. *Āsana*, *prāṇāyāma* and *dhyāna*, therefore, are essential to purify the body, stabilize the mind and clarify the intelligence. One must learn to use the body as a bow, and *āsana*, *prāṇāyāma* and *dhyāna* as arrows to be aimed at the target – the seer or the soul.

Mokṣa means liberation, freedom from the bondage of worldly pleasures. It is the experience of emancipation and beatitude, possible only when one is free from physical, psychological, intellectual and environmental afflictions (see I.30–31), and from poverty, ignorance and pride. In this state one realizes that power, knowledge, wealth and pleasure are merely passing phases. Each individual has to work hard to free himself from the qualities of nature (*guṇas*) in order to master them and become a *guṇātītan*. This is the very essence of life, a state of indivisible, infinite, full, unalloyed bliss.

These aims involve virtuous actions and are linked with the qualities of nature and the growth of consciousness. When the goal of freedom is attained, the restricting qualities of consciousness and nature cease to exist. At this point of fulfilment, the yogi realizes that the seeker, the seer and the instrument used to cognize the seer is *ātman*. This absoluteness of consciousness is nothing but the seer. Now, he is established in his own nature. This is *kaivalyāvasthā*.

The practice of yoga serves all aims of life. Through the proper use of the organs of action, senses of perception, mind, ego, intelligence and consciousness, their purpose of serving their Lord, the seer, comes to an end, and these vestments of the seer, along with the qualities of nature, involute and withdraw, to merge in the root of nature (*mūla-prakṛti*).

There, they are held and isolated. By this, the *citta* becomes pure and supreme. In this supreme state, *citta* divinely merges in the abode of the seer so that the seer can shine forth in his pristine, pure and untainted state of aloneness. Now, the yogi shines as a king amongst men. He is crowned with spiritual wisdom. He is a *kṛtārthan*, a fulfilled soul, who has learned to control the property of nature. He brings purity of intelligence (see III.56) into himself. He is now free from the rhythmic mutation of *guṇas*, of time, and thus free from aims and objects as his search for the soul ends. All the twenty-four principles of nature (see II.19) move back into nature and the twenty-fifth, the seer, stands alone, in *kaivalya*. He is one without a second, he lives in benevolent freedom and beatitude. With this power of pure consciousness, *citta śakti*, he surrenders completely to the seed of all seers, *Paramātmā* or God.

Lord Kṛṣṇa, in the *Bhagavad Gītā* XVIII.61–62, explains that 'the Supreme Ruler abides in the hearts of all beings and guides them, mounting them on wheels of knowledge for spiritual evolution'. He says: 'one who has earned this divine knowledge should seek refuge by surrendering all actions as well as himself to the Supreme Spirit or God', so that he journeys from Self-Realization towards God-Realization.

Patañjali began the journey towards the spiritual kingdom with the word *atha* meaning 'now'. He ends with the word *iti*, meaning 'that is all'. The yogi has reached his goal.

Here ends the exposition of *kaivalya*, the fourth *pāda* of Patañjali's *Yoga Sūtras*.

Epilogue

Here end the *Yoga Sūtras* of Patañjali, the greatest thinker India has ever known, speaking to us across the ages, at a time when mankind, with its technical and social progress, and its paucity of human and spiritual values, is at a crossroads.

With the ending of the sūtras comes the hope of a new beginning, a new age, a rekindling of interest in Patañjali's universal philosophy, which aims for the good of all mankind.

My words would indeed be in vain if, towards the end of this century, yoga had not become so resoundingly successful, and so widely practised. But yoga is no longer regarded as a 'fringe' subject merely for the elite few, though it deals in transcendentals. It is not a will-o'-the-wisp theory, but tangible, scientific and of proven value. The flame of yoga has lighted for *sādhakas* all over the world the way to physical health, mental strength and spiritual growth.

India is believed to be the mother of civilization. Patañjali is known as the father of yoga. In our own invocatory prayers, we call him a patriarch, spiritual father of many generations, and a revered sage.

His *Yoga Sūtras* is a concise work, eloquent in style, with a minimum of words and an unparalleled wealth of meaning.

The sūtras are terse. Yet they are full of gems of wisdom on which to ponder and by which to live. Patañjali has studied the human condition in depth and shown why man suffers, and how he may overcome his sufferings – how each of us can lead a fuller and happier life.

He was the analyst of consciousness, and its various states and moods. His methodology proves an original mind, a clear, penetrating intellect and an astounding analytical ability.

He offers us a total model of consciousness, both in its internal and external aspects; how it turns outwards, how it turns inwards, and how it may repose quietly within itself. He offers us a clear explanation of the natural and physical world wherever it relates to consciousness, sense awareness and human action. He offers a graduated method of evolution and transcendence of consciousness. He describes differences between individuals according to the three qualities of nature, and explains how each one, according to his aptitude and state of intelligence, may integrate himself through the quest for freedom. Interestingly, he does not consider people to be fundamentally different at heart. He leads us from the particular and differentiated to the Absolute and Indivisible.

Yet, he is not a dry psychologist or philosopher. He leads us not into the labyrinthine ramifications of the mind and consciousness but into our inner selves, where we may seek shelter and peace. This peace is eternally present in the core of our being, waiting for us, guiding us, sometimes hidden, sometimes chiding, sometimes welcoming. We find this inner peace through our yoga practice.

Patañjali does not omit India's unique traditional contribution to human upliftment, the techniques of *āsana* and *prāṇāyāma* which play their role in bringing about the states of *pratyāhāra, dhāraṇā, dhyāna* and *samādhi*, after the firm foundation has been laid through *yama* and *niyama*. A life which does not include these becomes mechanical, theoretical and static.

The *Yoga Sūtras* are set in a universal context as a guide to human existence, valid for all. Doesn't everyone seek to avoid pain and find pleasure? Patañjali's pedagogical method is uniquely practical: he provides a minimum of 'what' and a maximum of 'how'. He shows us, step by step, how to grow from our life's afflictions towards freedom. Reading and re-reading the sūtras, we notice how often he throws out a lifeline, so that everyone may catch it somewhere. Each chapter explains, sheds light on and integrates the other chapters.

Senses and mind are brought under control by practice. Through practice we overcome afflictions and develop stability and mature intelligence. Through mature intelligence comes renunciation. Patañjali is totally impartial in exploring how one succeeds or why one fails. 'Do this', he says 'and you will see for yourself.' He promises us no material rewards; the most alluring prizes are to be shunned.

Whether or not we reach the goal in this life, the journey in yoga to self-culture is itself worth the effort: we all want refinement in our intelligence and progress in our way of thinking. As we end the *kaivalya pāda*, our lasting impression is of light, fragrance, clarity, simplicity, and unrelenting resolve. Though Patañjali is an austere teacher, he is a wholly compassionate guide, always at our elbow.

Ultimately, the yoga system of Patañjali cannot be compared to other traditional or modern structures of thought, knowledge or wisdom. His work has absolute integrity and permanence and is not to be judged from the outside. Only the practitioner, if he practises with faith and renounces with love, will discover its truth.

If we follow Patañjali's teachings meticulously and diligently, and contemplate their inner meaning in the depths of our own inner selves, we will learn to understand both ourselves and others in a new light. Let us now briefly summarize how this comes about.

According to yoga, there are three qualities of nature (*guṇas*) which permeate the mind (*manas*), the intelligence (*buddhi*) and the consciousness (*citta*). Intelligence may in turn be categorized in three tiers – subtle (*sūkṣma*), subtler (*ati sūkṣma*) and the most subtle (*parama sūkṣma*). These can be interpreted as being 'average, sharp and intensely sharp' intellectual sensitivities.

Patañjali thus defines various states of intelligence and awareness of consciousness, so that one who practises yoga will be able to recognize his level of personal evolution and, through practice, transcend it till he reaches the very core of being – the seer. From then on he lives in the abode of the soul. This source has no beginning and no end. It is an eternal, uninterrupted flow of the life-force.

Consciousness (*citta*) has seven facets. They are: emerging, restraining, created, tranquil, attentive, fissured and finally pure, eternal or divine (*vyutthāna, nirodha, nirmāṇa, praśānta, ekāgratā, chidra* and finally, *śuddha, nitya* or *divya*).

If a practitioner uncovers these seven aspects of consciousness, he reaches that exalted, indivisible state of existence where the search for self ends and the seeker becomes the seer.

Patañjali addresses each type of *sādhaka* according to his level of intelligence and awareness. For those of average intellect, he explains five types of afflictions (*kleśas*) and the ways in which they cause disturbances in the *citta*. For those of sharp intellect, he stresses the study of the five fluctuations (*vṛttis*) which may lead to afflictions. In speaking to the most keenly sensitive, he explains the fissures which may occur in the very well of consciousness. He guides each level of practitioner, in ways appropriate to his own evolution, in overcoming the obstacles he encounters on his path of spiritual growth.

Patañjali threads his themes throughout the work, and certain ideas recur. Each time they recur, one is given a slightly different, and deeper, insight. For example, in discussing the effects of actions (*karmaphala*), he explains that though these may vary slightly, their content remains intact (compare II.13–14 with IV.1–2). Almost identical explanations are given in II.20 and IV.18. For those of average intellect, he speaks of sorrows and pains which have yet to come and can be avoided by discipline (II.16); for those of the most subtle and sensitive intellect, he explains that the effect of fissures created in the consciousness is experienced at once (IV.28). And he gives identical ways of overcoming afflictions and disturbances in I.23, 29; II.11 and IV.6 – but by now, one's understanding is deeper and more subtle.

These examples are not exhaustive. In the future, it will be fruitful to make a further comparative study of the sūtras and their relevance in various fields – for example, the education of children.

The initial disciplining of a child through the 'don'ts' and 'dos' is comparable to the *yamas* and *niyamas*. As he grows older he is encouraged to play games with other children. He learns to co-ordinate his organs of action with his organs of perception. In the process he develops friendliness, companionship and a sporting spirit. This corresponds to *āsana* and *prāṇāyāma*. When he starts going to school, his mind is turned from fun towards study: here we see the application of the principle of *pratyāhāra*. The process of immersing himself in his studies is *dhāraṇā*. Achieving the goal of his education is *dhyāna*. At this juncture, he starts to question whether this progress has been for selfish or selfless reasons, and realizes that only selflessness in his approach will lead to profundity of life.

However, the most important message of this inspired seer, coming to us through the ages, is that the real purpose of our life is to cross the ocean of illusion, from the shore of worldly pleasures to the other shore, of emancipation and eternal bliss.

APPENDIX I

A Thematic Key to the Yoga Sūtras

In this analytical appendix, I have covered Patañjali's entire *aṣṭāṅga yoga*, the methods of its practice, the causes of sorrows, the afflictions and disturbances and the means to overcome them, the renunciation of worldly pleasures, the properties and effects of yoga and the ways to emancipation.

The principal themes are arranged so as to provide a quick reference for the reader to understand and grasp them more easily.

→ = see entry

abhyāsa, anuṣṭhāna or *sādhana* (practice)
  I.1–2, 12–14, 20, 23, 32–39
  II.1, 25–26, 29–34, 43, 46–47, 49–51, 54
  II.1–3, 6, 9–12, 15
  IV.3
absorption → *samādhi* and *samapātti*
accomplishments or properties of yoga → *vibhūtis*
adepts → *siddha yogins*
afflictions → *kleśas*
antarāyas (obstacles)
  I.30–31
  II.33–34
  III.38, 52
  IV.4, 5, 10, 27
anuṣṭhāna (practice) → *abhyāsa, anusṭḥāna* and *sādhana*
aspirants → *sādhakas*
aṣṭāṅga yoga (eight limbs of yoga)
(i) eight aspects
  II.29
(ii) effects in general
  I.3, 17–19, 29, 41–51
  II.2, 11, 25, 27–28, 35–45, 48, 52–53, 55
  III.5, 13, 46–47, 51, 53, 55
  IV.5, 23, 25–26, 29–34
(iii) instant effects
  I.21
  III.54

(iv) time-bound effects
I.22
II.22
III.15
IV.6, 30
ātma jñāna (knowledge of the Self)
II.20
III.36
IV.18, 22
ātman (Self)
I.3, 16, 41, 47
II.20
III.35, 36, 56
IV.25, 29, 34
awareness (*prajñā*) → *sādhana*'s effect on the quality of awareness *cakras* (energy centres)
III.29 *dhruva* corresponding to *ājñā cakra*
30 *nābhicakra* corresponding to *maṇipūraka cakra*
31 *kaṇṭha kūpa* corresponding to *viṣuddhi cakra*
32 *kūrma nādi* corresponding to *svādhiṣṭhāna cakra*
33 *mūrdha jyoti* corresponding to *sahasrāra cakra*
35 *hṛdaya* corresponding to *anāhata cakra*
cause and effect theory → *karma cakra*
citta (consciousness)
(i) waves in the consciousness:
I.5–6, 30–31, 41
II.3–4, 11
III.9–13, 50
IV.4–5, 15–17, 20–27
(ii) control of the consciousness
I.2, 23, 32–39, 51
II.1, 11, 25–26, 28–32, 34, 46, 49–51, 54
III.1–3, 6, 9–12, 14–15, 53
IV.3–4, 13–22, 24
citta jñāna (knowledge of consciousness)
I.5–6, 30–31, 41
II.3–4, 11
III.9–13, 50
IV.4–5, 15–17, 19–24, 26–27
citta prasādanam (peace of consciousness)
I.33–39, 47
II.1, 52

III.5
IV.25
consciousness → *citta*
(fluctuations of the –) → *kleśas* and *vṛttis*
(knowledge of –) → *citta jñāna*
(peace of –) → *citta prasādanam*
energy centres → *cakras*
ethical discipline → *yama* and *niyama*
fluctuations (*vṛttis*) → *kleśas* and *vṛttis*
knowledge of consciousness → *citta jñāna*
knowledge of nature → *prakṛti jñāna*
knowledge of the self→ *ātma jñāna*
God → *Puruṣa viśeṣa* or *Īśvara*
kaivalya or *mokṣa* (liberation)
I.3, 47, 51
II.18, 25, 27, 29
III.36, 51, 56
IV.18, 25, 29, 32–34
kāla (time)
I.21–22, 51
II.47
III.9–10, 12–16, 53
IV.12–15, 20, 32–33
karma cakra (cause and effect theory)
(i) general
II.15, 22
IV.7–11, 13
(ii) cessation of cause and effect
I.41, 43, 45, 50
II.15, 22–23, 25–26
III.5, 53
IV.7, 29–30, 32
kleśas and *vṛttis* (afflictions and fluctuations of consciousness)
(these two aspects are inter-related and interwoven and they are also correlated to disease; see I.30–31)
(i) general
I.4, 30–31
II.3
(ii) causes
II.3, 11–14, 17, 21–24, 34
III.38, 52
IV.10, 27–28

(iii) different types
I.5–11, 30–31
II.3, 5–9
(iv) qualities
I.5–11
II.4–10
IV.13
(v) methods of minimizing or eradicating them
I.29, 39
II.2
III.5
IV.6, 29
(vi) methods of preventing them
I.32–33
II.16, 26, 33
III.51
IV.28
liberation → *kaivalya* or *mokṣa*
mokṣa → *kaivalya* or *mokṣa*
nature
(conjunction of – and seer) → *prakṛti puruṣa saṁyoga*
(knowledge of –) → *prakṛti jñāna*
niyama → *yama* and *niyama*
obstacles → *antarāyas*
peace of consciousness → *citta prasādanam*
practice → *abhyāsa*, *anuṣṭhāna* or *sādhana*
prajña → *sādhana*'s effect on the quality of awareness
prakṛti jñāna (gnosis of nature)
II.18–19
prakṛti puruṣa saṁyoga (conjunction of nature and seer)
I.4
II.17–18, 20–23
III.45–48
IV.7
puruṣa (seer)
Conjunction of nature and seer → *prakṛti puruṣa saṁyoga*
Puruṣa Viśeṣa or *Īśvara* (God)
(i) definition
I.24–26
IV.34
(ii) meditation on God
I.27–29

renunciation → detachment or *vairāgya*

sādhakas (aspirants)

Qualities of aspirants

I.20–22

sādhana (practice) → *abhyāsa, anuṣṭhāna* or *sādhana*

sādhana (it's effect on the quality of awareness)

I.48–49

III.6, 15

samādhi and *samapātti* (absorption)

I.17–19, 41–51

II.2, 45

III.3, 8, 11

IV.25, 29, 31

seer (*puruṣa*)

Conjunction with nature → *prakṛti puruṣa saṁyoga*

self→ *ātman*

siddha yogins (adepts)

I.19, 40

IV.1–3

time → *kāla*

vairāgya (renunciation or detachment)

(i) practice needed to develop renunciation

I.12–16, 23, 32–33

II.4, 11, 20, 29–30, 32–33, 43–47, 49, 51, 54

III.51

(ii) methods

I.2, 12–16, 23, 32–33, 40, 49–51

II.29, 33, 54

III.51

vibhūtis (accomplishments or properties of yoga)

II.27–28, 35–36

III.16–50, 54–55

vṛttis (fluctuations) → *kleśas* and *vṛttis*

yama and *niyama*

II.30–45

yoga (eight limbs of –) → *aṣṭāṅga yoga*

APPENDIX II

Interconnection of Sūtras

The reader will notice that many of Patañjali's ideas recur throughout the *Yoga Sūtras*. Certain key themes recur many times; each time, giving new insight that deepens our understanding. At the end of the commentary on each sūtra I have listed the sūtras that convey the same meaning. This cross-reference is a summary guide to these thematically interconnected sūtras. Readers who use it as an aid to their study will find their understanding of Patañjali's text, and of yoga, greatly enhanced.

Sūtra number	*Sūtras which convey the similar idea*	*Sūtras which help the understanding*
I.2	I.18; II.28	
I.3	I.16, 29, 47, 51; II.21, 23, 25; III.49, 56; IV.22, 25, 34	
I.4	II.20; IV.22	I.18–19, 23, 27–28, 33–39; II.12, 29
I.5	I.30–31; II.3, 12, 16–17	
I.7		I.49; III.55; IV.26
I.8	II.5	
I.11	II.5	
I.12	II.29–32, 35–53	I.4–6; II.28–29
I.13	I.20	
I.15		I.40; II.28, 53–55
I.16	I.17–51; III.51; IV.34	II.19; IV.29, 31
I.17	II.18–19, 21; III.45, 48	
I.18		I.50–51; II.9
I.19		I.10, 18; III.44
I.20		I.17–19
I.21		III.4
I.24		II.3; III.36
I.25	III.50; IV.31	
I.28	I.23, 41; II.1	
I.29		I.30–31
I.30		1.29
I.31	I.6; II.3, 17, 34	
I.33	II.30	

I.34		I.34–39
I.36	I.45	
I.38	III.11–12	
I.39		II.9
I.40	I.45	
I.44	I.41	
I.45	II.19	
I.46		I.18; IV.4
I.47	I.3	
I.49	I.7	
I.51		I.18, 50; III.56
II.1	II.29	
II.3	I.8	
II.6	IV.4	II.17, 21–23; III.36
II.9	III.10; IV.10	
II.10	II.3–4, 11, 48, 54	II.4
II.11	I.17	
II.12		I.5
II.14		I.33; II.30, 32–33
II.15		II.7–8
II.17		IV.4
II.19	III.13	
II.20	I.3; IV.22	
II.24		I.4, 8, 30–31; II.5
II.25	I.45	I.3, 5; IV.34
II.27		III.9–11; IV.27, 29
II.32		I.33
II.40	II.43	
II.45	I.16; IV.29	
II.46	I.20	II.48; III.1–2
II.49	III.40	
II.54		IV.19
III.1	II.53	
III.2	II.1, 11	
III.3	I.27–28, 41, 43	
III.5	I.47; III.36; IV.29	
III.6	I.17, 40; II.27	
III.8	I.16–18, 41–45; III.13	I.2; III.7–8
III.9	I.18, 20	I.34
III.10	I.12, 33, 47; II.9, 47; IV.29, 32	

III.11	I.2, 5, 32, 43, 50	
III.12	I.47, 51; II.19–20	
III.13	I.3; II.15, 18–20; III.5, 45, 48 II.26	
III.15	I.18, 19; IV.32	
III.16	IV.1, 28	
III.17	IV.1; 28	
III.18	II.12–13, 39; IV.33	
III.23	II.12; III.14–15, 18; IV.7	
III.24	I.33	
III.27		II.27
III.32	I.18–19	
III.36	I.3; II.18, 20; III.35; IV.34	
III.37	III.26, 34	
III.44	I.19	
III.45	II.18–19	I.27
III.46	I.30–31, 40; II.55	
III.48	II.6, 21–22; IV.4	III.45
III.49	I.41, 48; III.26, 37	
III.50	I.36, 47; II.18, 20; III.36; IV.25	
III.51	I.3; II.25; IV.27–30	IV.28
III.52	I.16, 21, 48; II.27	
III.53	IV.12–13	I.20
III.55	I.36; II.52; III.34, 36	
III.56	II.23; III.49; IV.26	
IV.3	I.2, 18, 29–39; II.2, 12–13, 18, 29–22; III.15	
IV.4	I.2; II.6; III.12–13	
IV.5	I.2, 17; II.6; III.13–14; IV.1, 3	
IV.6	I.23, 29, 32; II.11–12; III.51 IV.1	
IV.7	II.12–15; IV.4	
IV.8	I.12, 43; II.12–13, 28; III.18, 23, 38	
IV.10	I.35; II.1, 9; III.51	
IV.11	I.4; II.3–9, 12–14, 18	
IV.12	III.14, 16; IV.33	
IV.13	II.18–19	
IV.14	II.18–19	
IV.15	I.41–43	I.41–43; III.56
IV.16	I.43; II.22; IV.22, 31–32	
IV.17	I.2–4, 41; II.3, 12–14, 20	

IV.18	II.17, 20, 22–24; IV.30	
IV.19	II.19–20	
IV.20	I.2, 33, 38, 47; III.10	
IV.21	I.4–6, 17, 48; II.3–4	I.6; II.3
IV.23	I.41; II.18, 23; IV.4	
IV.24	I.41; II.18–19, 22–23; IV.27	
IV.25	I.47; II.10–12; III.56	
IV.26	I.49; II.25–26; III.55; IV.29	
IV.27	I.50; III.55–56	
IV.29	I.16, 49, 50; III.50, 55–56	
IV.30	I.3–5, 47; II.12, 20–21, 24, 52; III.55–56; IV.3–4, 25	
IV.31	I.3, 47; II.22, 52; III.49, 56	
IV.32	II.18, 22–24	
IV.33	II.18; III.13, 15, 53	

APPENDIX III

Alphabetical Index of Sūtras

abhāvapratyayālambanā vṛttirnidrā	I.10
abhyāsavairāgyābhyām tannirodhaḥ	I.12
ahiṁsāpratiṣṭhāyām tatsannidhau vairatyāgaḥ	II.35
ahiṁsāsatyāsteyabrahmacaryāparigrahāḥ yamāḥ	II.30
anityāśuciduḥkhānātmasu nityaśucisukhātmakhyātiravidyā	II.5
anubhūtaviṣayāsaṁpramoṣaḥ smṛtiḥ	I.11
aparigrahasthairye janmakathaṁtāsaṁbodhaḥ	II.39
asteyapratiṣṭhāyāṁ sarvaratnopasthānam	II.37
atha yogānuśāsanam	I.1
atītānāgataṁ svarūpato styadhvabhedāddharmāṇām	IV.12
avidyāsmitārāgadveṣābhiniveśāḥ kleśāḥ	II.3
avidyā kṣetramuttareṣāṁ prasuptatanuvicchinnodārāṇām	II.4
bahirakalpitā vṛttirmahāvidehā tataḥ prakāśāvaraṇakṣayaḥ	III.44
bāhyābhyantarastambhavṛttirdeśakālasaṁkhyābhiḥ paridṛṣṭo dīrghasūkṣmaḥ	II.50
bāhyābhyantaraviṣayākṣepī caturthaḥ	II.51
baleṣu hastibalādīni	III.25
bandhakāraṇaśaithilyāt pracārasaṁvedanācca cittasya paraśarīrāveśaḥ	III.39
bhavapratyayo videhaprakṛtilayānām	I.19
bhuvanajñānaṁ sūrye saṁyamāt	III.27
brahmacaryapratiṣṭhāyāṁ vīryalābhaḥ	II.38
candre tārāvyūhajñānam	III.28
citerapratisaṁkramāyāstadākārāpattau svabuddhisaṁvedanam	IV.22
cittāntaradṛśye buddhibuddheratiprasaṅgaḥ smṛtisaṅkaraśca	IV.21
deśabandhaścittasya dhāraṇā	III.1
dhāraṇāsu ca yogyatā manasaḥ	II.53
dhruve tadgatijñānam	III.29
dhyānaheyāstadvṛttayaḥ	II.11
draṣṭā dṛśimātraḥ śuddhopi pratyayānupaśyaḥ	II.20
draṣṭṛdṛśyayoḥ saṁyogo heyahetuḥ	II.17
draṣṭṛdṛśyoparaktaṁ cittaṁ sarvārtham	IV.23
dṛkdarśanaśaktyorekātmatevāsmitā	II.6
dṛṣṭānuśravikaviṣayavitṛṣṇasya vaśīkārasaṁjñā vairāgyam	I.15

duḥkhadaurmanasyaṅgamejayatvaśvāsapraśvāsā vikṣepasahabhuvaḥ	I.31
duḥkhānuśayī dveṣaḥ	II.8
ekasamaye cobhayānavadhāraṇam	IV.20
etayaiva savicārā nirvicārā ca sūkṣma viṣayā vyākhyātā	I.44
etena bhūtendriyeṣu dharmalakṣaṇāvasthāpariṇāmaḥ vyākhyātāḥ	III.13
etena śabdādyantardhānamuktam	III.22
grahaṇasvarūpāsmitānvayārthavattvasaṁyamādindriyajayaḥ	III.48
hānameṣāṁ kleśavaduktam	IV.28
hetuphalāśrayālambanaiḥ saṅgṛhītatvādeṣāmabhāve tadabhāvaḥ	IV.11
heyaṁ duḥkhamanāgatam	II.16
hṛdaye cittasaṁvit	III.35
Īśvarapraṇidhānādvā	I.23
janmauṣadhimantratapaḥ samādhijāḥ siddhayaḥ	IV.1
jātideśakālasamayānavacchinnāḥ sārvabhaumāḥ mahāvratam	II.31
jātideśakālavyavahitānāmapyānantaryaṁ smṛtisaṁskārayorekarūpatvāt	IV.9
jātilakṣaṇadeśairanyatānavacchedāt tulyayostataḥ pratipattiḥ	III.54
jātyantarapariṇāmaḥ prakṛtyāpūrāt	IV.2
kaṇṭhakūpe kṣutpipāsānivṛttiḥ	III.31
karmāśuklākṛṣṇaṁ yoginastrividhamitareṣām	IV.7
kāyākāśayoḥ saṁbandhasaṁyamāllaghutūlasamāpatteścā kāśagamanam	III.43
kāyarūpasaṁyamāt tadgrāhyaśaktistambhe cakṣuṣprakāśāsaṁprayoge antardhānam	III.21
kāyendriyasiddhiraśuddhikṣayāttapasaḥ	II.43
kleśakarmavipākāśayairaparāmṛṣṭaḥ puruṣaviśeṣa Īśvaraḥ	I.24
kleśamūlaḥ karmāśayo dṛṣṭādṛṣṭajanmavedanīyaḥ	II.12
kramānyatvaṁ pariṇāmānyatve hetuḥ	III.15
kṛtārthaṁ pratinaṣṭamapyanaṣṭaṁ tadanyasādhāraṇatvāt	II.22
kṣaṇapratiyogī pariṇāmāparāntanirgrāhyaḥ kramaḥ	IV.33
kṣaṇatatkramayoḥ saṁyamādvivekajaṁ jñānam	III.53
kṣīṇavṛtterabhijātasyeva maṇergrahītṛgrahaṇagrāhyeṣu tatsthatadañjanatā samāpattiḥ	I.41
kūrmanāḍyāṁ sthairyam	III.32
maitrīkaruṇāmuditopekṣāṇāṁ sukhaduḥkhapuṇyāpuṇya viṣayāṇāṁ bhāvanātaścittaprasādanam	I.33
maitryādiṣu balāni	III.24
mṛdumadhyādhimātratvāt tato 'pi viśeṣaḥ	I.22
mūrdhajyotiṣi siddhadarśanam	III.33
nābhicakre kāyavyūhajñānam	III.30
na caikacittatantraṁ cedvastu tadapramāṇakaṁ tadā kiṁ syāt	IV.16

na ca tatsālambanaṁ tasyāviṣayībhūtatvāt	III.20
na tat svābhāsaṁ dṛśyatvāt	IV.19
nimittamaprayojakaṁ prakṛtīnāṁ varaṇabhedastu tataḥ kṣetrikavat	IV.3
nirmāṇa cittānyasmitāmātrāt	IV.4
nirvicāravaiśāradye adhyātmaprasādaḥ	I.47
paramāṇuparamamahattvānto asya vaśikāraḥ	I.40
pariṇāmaikatvādvastutattvam	IV.14
pariṇāmatāpasaṁskāraduḥkhairguṇavṛttivirodhācca duḥkhameva sarvaṁ vivekinaḥ	II.15
pariṇāmatrayasaṁyamādatītānāgatajñānam	III.16
pracchardanavidhāraṇābhyāṁ vā prāṇasya	I.34
prakāśakriyāsthitiśīlaṁ bhūtendriyātmakaṁ bhogāpavargārthaṁ dṛśyam	II.18
pramāṇaviparyayavikalpanidrāsmṛtayaḥ	I.6
prasaṁkhyāne api akusīdasya sarvathā vivekakhyāterdharmameghaḥ samādhiḥ	IV.29
prātibhādvā sarvam	III.34
pratyakṣānumānāgamāḥ pramāṇāni	I.7
pratyayasya paracittajñānam	III.19
pravṛttibhede prayojakaṁ cittamekamanekeṣām	IV.5
pravṛttyālokanyāsāt sūkṣmavyavahitaviprakṛṣṭajñānam	III.26
prayatnaśaithilyānantasamāpattibhyām	II.47
puruṣārthaśūnyānāṁ guṇānāṁ pratiprasavaḥ kaivalyaṁ svarūpapratiṣṭhā vā citiśaktiriti	IV.34
ṛtaṁbharā tatra prajñā	I.48
rūpalāvaṇyabalavajrasaṁhananatvāni kāyasampat	III.47
śabdajñānānupātī vastuśūnyo vikalpaḥ	I.9
śabdārthapratyayānāmitaretarādhyāsāt saṅkarastatpravibhāgasaṁyamāt sarvabhūtarutajñānam	III.17
sadā jñātāścittavṛttayastatprabhoḥ puruṣasyāpariṇāmitvāt	IV.18
sa eṣa pūrveṣāmapi guruḥ kālenānavacchedāt	I.26
samādhibhāvanārthaḥ kleśatanūkaraṇārthaśca	II.2
samādhisiddhirīśvarapraṇidhānāt	II.45
samānajayājjvalanam	III.41
saṁskārasākṣātkaraṇāt pūrvajātijñānam	III.18
śāntoditāvyapadeśyadharmānupātī dharmī	III.14
santoṣādanuttamaḥ sukhalābhaḥ	II.42
sarvārthataikāgratayoḥ kṣayodayau cittasya samādhipariṇāmaḥ	III.11
sati mūle tadvipāko jātyāyurbhogāḥ	II.13
sattvapuruṣānyatākhyātimātrasya sarvabhāvādhiṣṭhātṛtvaṁ sarvajñātṛtvaṁ ca	III.50

sattvapuruṣayoḥ śuddhisāmye kaivalyamiti III.56
sattvapuruṣayoratyantāsaṁkīrṇayoḥ pratyayāviśeṣo bhogaḥ parārthatvāt svārthasaṁyamāt puruṣajñānam III.36
sattvaśuddhisaumanasyaikāgryendriyajayātma-darśanayogyatvānica II.41
sa tu dīrghakālanairantaryasatkārāsevito dṛḍhabhūmiḥ I.14
satyapratiṣṭhāyāṁ kriyāphalāśrayatvam II.36
śaucasaṅtoṣatapaḥsvādhyāyeśvarapraṇidhānāni niyamāḥ II.32
śaucāt svāṅgajugupsā parairasaṁsargaḥ II.40
smṛtipariśuddhau svarūpaśūnyevārthamātranirbhāsā nirvitarkā I.43
sopakramaṁ nirupakramaṁ ca karma tatsaṁyamādaparāntajñānamariṣṭebhyo vā III.23
śrāddhāvīryasmṛtisamādhiprajñāpūrvaka itareṣām I.20
śrotrākāśayoḥ saṁbandhasaṁyamāddivyaṁ śrotram III.42
śrutānumānaprajñābhyāmanyaviṣayā viśeṣārthatvāt I.49
sthānyupanimantraṇe saṅgasmayākaraṇaṁ punaraniṣṭaprasaṅgāt III.52
sthirasukhamāsanam II.46
sthūlasvarūpasūkṣmānvayārthavatvasaṁyamādbhūtajayaḥ III.45
sukhānuśayī rāgaḥ II.7
sūkṣmaviṣayatvaṁ cāliṅgaparyavasānam I.45
svādhyāyādiṣṭadevatāsaṁprayogaḥ II.44
svapnanidrājñānālambanaṁ vā I.38
svarasavāhī viduṣopi tathārūḍhōbhiniveśaḥ II.9
svasvāmiśaktyoḥ svarūpopalabdhihetuḥ saṁyogaḥ II.23
svaviṣayāsaṁprayoge cittasya svarūpānukāra ivendriyāṇāṁ pratyāhāraḥ II.54
tacchidreṣu pratyayāntarāṇi saṁskārebhyaḥ IV.27
tadabhāvāt saṁyogābhāvo hānaṁ taddṛśeḥ kaivalyam II.25
tadā draṣṭuḥ svarūpevasthānam I.3
tadapi bahiraṅgaṁ nirbījasya III.8
tadartha eva dṛśyasyātmā II.21
tadasaṅkhyeya vāsanābhiścitramapi parārthaṁ saṁhatyakāritvāt IV.24
tadā sarvāvaraṇamalāpetasya jñānasyānantyāt jñeyamalpam IV.31
tadā vivekanimnaṁ kaivalyaprāgbhāraṁ cittam IV.26
tadevārthamātranirbhāsaṁ svarūpaśūnyamiva samādhiḥ III.3
taduparāgāpekṣitvāccittasya vastu jñātājñātam IV.17
tadvairāgyādapi doṣabījakṣaye kaivalyam III.51
tā eva sabījaḥ samādhiḥ I.46
tajjaḥ saṁskāro 'nyasaṁskārapratibandhī I.50
tajjapastadarthabhāvanam I.28

tajjayāt prajñālokaḥ III.5
tapaḥsvādhyāyeśvarapraṇidhānāni kriyāyogaḥ II.1
tārakaṁ sarvaviṣayaṁ sarvathāviṣayamakramaṁ ceti vivekajaṁ jñānam III.55
tāsāmanāditvaṁ cāśiṣo nityatvāt IV.10
tasminsati śvāsapraśvāsayorgativicchedaḥ prāṇāyāmaḥ II.49
tasya bhūmiṣu viniyogaḥ III.6
tasya heturavidyā II.24
tasya praśāntavāhitā saṁskārāt III.10
tasyāpi nirodhe sarvanirodhānnirbījaḥ samādhiḥ I.51
tasya saptadhā prāntabhūmiḥ prajñā II.27
tasya vācakaḥ praṇavaḥ 1.27
tataḥ kleśa karma nivṛttiḥ IV.30
tataḥ kṛtārthānāṁ pariṇāma krama samāpattirguṇānām IV.32
tataḥ kṣīyate prakāśāvaraṇam II.52
tataḥ paramā vaśyatendriyāṇām II.55
tataḥ prātibhaśrāvaṇavedanādarśāsvādavārtā jāyante III.37
tataḥ pratyakcetanādhigamoṕyantarāyābhāvaśca I.29
tataḥ punaḥ śāntoditau tulyapratyayau cittasyaikāgratāpariṇāmaḥ III.12
tatastadvipākānuguṇānāmevābhivyaktirvāsanānām IV.8
tato dvandvānabhighātaḥ II.48
tato manojavitvaṁ vikaraṇabhāvaḥ pradhānajayaśca III.49
tato 'ṇimādiprādurbhāvaḥ kāyasaṁpat taddharmānabhighātaśca III.46
tatparaṁ puruṣakhyāterguṇavaitṛṣṇyam I.16
tatpratiṣedhārthamekatattvābhyāsaḥ 1.32
tatra dhyānajamanāśayam IV.6
tatra niratiśayaṁ sarvajñabījam I.25
tatra pratyayaikatānatā dhyānam III.2
tatra śabdārthajñānavikalpaiḥ saṅkīrṇā savitarkā samāpattiḥ I.42
tatra sthitau yatnoḃhyāsaḥ 1.13
te hlādaparitāpaphalāḥ puṇyāpuṇya hetutvāt II.14
te pratiprasavaheyāḥ sūkṣmāḥ II.10
te samādhāvupasargā vyutthāne siddhayaḥ III.38
te vyaktasūkṣmā guṇātmānaḥ IV.13
tīvrasaṁvegānāmāsannaḥ I.21
trayamantaraṅgaṁ pūrvebhyaḥ III.7
trayamekatra saṁyamaḥ III.4
udānajayājjalapaṅkakaṇṭakādiṣvasaṅga utkrāntiśca III.40
vastusāmye cittabhedāt tayorvibhaktaḥ panthāḥ IV.15
viparyayo mithyājñānamatadrūpapratiṣṭham I.8

virāmapratyayābhyāsapūrvaḥ saṁskāraśeṣo 'nyaḥ	I.18
viṣayavatī vā pravṛttirutpannā manasaḥ sthitinibandhanī	I.35
viśeṣadarśina ātmabhāvabhāvanānivṛttiḥ	IV.25
viśeṣāviśeṣaliṅgamātrāliṅgāni guṇaparvāṇi	II.19
viśokā vā jyotiṣmatī	I.36
vītarāgaviṣayaṁ vā cittam	I.37
vitarkabādhane pratipakṣabhāvanam	II.33
vitarkā hiṁsādayaḥ kṛtakāritānumoditā lobhakrodhamohapūrvakā mṛdumadhyādhimātrā duḥkhājñānānantaphalā iti pratipakṣabhāvanam	II.34
vitarkavicārānandāsmitārūpānugamāt saṁprajñātaḥ	I.17
vivekakhyātiraviplavā hānopāyaḥ	II.26
vṛttayaḥ pañcatayyaḥ kliṣṭākliṣṭāḥ	I.5
vṛttisārūpyamitaratra	I.4
vyādhistyānasaṁśaya pramādālasyāvirati bhrāntidarśanālabdha bhūmikatvānavasthitatvāni cittavikṣepāste 'ntarāyāḥ	I.30
vyutthānanirodhasaṁskārayor abhibhavaprādurbhāvau nirodhakṣaṇacittānvayo nirodhapariṇāmaḥ	III.9
yamaniyamāsanaprāṇāyāmapratyāhāradhāraṇādhyāna-samādhayo 'ṣṭāvaṅgāni	II.29
yathābhimatadhyānādvā	I.39
yogāṅgānuṣṭhānādaśuddhikṣaye jñānadīptirāvivekakhyateḥ	II.28
yogaścittavṛtti nirodhaḥ	I.2

APPENDIX IV

Yoga in a Nutshell

Table 15: *Cosmogony*

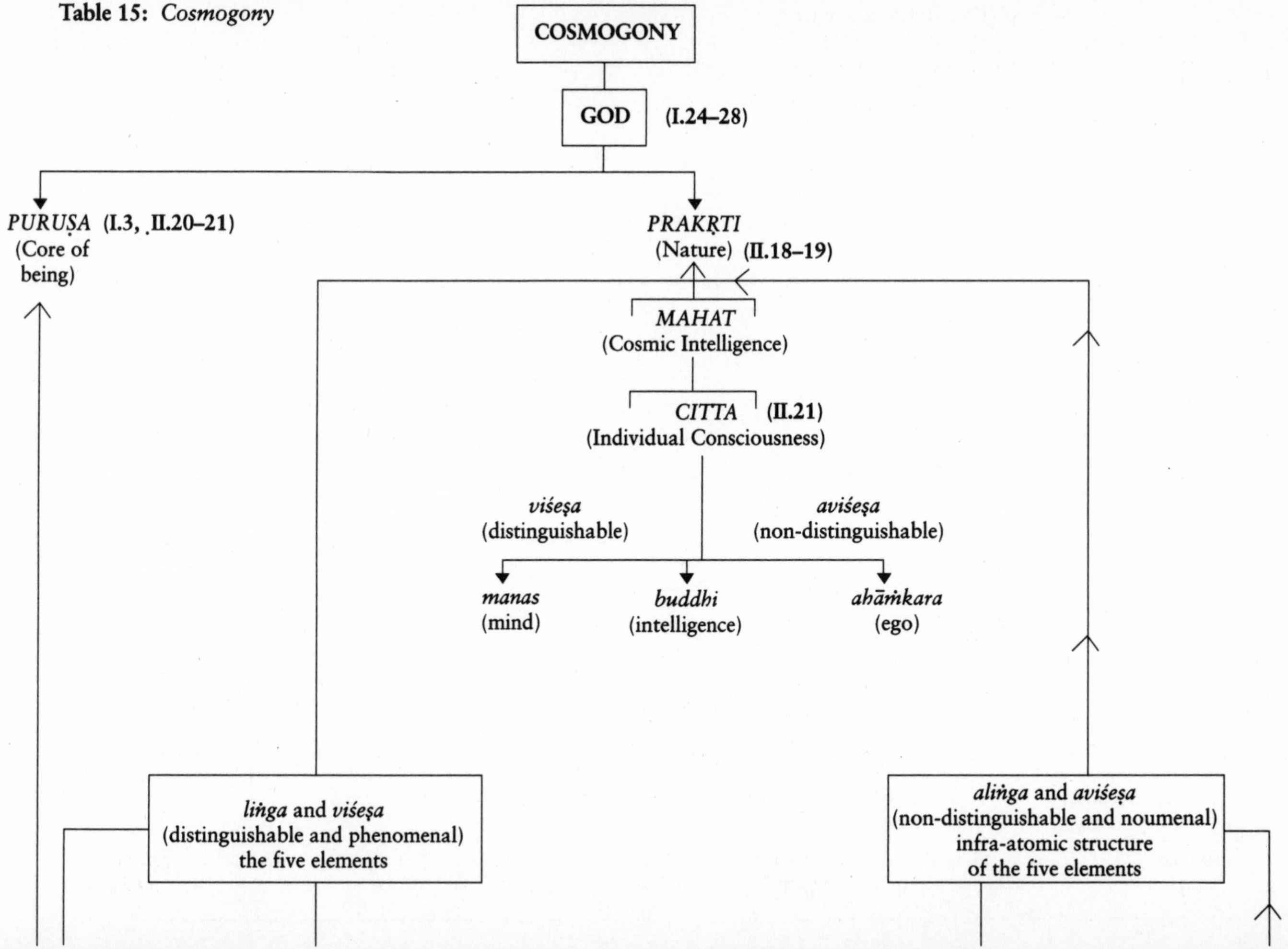

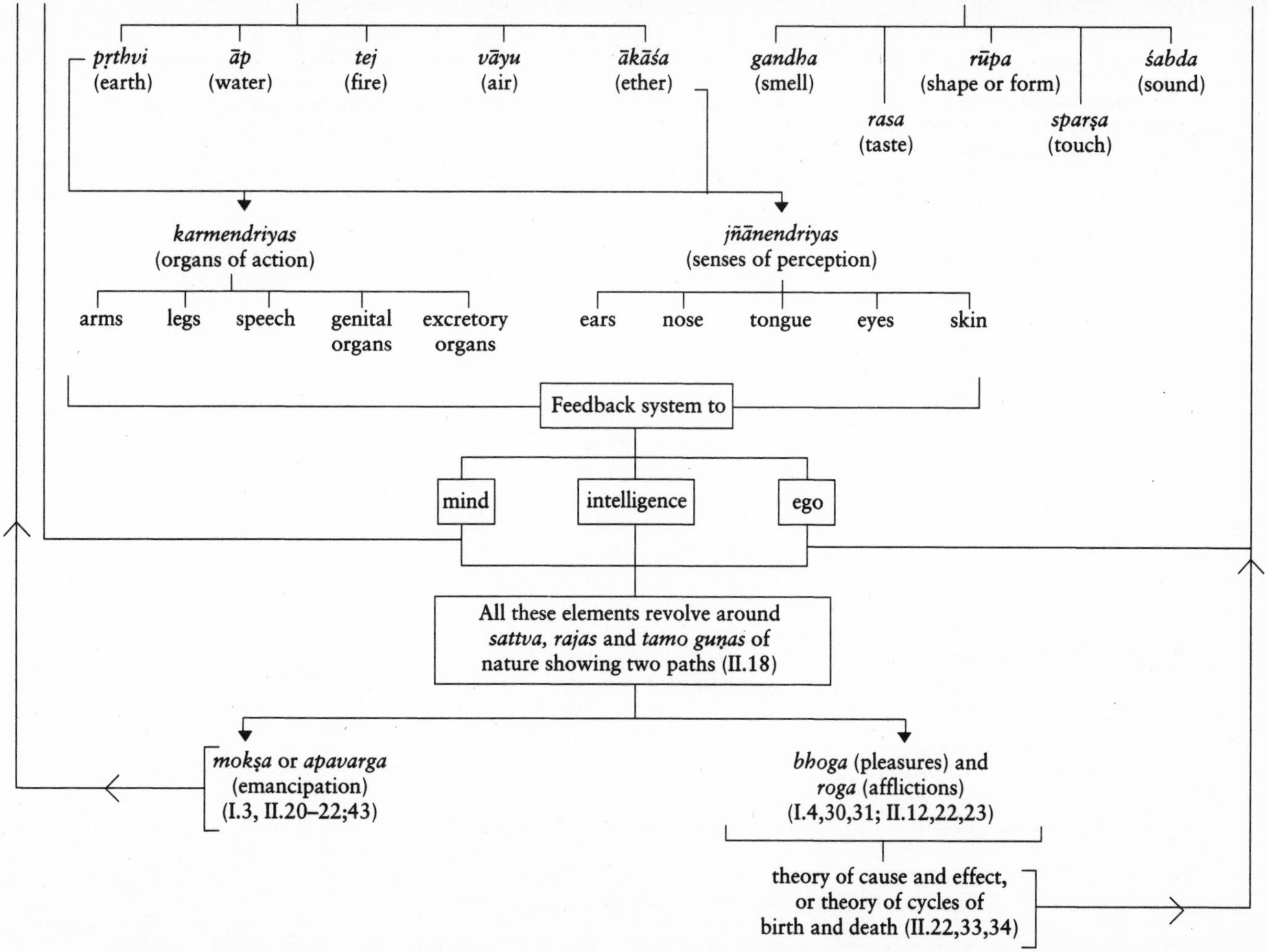

prthvi (earth)
āp (water)
tej (fire)
vāyu (air)
ākāśa (ether)
gandha (smell)
rasa (taste)
rūpa (shape or form)
sparṣa (touch)
śabda (sound)
karmendriyas (organs of action)
jñānendriyas (senses of perception)
arms
legs
speech
genital organs
excretory organs
ears
nose
tongue
eyes
skin
Feedback system to
mind
intelligence
ego
All these elements revolve around sattva, rajas and tamo guṇas of nature showing two paths (II.18)
mokṣa or apavarga (emancipation) (I.3, II.20–22;43)
bhoga (pleasures) and roga (afflictions) (I.4,30,31; II.12,22,23)
theory of cause and effect, or theory of cycles of birth and death (II.22,33,34)

Causes for Fluctuations and Absoluteness

- intellectual (*vṛttis*) (I.6)
  - *pramāṇa* (I.7) (valid knowledge)
    - *pratyakṣa* (direct perception)
    - *anumāna* (interference)
    - *āgama* (testimony)
  - *viparyaya* (I.8) (mistaken identity)
  - vikalpa (I.9) (knowledge devoid of substance)
  - *nidrā* (I.10)
  - (sleep or inert state)
  - *smṛti* (I.11) (memory, instant colourization)

- emotional or mental (*kleśas*) (II.3)
  - *avidyā* (II.5) (want of spiritual knowledge)
  - *asmitā* (II.6) (I or me or mine)
  - *rāga* (II.7) (desire and attachment)
  - *dveṣa* (II.8) (pain and hatred)
  - *abhiniveśa* (II.9) (attachment to life and fear of death)

- environmental (*citta vikśepa*) (impediments that scatter consciousness) (I.31–32)
  - *vyādhi* (disease)
  - *styāna* (mental laziness)
  - *saṁśaya* (doubt)
  - *pramāda* (carelessness)
  - *ālasya* (idleness)
  - *avirati* (incontinence)
  - *bhrāntidarśana* (mistaken notion)
  - *alabdhabhūmikatva* (missing the point)
  - *anavasthitva* (inability to maintain progress)
  - *duḥkha* (pain)
  - *daurmanasya* (dejection)
  - *aṅgamejayatva* (unsteadiness in the body)
  - *śvāsapraśvāsa* (irregular breathing)

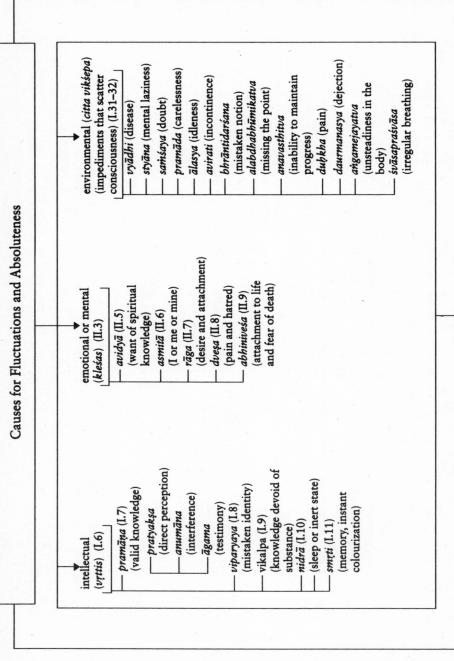

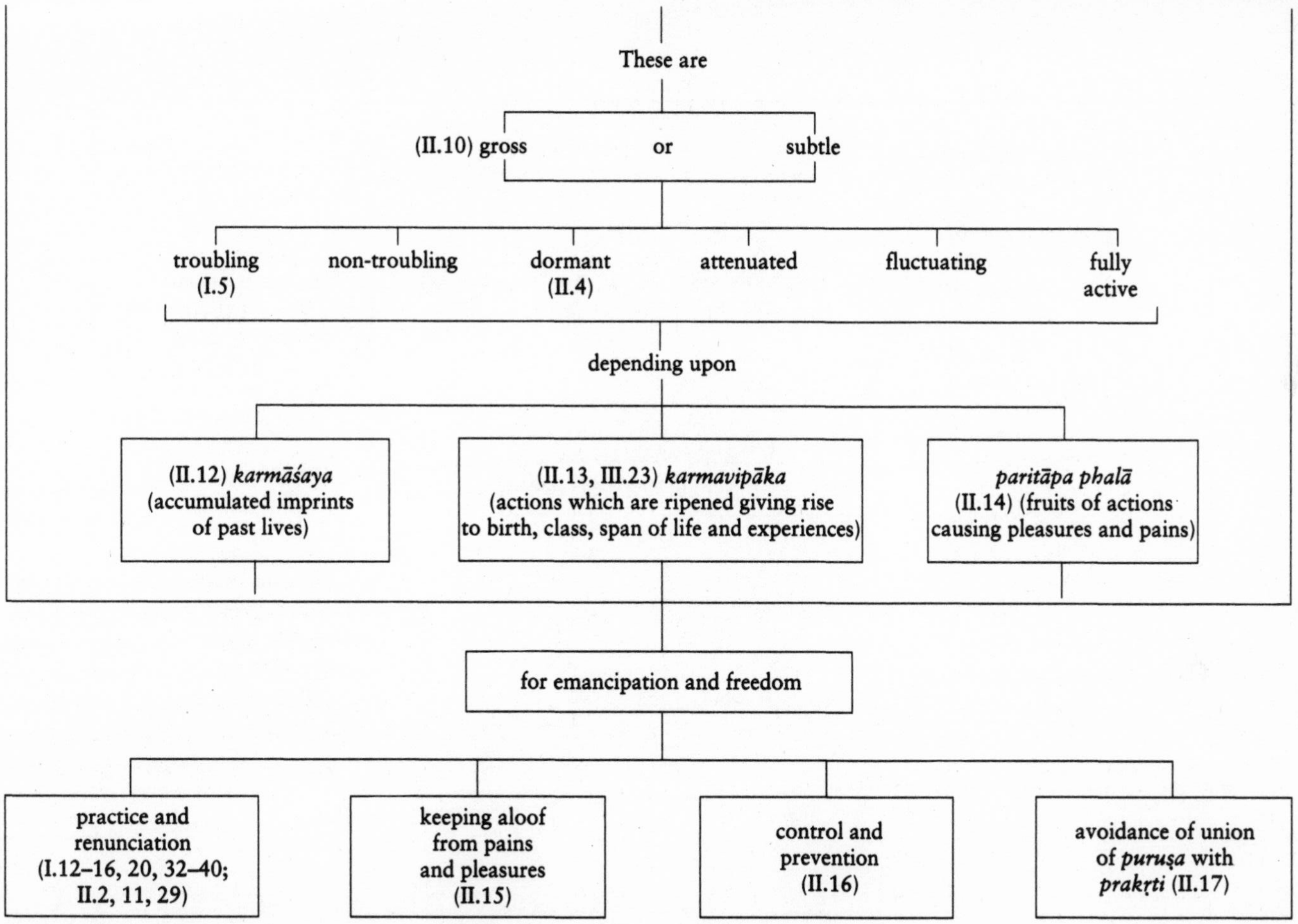

Table 16: *Causes for fluctuations and absoluteness, emancipation and freedom*

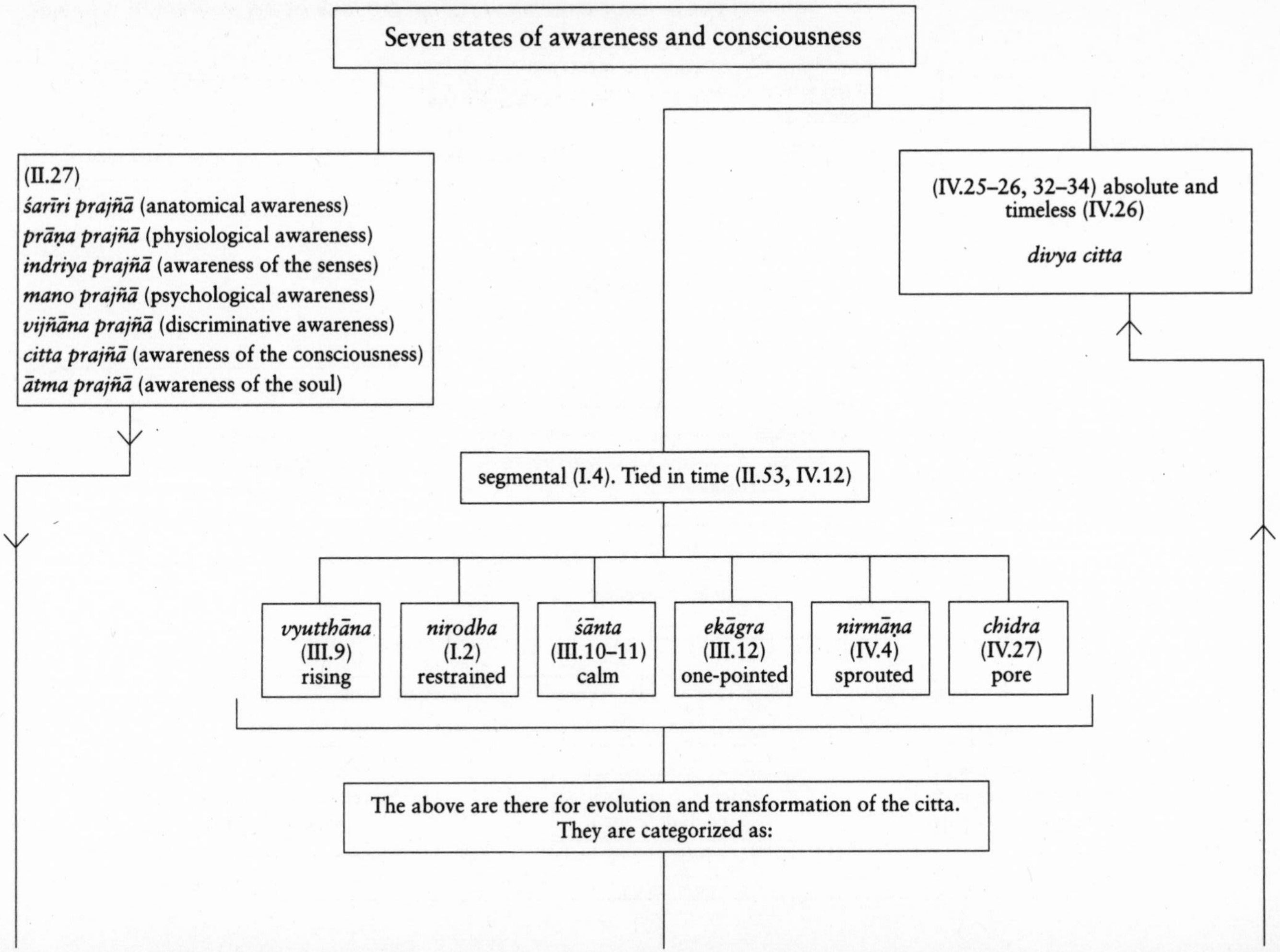

Seven states of awareness and consciousness
(II.27)
śarīri prajñā (anatomical awareness)
prāṇa prajñā (physiological awareness)
indriya prajñā (awareness of the senses)
mano prajñā (psychological awareness)
vijñāna prajñā (discriminative awareness)
citta prajñā (awareness of the consciousness)
ātma prajñā (awareness of the soul)
(IV.25–26, 32–34) absolute and timeless (IV.26)
divya citta
segmental (I.4). Tied in time (II.53, IV.12)
vyutthāna (III.9) rising
nirodha (I.2) restrained
śānta (III.10–11) calm
ekāgra (III.12) one-pointed
nirmāṇa (IV.4) sprouted
chidra (IV.27) pore
The above are there for evolution and transformation of the citta. They are categorized as:

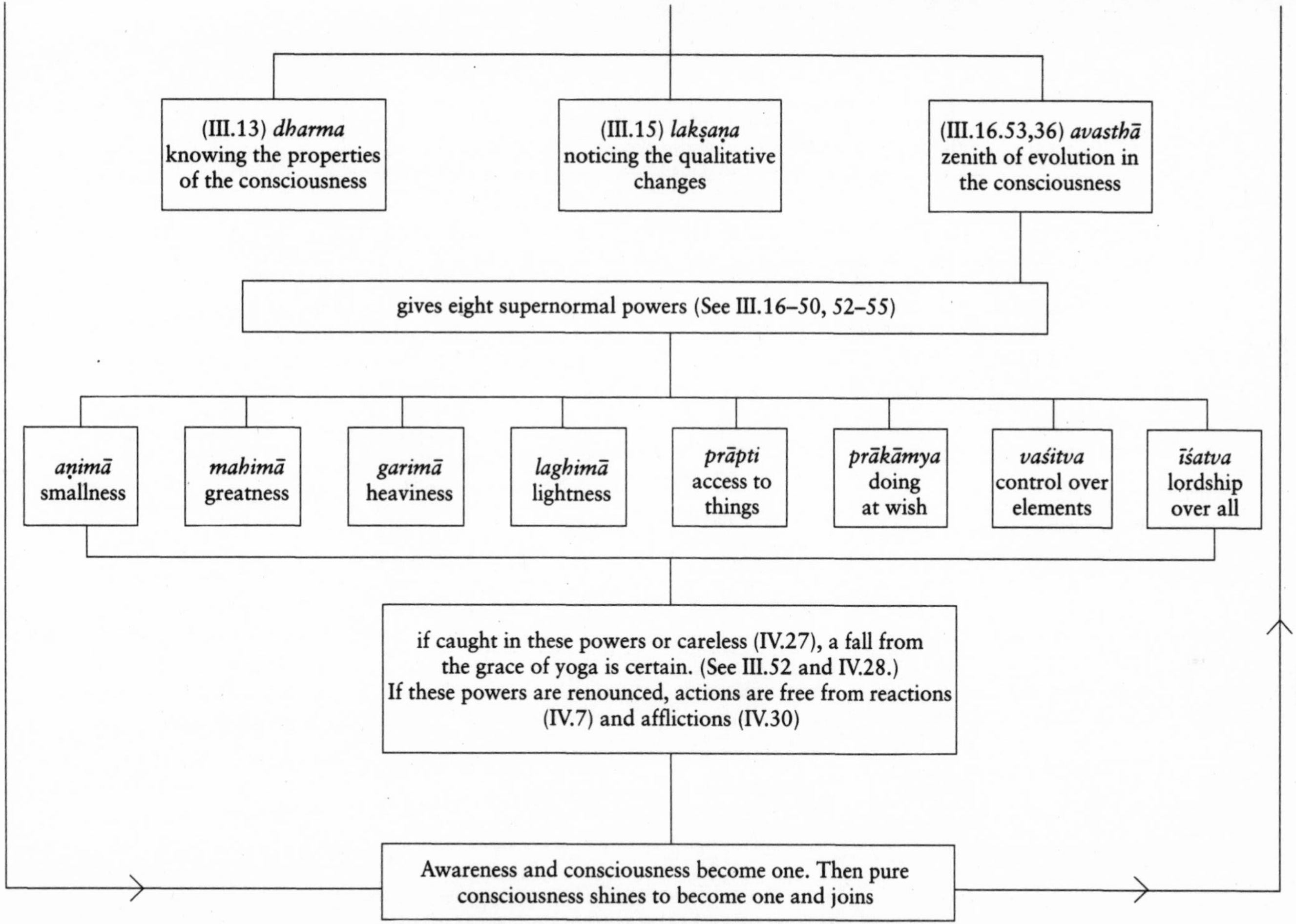

Table 17: *The cycle of the seven states of awareness and consciousness*

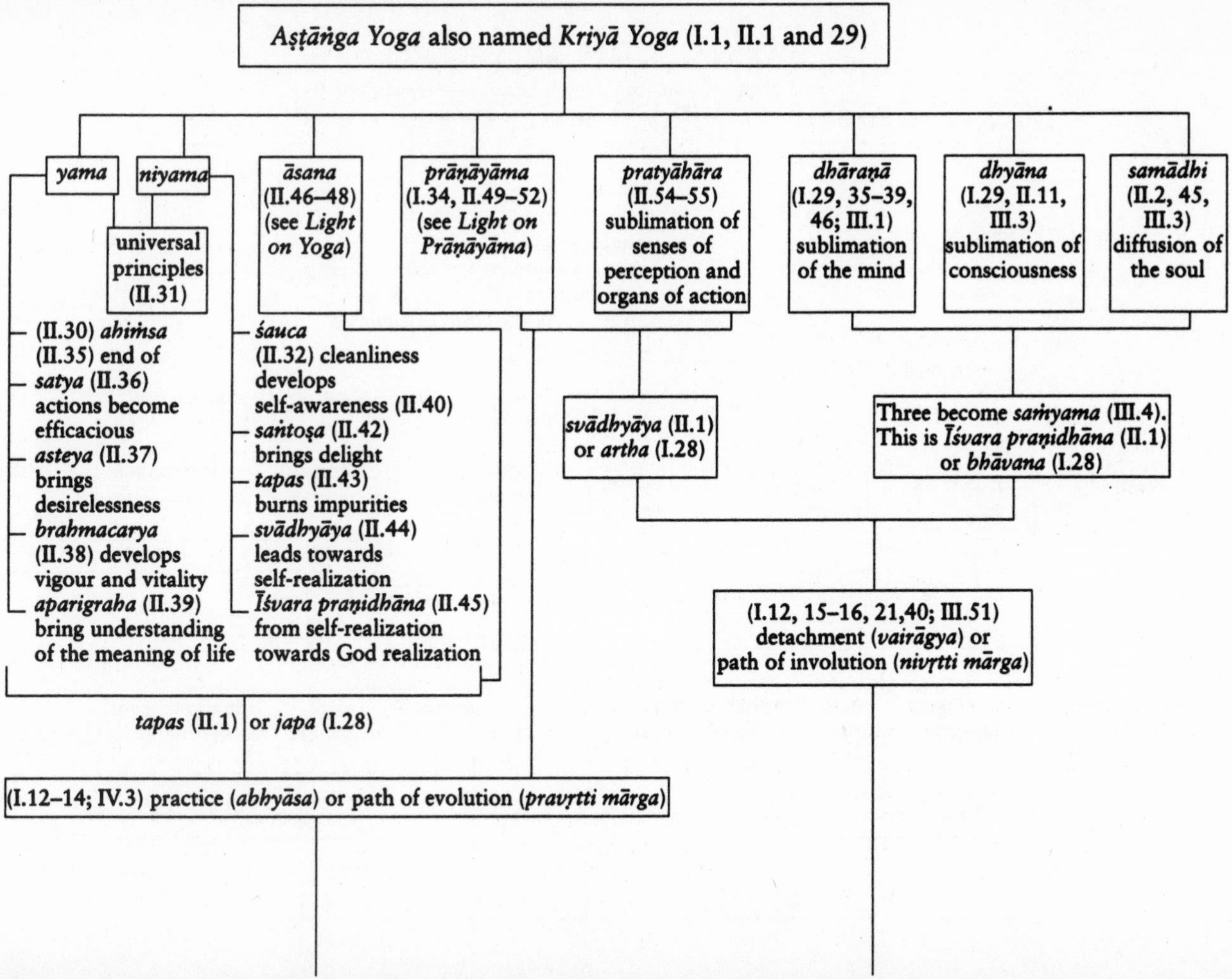
Aṣṭāṅga Yoga also named Kriyā Yoga (I.1, II.1 and 29)
yama
niyama
universal principles (II.31)
āsana (II.46–48) (see Light on Yoga)
prāṇāyāma (I.34, II.49–52) (see Light on Prāṇāyāma)
pratyāhāra (II.54–55) sublimation of senses of perception and organs of action
dhāraṇā (I.29, 35–39, 46; III.1) sublimation of the mind
dhyāna (I.29, II.11, III.3) sublimation of consciousness
samādhi (II.2, 45, III.3) diffusion of the soul
(II.30) ahiṁsa (II.35) end of
satya (II.36) actions become efficacious
asteya (II.37) brings desirelessness
brahmacarya (II.38) develops vigour and vitality
aparigraha (II.39) bring understanding of the meaning of life
śauca (II.32) cleanliness develops self-awareness (II.40)
saṅtoṣa (II.42) brings delight
tapas (II.43) burns impurities
svādhyāya (II.44) leads towards self-realization
Īśvara praṇidhāna (II.45) from self-realization towards God realization
svādhyāya (II.1) or artha (I.28)
Three become saṁyama (III.4). This is Īśvara praṇidhāna (II.1) or bhāvana (I.28)
tapas (II.1) or japa (I.28)
(I.12, 15–16, 21,40; III.51) detachment (vairāgya) or path of involution (nivṛtti mārga)
(I.12–14; IV.3) practice (abhyāsa) or path of evolution (pravṛtti mārga)

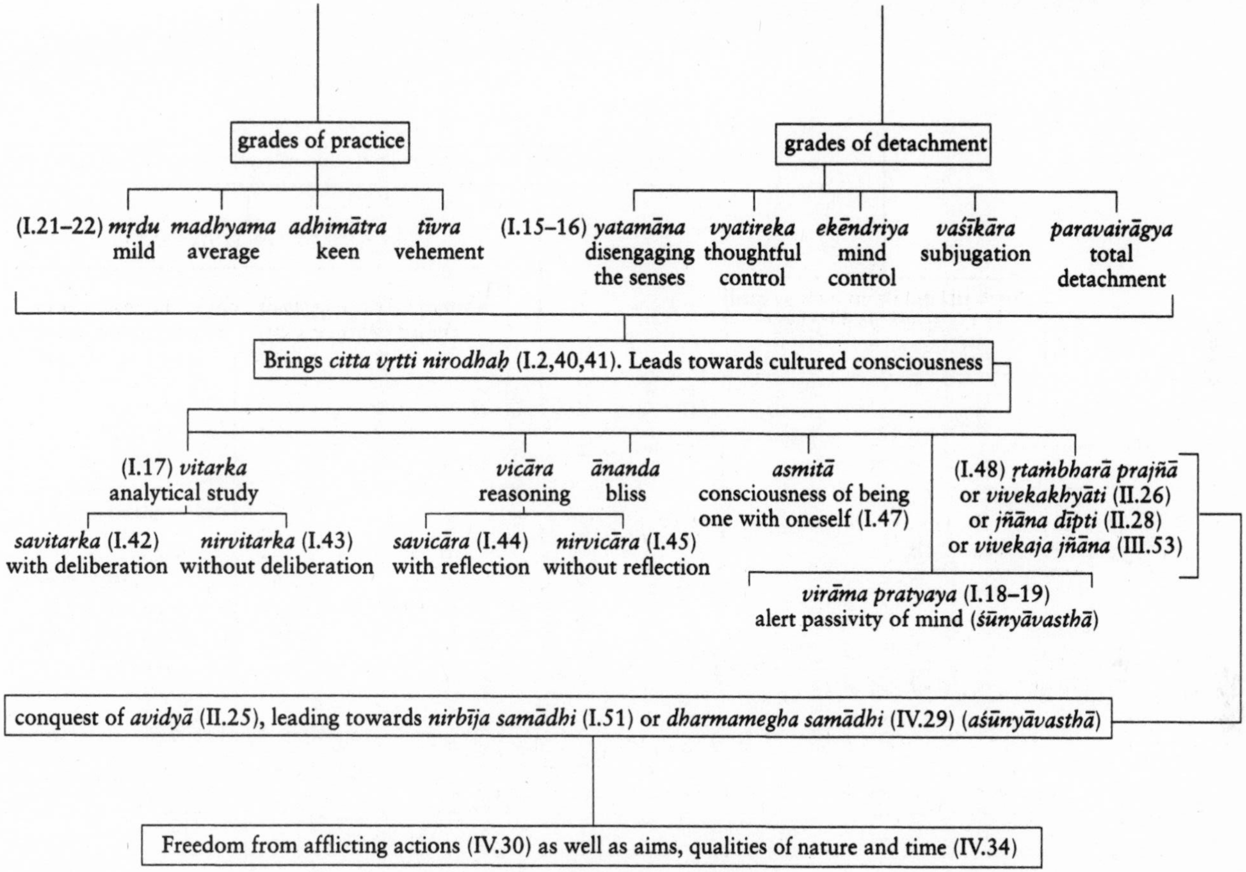
grades of practice
(I.21–22) mṛdu mild
madhyama average
adhimātra keen
tīvra vehement
grades of detachment
(I.15–16) yatamāna disengaging the senses
vyatireka thoughtful control
ekēndriya mind control
vaśīkāra subjugation
paravairāgya total detachment
Brings citta vṛtti nirodhaḥ (I.2,40,41). Leads towards cultured consciousness
(I.17) vitarka analytical study
savitarka (I.42) with deliberation
nirvitarka (I.43) without deliberation
vicāra reasoning
savicāra (I.44) with reflection
nirvicāra (I.45) without reflection
ānanda bliss
asmitā consciousness of being one with oneself (I.47)
(I.48) ṛtambharā prajñā or vivekakhyāti (II.26) or jñāna dīpti (II.28) or vivekaja jñāna (III.53)
virāma pratyaya (I.18–19) alert passivity of mind (śūnyāvasthā)
conquest of avidyā (II.25), leading towards nirbīja samādhi (I.51) or dharmamegha samādhi (IV.29) (aśūnyāvasthā)
Freedom from afflicting actions (IV.30) as well as aims, qualities of nature and time (IV.34)

✳ THUS ENDS THE SPIRITUAL JOURNEY ✳

Table 18: *The tree of* aṣṭāṅga *yoga*

List of Tables and Diagrams

1. Levels of *sādhaka*, levels of *sādhana* and stages of evolution, p. 19
2. Stages of *vairāgya* (detachment) and the involution of *prakṛti*, p. 66
3. Levels of *sādhakas* and types of awareness, p. 77
4. Stages in the purification of *citta*, p. 92
5. The stages of *samādhi*, p. 100
6. The acts of *kriyāyoga* and the paths of the *Bhagavad Gītā*, p. 110
7. The five *kleśas* (afflictions) and the brain, p. 112
8. The evolution of *citta*, p. 127
9. The evolution and involution of *prakṛti*, pp. 132–3
10. The seven states of consciousness, p. 138
11. The seven *kośas* (body sheaths) and corresponding states of consciousness, p. 141
12. The order of transformations of *citta* and *prakṛti*, p. 190
13. The four planes of consciousness, p. 197
14. The elements and their properties, p. 227
15. Cosmogony, pp. 310–11
16. Causes for fluctuations and absoluteness, freedom and emancipation, pp. 312–13
17. The cycle of the seven states of awareness and consciousness, pp. 314–15
18. The tree of *aṣṭāṅga* yoga, pp. 316–17

Glossary

a-	Non-
abhāva	Non-existence, non-occurrence, absence of feeling
abhedhya	Indivisible existence
abhibhava	Overpowering, subjugating
abhijāta	Transparent, learned, inborn, distinguished, noble
abhiniveśa	Clinging to life, fear of death, intentness of affection
abhivyakti	Manifestation, revelation
abhyantara	Internal
abhyāsa	Practice, repetition
ādarśa	Faculty of vision, mirror
ādhibhautika roga	Diseases caused by the imbalance of elements in the body
ādhidaivika roga	Genetic, allergic diseases
adhigama	To find, discover, acquire mastery
adhimātra	Intense, sharp in understanding
adhimātratama	Supremely intense
adhiṣṭhatṛtvam	Over-lordship, omnipotent
adhvabheda	Different condition
ādhyaḥ	Stands for
adhyāsa	Superimposition
adhyātma	Supreme Soul (manifested as an individual soul)
adhyātma prasādanam	Expansion of the seer, diffusion of the soul, sight of the soul
ādhyātmika roga	Self-inflicted diseases
ādi	So forth
ādīni	The others
Ādiśeṣa	The Lord of serpents, couch of Lord Viṣṇu
adṛṣṭa	Unperceived, invisible, fate, destiny
advaitā	Monism expounded by Śrī Śaṅkarācārya
āgama	Spiritual doctrines testimony
Agastya	Name of a sage
Ahalyā	Wife of sage Gautama
aham	Personal pronoun 'I'
ahaṁkāra	Ego, pride, the making of self, sense of self

ahiṁsā	Non-violence, non-injury, harmlessness
ajñā cakra	Energy centre situated between the centre of the two eyebrows
ajñāna	Ignorance
ajñāta	Unknown
akalpita	Unimaginable
ākāṅkṣā	Ambitions
ākāra	Form
akaraṇam	Non-performance, non-accomplishment
ākāśa	Ether, space, one of the five elements of nature
akliṣṭā	Incognizable, non-disturbing, non-painful
akrama	Without succession, without sequence
akṛṣṇa	Non-black
akusīda	Free from desires and aversions
alabdha bhūmikatva	Not being able to hold on to what is undertaken, missing the point
ālaṁbana	Support, dependent upon
ālasya	Laziness
aliṅga	(*a* = not; *liṅga* = mark) without mark, an unmanifested form, having no characteristic mark
āloka	Looking, seeing, sight, light, lustre, splendour
ālokya	Insight
alpam	Small, little, trivial
amaṇaskatva	(*a* = not; *manas* = mind) a state of being, that is, without the influence of the mind
Amaraka	Name of a king
amṛta	Nectar
amṛta manthana	Nectar, produced at the time of churning of the ocean by the demons and angels
anabhighāta	Non-resistance, indestructibility, cessation of disturbances
anāditvam	Time immemorial, existing from eternity
anāgata	Unknown, future
anāhata cakra	Energy centre situated in the seat of the heart
ānanda	Bliss, elation, felicity
ānandamaya kośa	The blissful sheath
ānanda prajñā	Knowledge of elation
ananta	Infinite, eternal, boundless, inexhaustible
anantaryam	Uninterrupted sequence
anāśayam	Freedom from impressions or influences
anaṣṭam	Not destroyed, not lost
anātma	Non-self, something different from the Soul

anavaccheda	Not bound, continuous, undefined, without a limit
anavadhāraṇam	Not comprehensible
anavasthitattva	Inability to maintain the achieved progress
anekeṣām	Innumerable
aṅga	A component aspect, limb, body, constituent part, member, division
aṅgamejayatva	Tremors or unsteadiness in the body
Āṅgīrasa	Author of *Ṛgveda*
aṇimā	As minute as an atom, atomization, the capacity to make oneself infinitely small, one of the eight supernatural powers
aniṣṭa	Undesirable, unfavourable
anitya	Non-eternal
annamaya kośa	Anatomical body of man
antaḥkaraṇa	Conscience
antara	Internal
antara kuṁbhaka	(*antara* = internal; *kuṁbhaka* = retention of breath) retention of breath after inhalation
antarāṅga	(*antara* = internal; *aṅga* = limb) internal, interior part
antaraṅga sādhana	Practice concerning the internal quest
antarātmā	Universal Self
antarātma sādhana	Practice concerning the innermost quest
antara vṛtti	Inhalation, internal thought waves
antarāyā	Impediment, hindrance, obstacle
antardhānam	Invisibility, disappearance
antardṛśya	Intuitive vision
ānubhāvikajñāna	Knowledge gained by experience
anubhūta	Perception
anugamāt	By following, approaching
anuguṇānām	Accordingly
anukāraḥ	Imitation, following
anumāna	Logic, doubt, reflection, inference
anumodita	By compliancy, abetment
anupaśya	Seeing, perceiving, one who sees
anupātī	Following a sequence, closely followed
anuśāsanam	Instructions, directions, code of conduct, advice, order, command, introduction or guidelines given in procedural form
anuśayī	(*anu* = close; *śayī* = connection) close connection, close attachment

ānuśravika	Listening or heard, resting on the *Vedas* or tradition
anuṣṭhāna	Devoted practice
anuttama	Supreme
anvaya	All-pervasiveness, association, interpenetration
anya	Other, another, otherwise, distinct
anyaḥ	Different
āp	Water, one of the five elements of nature
apāna	One of five vital energies which moves in the lower trunk controlling elimination of urine, semen and faeces
aparānta	Death, at the end
aparigraha	Freedom from avarice, without greed, non-acceptance of gifts
apariṇāmitva	Changelessness
āpattau	Identical, identified, assumed, having accomplished
apavarga	Emancipation, freedom, beatitude, liberation
āpetasya	Bereft of, devoid of, removed
api	Also, in addition to, although
apramāṇakam	Unrecognized, unobserved
apratisaṁkramāyāḥ	Changeless, non-moving
aprayojakam	Useless, unserviceable
apuṇya	Vice
āpūrāt	Becoming full, being full
āraṁbhāvasthā	Beginner's stage
ariṣṭa	Omens, portents
Arjuṅa	Hero of *Mahābhārata*, receiver of knowledge of yoga from Lord Kṛṣṇa in *Bhagavad Gītā*
artha	Means of livelihood, purpose, means, the second of the four aims of life
arthamātra nirbhāsā	(*artha* = cause, aim, purpose, means, reason; *mātra* = alone; *nirbhāsā* = manifestation) shining alone in its purest form
arthavatva	Purposefulness, fullness
āśā	Desire
asaṁprajñātā	(*a* = non; *saṁprajñāta* = distinction) a non-distinguishable state
asaṁpramoṣaḥ	Without stealing from anything else, not slipping away
asaṁprayogaḥ	Not coming in contact
asaṁsaktaḥ	Indifference to praise and revilement, non-attachment

asaṁsargaḥ	Non-contact, non-intercourse
āsana	A seat, posture, position; third of the eight aspects of *aṣṭāṅga yoga*
asaṅgaḥ	Non-contact
asaṅkhyeya	Innumerable
asaṅkīrṇayoḥ	Distinction from each other
āsannaḥ	Drawn near, approached
asat	Non-being
āśayaḥ	A chamber, reservoir
āsevitaḥ	Zealously practised, performed assiduously
āśīṣaḥ	Desires
asmitā	Pride, egoism, 'I' consciousness
āśrama	Stages of development, hermitage
āśraya	Support
āśrayatvam	Substratum, foundation, dependence
aṣṭāṅga yoga	Eightfold disciplines or aspects of yoga: *yama*, *niyama*, *āsana*, *prāṇāyāma*, *pratyāhāra*, *dhāraṇā*, *dhyāna* and *samādhi*
aṣṭa siddhi	Eight supernatural powers: *aṇimā*, *mahimā*, *laghimā*, *garimā*, *prāpti*, *prākāmya*, *īśatva* and *vaśitva*
aṣṭau	Eight
asteya	Non-stealing, non-misappropriation
asthi	Bones
asti	Exists
aśuci	Impure
aśuddhi	Impurities
aśukla	Non-white
asura	Demon
āsvāda	Faculty of taste
asya	Of this
atadrūpa	Not in its own form
atala	Nether world or lower region, one of the seven *pātālas*, being the first among them
atha	Now
atikrānthi bhāvanīya	Feeling of the highest knowledge of the seer and having attained the strength of *paravairāgya*
atiprasaṅgaḥ	Too many, superfluity
atīta	The past
ātmā, *ātman*	The individual, individual spirit
ātmabhāva	Feeling the soul
ātmabīja	Seed of the soul

ātmadarśana	Reflection of the soul
ātmajñāna	Knowledge of the self
ātmajyoti	Light of the soul
ātmakam	Being one with the self
ātma prasādanam	A glimpse or the reflection of the soul
ātma sākṣātkāra	Realization of the soul, dwelling in the abode of the soul
atyanta	Absolute, extreme
āuṁ	Sacred syllable, Śabda Brahman
aura	spiritual lustre
Aurobindo	Sage of Pondicherry
auṣadha	A drug, herb, medicine, remedy
auṣadhi	Herbs
āvaraṇa	Veil, covering
avasthā	A condition, state
avasthānam	Stand, rest, dwell, abide, reside
avasthā pariṇāma	Transformation towards the final state of refinement
āveśaḥ	Occupation, entrance
avidyā	Want of spiritual knowledge, lack of wisdom, ignorance
aviplavā	Unfluctuating, undisturbed
avirati	Desires, gratifications
aviṣayī	Unperceived, beyond the reach of the mind
aviśeṣa	(*ā* = tall, reaching up to; *viveka* = discriminative understanding; *khyāte* = summit of knowledge) the glory or the essence of knowledge
avyapadeśya	Latent, lying in potential form
āyāma	Ascension, expansion, extension
āyuḥ	Span of life
āyurveda	Science of life and health, Indian medicine
bādhana	Obstruction
bahiraṅga	External part, external limb
bahiraṅga sādhana	External quest
bāhya	Outside, external
bāhya vṛtti	Exhalation, movement of the outbreath, external thought waves
bala	Moral and physical strength
bandha	Block, lock, a practice of *haṭha yoga*
Bhagavad Gītā	A classical text of yoga, a dialogue between Lord Kṛṣṇa and Arjuṅa, containing the celestial sayings of Lord Kṛṣṇa

bhaktan	Devotee
bhakti	Devotion
bhakti mārga	Path of devotion
bhakti yoga	Yoga of devotion
bhāram	Gravitation
Bhārata	India
Bhāratī	Wife of Mandana Miśra, a staunch practitioner of *pūrva mīmāṁsa*
bhāṣya	Commentary
bhava	In a state of being, existence
bhāvanā	Feeling, understanding, reflection
bhāvanārthaḥ	Contemplating with meaning and feeling
bhedaḥ	Division
bhedāt	Being different
Bhīma	Hero of Mahābhārata, brother of Arjuṅa
bhoga	Enjoyment, pleasure, experience of sensual joys
bhogāsana	*Āsanas* of pleasure
bhrānti darśana	Delusion, false idea, supposition, bewilderment, perplexity, confusion
bhraṣṭa	Fallen down, fallen out, stamped from, depraved, fallen from grace
bhū	Being, becoming, land, ground
bhūloka	The terrestrial world, the earth
bhūmiṣu	Degree, stage
bhūta	Living beings
bhūtatvāt	In life
bhūtendriyeṣu	In case of elements, body, senses of perception, organs of action
bhuvarloka	Aerial region, one of the divisions of the Universe, the space between earth and heaven
bīja	A seed, source, origin, beginning
biṁba-pratibiṁba vāda	(*biṁba* = reflector; *pratibiṁba* = reflected image; *vāda* = exposition) exposition of double reflection
Brahma	The first deity of the Hindu Triad, the Creator
brahmacārī	Celibate
brahmacarya	Celibacy, continence, chastity, stage of studentship to learn wordly as well as spiritual knowledge, first of the four stages of life
brahmacaryāśrama	The first of the four religious stages or orders
Brahmajñāna	The realization of the Supreme, the highest knowledge

brahmakapāla	Energy centre, intelligence of the head, thousand-petalled cakra
Brahman	The Universal Spirit, Universal Soul
brāhmaṇa	Priest class, one who has realized the Self, one of the four *varṅas* or classes of Hinduism
Brahma Sūtra	Treatise on the knowledge of the Self
brahmavariṣṭa	Living in the vision of the soul
brahmavid variṣṭa	Vision of the soul, beyond words
Brahmendra Swāmi	Guru of Bājirao I of Mahārāṣṭra (India), who used to sit on a palm leaf to float on water
Bṛhaspati	Preceptor of Indra, Lord of heavens
Buddha	The founder of Buddhism
buddhi	Intelligence
buddhi buddheḥ	Cognition of cognitions
ca	And, both, as well as, also
Caitanya	Saint from Bengal (India)
cakra	Energy centres situated inside the spinal column
cakṣu	Eye
candra	Moon, referred to the mind
candra sthāna	Centre of para-sympathetic nervous system
caritādhikāra	Power of attaining one's object, serving a purpose
caturthaḥ	The fourth
ced	If
chidra	A pore, a fissure, a rent, a flaw
cintā	Disturbed thought, anxious thought
cintana	Deliberate thinking
cit	Thought, emotion, intellect, feeling, disposition, vision, to perceive, to notice, to know, to understand, to desire
citi	The self, the seer
citiśakti	Power of the self
citram	Bright, diversified, equipped
citra nāḍī	One of the *nāḍīs* sprouting from the heart
citta	Consciousness, a composite word for mind, intellect and ego (pride or the sense of self)
citta bhāva	Feeling of consciousness
citta jñāna	Knowledge of the consciousness
citta laya	Reposed consciousness, dissolution of consciousness
citta maya	Full of consciousness
citta prasādanam	Diffusion of the consciousness, favourable disposition of the consciousness

citta śakti	Power of consciousness
citta śuddhi	Purity of the consciousness
citta vikṣepa	Scattered consciousness, distraction
citta vṛtti	Movement in the consciousness
dairghyatā	Expansion, expansive
darśana	Seeing, looking, seeing the mind, perception, sight, vision, knowledge
darśinaḥ	The seer
daurmanasya	Fickle-mindedness, despair
dehābhimānatva	Believing that the perishable body is the self (*ātman*)
deśa	Place, spot, region
deva	Angel
devadatta	*Upavāyu* which causes yawning and induces sleep
Devayāni	Daughter of Śukrācārya – the preceptor of demons, wife of king Yayāti
dhairya	Courage
Dhammapāda	Treatise of Buddhism
dhanaṁjaya	*Upavāyu* which produces phlegm, nourishes and remains in the body even after the death and inflates the corpse
dhāraṇā	Concentration, attention, focusing, sixth of the eight aspects of *aṣṭāṅga yoga*
dharma	First of the four aims of life, science of duty, religious duty, virtue
dharma megha	(*dharma* = duty; *megha* = cloud) rain-cloud of justice, delightful fragrance of virtue
dharma pariṇāma	Transformation towards that which is to be held fast or kept, virtue, justice
dharmendriya	The sense of virtuousness, the inner voice
dharmī	Virtuous, religious, pious, characteristic
dhārmic	Pertaining to *dharma*
dhātu	Constituent element or an essential ingredient of the body
Dhruva	Son of Uttānapāda, who became the king of *dhruvaloka*; stable, constant, permanent, tip of the nose
dhruva nakṣatra	The Polar Star, the North Pole
dhyāna	Meditation, reflection, observation, contemplation, seventh of the eight aspects of *aṣṭāṅga yoga*
dhyānajam	Born of meditation
dīpti	Radiation, brilliancy, lustre

dīrgha	Long (as space or time), lasting long
divya	Divine
divya citta	Divine consciousness
draṣṭā	*Puruṣa*, seer, one who sees
dṛdhabhūmi	(*dṛdha* = firm; *bhūmi* = ground) firm ground
dṛk	Power of consciousness
dṛśam	Seen object
dṛṣṭa	Visible, perceptible
dṛṣṭrā	The knower, the seer
dṛśya	To be seen, to be looked at, visible
dṛśyatvāt	On account of its knowability or perceptibility
duḥkha	Sorrow, pain, grief, distress
dvandvaḥ	Dualities, opposite
dveṣa	Aversion, hate, dislike
eka	One, singular, alone, unique
ekāgra	Intent upon one object, one-pointed attention, concentration, fixity. Also *eka* = one without a second; *agra* = prominent, root, base, excellent, summit, i.e. indivisible soul
ekāgratā	One-pointed attention on the indivisible self
ekāgratā pariṇāma	Mode of transformation towards one-pointed attention
eka rūpatva	One in form
eka samaya	Same time
ekatānatā	Uninterrupted flow of attentive awareness
ekātmatā	Having same nature
ekatra	Together, jointly
ekatvāt	Due to oneness, on account of oneness
ekendriya	One sense, that is the mind
ēṣa	God
eṣām	Of these
etena	By this
eva	Also, alone, only
gamana	Passage, going, movement, motion
gandha	Smell
garimā	Becoming heavier, one of the eight supernatural powers
gati	Movement, motion, path, cause of event
ghaṭāvasthā	(*ghaṭa* = body compared to pot; *avasthā* = stage) the second stage of practice where one has to understand the functions of the body
Goṇikā	Mother of Patañjali

grahaṇa	Seizing, perceiving, understanding, comprehension
grāhya	To be seized, perceivable, understood
gṛhasthāśrama	The second of the four religious stages of life, that of the householder
gṛhītṛ	One disposed to seize or take, the perceiver
guṇa	Qualities of nature: *sattva*, *rajas* and *tamas*
guṇaparvāṇi	Changes or stages in qualities
guṇātītan	Free from the qualities of nature
guṇātmānaḥ	Nature of qualities
guṇavaitṛṣṇyam	Indifference to the qualities of nature
guru	(*gu* = darkness; *ru* = light) a preceptor who removes ignorance and gives knowledge
ha	The seer, sun. In *Haṭha Yoga Pradīpikā* it represents *prāṇa*
halāhala	A sort of deadly poison
hānam	Act of leaving, stopping, quitting
hānopāyaḥ	Means to remove deficiency
Hanumān	Name of a monkey chief, son of the wind
hasti	Elephant
haṭha	Willpower, force
haṭhayoga	A particular path of yoga that leads towards Self-Realization through vigorous and rigorous discipline
haṭhayogī	One who practises *haṭhayoga*, a master of *haṭhayoga*
hetu	Motive, cause, ground, reason, purpose
hetutvāt	Caused by, on account of
heya	Grief, dislike
heyakṡīṇa	Grief to be discarded, eliminated, destroyed
Himālayā	Abode of snow
hiṁsā	Violence, injury
Hiraṇyagarbha	Golden womb, Brahman
hlāda	Pleasant
hṛdaya	The heart, the mind, the soul
hṛdaya puṇḍarīka	The lotus of the heart
icchā	To cause to desire, will
icchā prajñā	Knowledge of the will
iḍā	A *nāḍī* corresponding to the sympathetic nervous system
Indra	The Lord of the Heaven
indriya	Senses of perception, organs of action, mind
indriyamaya	Oneness with the senses

Īśaḥ	God
īśatva	Supremacy over all, one of the eight supernatural powers
Iṣṭa devatā	The desired deity
Īśvara	God, Lord
Īśvara praṇidhāna	(*pra* = fullness; *ni* = under; *dhāna* = placement) surrender of oneself to God
itaratra	At other times, elsewhere
itareṣām	Another, rest, whereas, different from, for others
itaretara	One for the other
iti	That is all, thus
iva	Like, as it were, as if, appearance
jaḍa	Cold, slow, dull, foolish, unemotional
Jaḍa Bhārata	Name of a sage
jaḍa citta	Unintelligent or dull state of consciousness
jāgrata	Conscious, careful, wakefulness
jāgratāvasthā	Wakeful state
jaḥ	Born
jala	Water
janma	Birth, existence, life, life-time
jātyantara pariṇāma	Transformation in the state of birth
jaya	Conquest, mastery
jāyante	Produced
Jayavantiyāmbikā	Jaḍa Bhārata's mother
jihvāgra	Root of the tongue
jijñāsā	To know, to enquire
jīvāmṛta	Nectar of life
jīvātmā	The living or individual soul enshrined in the human body, the vital principle, that principle of life which renders the body capable of motion and sensation
jñāna	Knowing, knowledge, cognizance, wisdom
jñāna Gaṅgā	Ganges of wisdom, river of knowledge
jñānamārga	Path of knowledge
jñāna yoga	Yoga of knowledge
jñānendriya	Senses of perception
Jñāneśwar	13th century saint of Mahārāṣtra
jñānī	A learned man, a wise person
jñātā	Known, perceived, understood
jñeyam	The state of being cognizable
jugupsā	Disgust, censure, abuse, reproach
jvalanam	Shining, burning, blazing

jyotiṣi	Light
jyotiṣmati	Luminous, brilliant
Kabīr	15th- and 16th-century poet, devotee of Lord Rāma
kaivalya	Absolute state of aloneness, eternal emancipation
kaivalya pāda	Fourth part of the *Yoga Sūtras* on perfect emancipation
kāka mudrā	(*kāka* = crow; *mudrā* = seal) one of the seals, wherein the tongue is rolled to touch the upper palate
kāla	Time, period of time
kāla cakra	Wheel of time, movement of moments
kāla phala	Fruit of time
Kālimātā	Goddess of destruction
kāma	Wish, desire, love, lust, the third of the four aims of life
kanda	A bulbous root
kandasthāna	Root centre of *nāḍīs* in the region of the navel
kaṇṭaka	A thorn, the point of a needle or pin
kaṇṭha	Throat
kaṇṭha kūpa	Pit of the throat (*viṣuddhi cakra*)
Kapila	Name of a sage, the founder of Sāṁkhya philosophy
kāraṇa	Cause
kāraṇa śarīra	Causal body
kārita	To provoke
kāritvāt	On account of it, because of it
karma	An act, action, performance, duty, universal law of cause and effect
karma mārga	Path of action
karma phala	Fruit of action
karmayoga	Yoga of action
karmendriya	Organs of action
karuṇā	Compassion
kārya śarīra	Gross body
kārya śuddhi	Clean of action
kathaṁtā	How, in what way, whence
kauśalam	Well-being, skillfulness, cleverness
kāyā	Body, bodily action, deed
kevala	Alone, pure, unmingled, perfect in one's self
kevala kuṁbhaka	Non-deliberate retention of breath
khecarī mudrā	Cutting the frenum of the tongue and increasing its length to touch the eye-brow and then to fold it back to close the wind and food pipes

kiṁ	What
kleśa	Affliction, pain, distress
kliṣṭā	Afflicted, tormented, pained, hurt
kośa	Sheath, layer
krama	Regular course, regular succession, order, sequence
kriyā	Action, execution, practice, accomplishment
kriyāmāṇa karma	Action which generates fruit in future lives
kriyā yoga	Yoga of action
kṛkara	One of the five *upavāyus* which prevents substances from passing through the nasal passages and makes one sneeze or cough
krodha	Anger
Kṛṣṇa	The eighth incarnation of Lord Viṣṇu, who recited *Bhagavad Gītā*; it also means black
kṛta	Directly done
kṛtārtham	Whose purpose has been fulfilled
kṛtārthan	A fulfilled soul
kṣaṇa	A moment, an infinitesimal unit in time
kṣaṇa cakra	Orderly rhythmic procession of moments
kṣatriya	Warrior class, martial race, one of the four *varṇas* or classes of Hinduism
kṣaya	Diminish, destroy, decay, destruction
kṣeṭram	A place, field, origin
kṣetrika	A farmer, peasant
kṣetrikavat	Like a farmer
kṣīṇa	Discarded, destroyed
kṣiptā	Neglected or distracted
kṣīyate	Destroyed, dissolved
kṣut	Hunger
kumbhaka	Retention of breath
kuṇḍalini	Divine cosmic energy
kūpa	Pit, well
kūrma	Tortoise, second incarnation of Lord Viṣṇu, one of the *upavāyus* which controls the movements of the eyelids and regulates the intensity of light for sight by controlling the size of the iris
kūrmanāḍī	Name of a *nāḍī* in the epigastric region
kuśala	Proficiency
kūṭstha nityan	The changeless seer
lābhaḥ	Acquired, gained, obtained, profit
laghimā	Weightlessness, one of the eight supernatural powers

laghu	Light
lakṣaṇa	Character, quality, distinctive mark
lakṣaṇa pariṇāma	Transformation towards qualitative change
lāvanya	Grace, loveliness, complexion
laya	Dissolution, rest, repose
liṅga	With mark
liṅgamātra	Mark, indicator
lobha	Greed
mada	Pride
madhu	Sweet, pleasant, agreeable, delightful
madhu bhūmika	A yogin of the second order
madhu pratīka	Turned towards the delightful state of pleasantness
Madhva	The *acārya* of the 13th century, who expounded the *dvaita* (dualism) philosophy
madhya	Moderate, middle, centre
madhyama	Moderate
mahā	Great
Mahābhāsya	A treatise on grammar
mahāloka	One of the aerial regions
mahat	Great, mighty, the great principle, cosmic intelligence, universal consciousness
mahātmā	Great soul
mahāvideha	Great discarnation, disembodied state
mahāvidyā	Exalted knowledge
mahāvratam	Mighty vow
mahimā	Greatness, majesty, glory, one of the supernatural powers of increasing the size at will, illimitable bulk
maitrī	Friendliness
majjā	Marrow, one of the seven constituents of the body
mala	Impurity
māṁsa	Flesh, one of the seven constituents of the body
manas	Mind
manasā	Thought
manas cakra	Seat of mind
Maṇḍana Miśra	A follower of *Pūrva Mīmāṁsā* (known as Karmakāṇḍa)
Māṇḍavya	A sage who had supernatural powers
maṇi	Jewel, a gem, a flawless crystal
maṇipūraka cakra	Energy centre at the navel area
manojavitvam	Speed of mind, quickness in mind
manojñāna	Knowledge of the mind

manolaya	Alert passive state of mind
manomaya kośa	The mental or the emotional sheath
manoprajñā	Awareness of mind
manovṛtti	Thought-waves
mantra	Incantation
manuśya	Man
mārga	Path
mātrā	Alone, only
mātsarya	Malice
matsya	Fish
Matsyendranāth	Father of *haṭha yoga*
meda	Fat, one of the seven constituents of the body
meru	Name of a mountain
mithyā jñāna	(*mithyā* = false, sham, illusory; *jñāna* = knowledge) false knowledge
moha	Delusion, frenzy, infatuation, error, the state of being enamoured
mokṣa	Liberation, deliverance, release, the fourth religious stage or order of life
mṛdu	Mild, feeble
mūḍa	Stupid, dull, ignorant
muditā	Joy
mudrā	Seal, a practice of *haṭha yoga*
mūlādhāra cakra	Energy centre situated at the root of the spine
mūla prakṛti	Root of nature
Muṇḍakopaniṣad	One of the important *Upaniṣads*
mūrdha	The head, the top
mūrdhajyoti	Energy centre at the seat of *ājñā cakra*
mūrdhani	The centre of the head
na	Not
nābhi	Navel
nābhi cakra	Energy control at the navel area (also known as *manipūraka cakra*)
nāḍī	Energy channel, channel through which energy flows in the subtle body (main *nāḍīs* are *iḍā*, *piṅgalā*, *suṣumnā*, *citrā*, *gāndhāri*, *hastijihvā*, *pūṣā*, *yaśasvīnī*, *ālambusā*, *kuhū*, *sarasvatī*, *vārunī*, *visvodharī*, *payasvinī*, *śaṁkhiṇī*, *kauśikī*, *sūrā*, *rākā*, *vijñāna* and *kūrma*)
nāga	One of the five *upavāyus*. It relieves pressure of the abdomen by belching
Nahūṣa	King who became the Lord of the heavens

Nandanār	A devotee of South India
Nandī	Son of Kāmadhenu, giver of plenty, vehicle of Lord Śiva
Nārada	Sage and author of aphorisms of bhakti or devotion (*Nārada Bhakti Sūtras*)
Nara Nārāyaṇa	Son of Dharma and grandson of Brahma
Narasiṁha	Incarnation of Viṣṇu as half man and half lion
nāsāgra	Tip of the nose
naṣṭam	Lost, destroyed, disappeared
nibandhanī	Foundation, origin
nidrā	Sleep, sleepy state
nimittam	Efficient cause
nirantara	Without interruptions
nirbhāsam	Shining, appearing
nirbīja	Seedless, without a seed
nirgrāhya	Distinctly recognizable
nirmāṇa	Forming, creating, fabricating
nirmāṇa citta	Cultured consciousness
nirmita	Measured out, formed, made, created
nirmita citta	Created or cultivated consciousness
nirodha	Restraint, check, obstruction
nirodha citta	Restraining consciousness
nirodha kṣaṇa	Moment of restraint
nirodha pariṇāma	Transformation towards restraint
nirodha saṁskāra	Suppression of emerging thought-waves
niruddha	Stopped, restrained, obstructed
nirupakrama	Actions which do not give quick results
nirvicāra	Without reflection
nirvitarka	Without analysis
niśpatti avasthā	State of becoming one with body, mind and self
nitya	Eternal
nivṛtti	Resigning, abstinence, cessation
nivṛtti mārga	Path of abstention from worldly concerns and engagements
niyama	Five individual ethical observances, second of the eight aspects of *aṣṭāṅga yoga*, purity, contentment, self-discipline, Self-study, and surrender to God
nyāsāt	Directing, projecting, extending
ojas	Vitality, power, strength, virility, energy, light, splendour

pāda	A quarter, a part, a chapter
pakṣa	To go with the current, to side with, to espouse a side
pañcamahābhūtaḥ	Five elements of nature; earth, water, fire, air and ether
pañcatayyaḥ	Fivefold
paṅka	Mud, mire
panthaḥ	Path, way of being
para	Of others, another's
parakāya	Another's body
parakāya praveśa	Entering the body of others (one of the supernatural powers)
parama	Highest, most excellent, best
paramamahatvā	Infinitely great, most distant
paramāṇu	An infinitesimal particle
paramātmā	God, Supreme Soul
paramātman	Supreme Soul, Universal Self
paraṁparā	Bound by tradition, lineage, one following the other, proceeding from one to another
parārthabhāvana	Re-absorption of phenomenal creation, non-perception of objects
parārthaṁ	For the sake of another
parārthatvāt	Apart from another
paravairāgya	The highest and purest form of renunciation
paricaya	Acquaintance, intimacy
paricayāvasthā	State of acquisition
paridṛṣṭaḥ	Regulated, measured
parijñāta	Known
pariṇāma	Change, alteration, transformation
pariṇāma nitya	Termination of mutation or transformation
paripakva	Highly cultivated, quite ripe
paripakva citta	Matured consciousness, ripe consciousness
paripūrṇa	Completely filled, quite full, perfect
pariśuddhi	Complete purification, purity
paritāpa	Pain, anguish, affliction, grief
paryāvasānam	End, termination, conclusion
pātāla	One of the seven regions under the earth
Patañjali	(*pata* = falling; *añjali* = prayer) the author of the *Yoga Sūtras*
phala	Fruit, result
piṅgalā	One of the main *nāḍīs*, controller of sympathetic nervous system

pipāsa	Thirst
pracāra	Coming forth, becoming manifest, being used or applied
pracchardana	Expelling
pradhāna	Primary matter, first cause, first principle
prādurbhāva	Coming into existence, manifestation
prāg	Towards
prāgbhāraṁ	Gravitational pull
Prahlāda	Son of the demon Hiraṇyakaśipu
prajñā	Awareness
prajñā jyoti	Light of wisdom
prajñātan	Wise person, learned person
prākāmya	Freedom of will, attainment of every wish, one of the eight supernatural powers
prākāśa	Evident, luminosity, brilliance, splendour
prakṛti	Nature
prakṛtijaya	Conquest of nature
prakṛti jñāna	Knowledge of nature
prakṛti laya	Merging in nature
prakṛtīnām	Potentialities of nature
pramāda	Carelessness
pramāṇa	Correct notion, right conception
prāṇa	Life force, vital energy, breath
prāṇa jñāna	Knowledge of vital energy
prāṇamaya kośa	The vital body, organic sheath of the body
prāṇa prajñā	Awareness of energy
praṇava	The sacred syllable *āuṁ*
prāṇavāyu	One of the five types of vital energy causing respiration; its seat is the top thoracic region
prāṇa vṛtti	Regulation of breath or energy
prāṇāyāma	(*prāna* = vital energy; *āyama* = expansion, extension). Expansion of the vital energy or life force through restraint of the breath. Fourth of the eight aspects of *aṣṭāṅga yoga*
praṇidhāna	Laying on, directing upon, profound religious meditation, surrender
prānta bhūmi	(*prānta* = edge, border, boundary; *bhūmi* = province, region, place) stages of growth in the field of yoga
prāpti	The power of obtaining everything, one of the supernatural powers
prāpya	To attain

prārabdha karma	Merit or demerit from previous life to experience in the present life
prasādaḥ	Settling down, becoming clear, purity, serenity of disposition
prasaṅga	Event, connection
prasaṅkhyena	Highest form of intelligence
praśānta	Tranquillity
praśānta citta	Tranquil consciousness
praśānta vāhinī	Flow of tranquillity
praśānta vṛtti	Movement of tranquillity
prasava	Bringing forth, procreation, evolution
prasupta	Dormant, asleep
praśvāsa	Outbreath, exhalation
prathamā	First, foremost
prathamā kalpita	First progress, just begun
prati	Against, opposite to
pratibandhī	Contradicting, objecting, impeaching
prātibhā	Light, brilliant conception, genius
prātibhāt	The effulgent light of wisdom
pratipakṣa	The opposite side, to the contrary
pratipattiḥ	Understanding, knowledge
pratiprasavaḥ	Involution, going back into the original state
pratiṣedha	Keeping or warding off
pratiṣṭhā	Establishment, consecration
pratiṣṭham	Occupying, seeing
pratiṣṭhāyām	To stand firmly
pratiyogi	Uninterrupted sequences, equally matched
pratyāhāra	Fifth of the eight aspects of *aṣṭāṅga* yoga, withdrawal of senses into the mind
pratyakcetana	The seer
pratyakṣa	Real, self-evident
pratyaya	Means, device, firm conviction, faith
pravibhāga	Distinction, differentiation
pravṛtti	Evolution, going forwards
pravṛtti mārga	Path of evolution
prayatna	Persevering effort, great exertion
prayojakam	Usefulness, effect
pṛthvī	One of the five elements, the earth
punaḥ	Again
puṇya	Virtue
puṇyāpuṇya	Virtues and vices
purāṇa	Legend, belonging to ancient times

Puru	Son of king Yayāti
puruṣa	The Seer, the Soul
puruṣa jñāna	Knowledge of the Soul
puruṣa khyāti	Perception of the Seer
puruṣārtha	Four objects or aims of life: *dharma* (discharge of duty), *artha* (acquirement of wealth), *kāma* (gratification of desires) and *mokṣa* (final emancipation)
puruṣārtha śūnya	Devoid of four aims of life
puruṣa viśeṣaḥ	Special entity, distinct puruṣa, God
puruṣayoḥ	Of the soul
pūrva	Earlier than, former, previous, prior
Pūrva Mīmāṁsā	A systematical inquiry into the ritual portion of the *Veda* founded by Jaimini
pūrvebhyaḥ	In relation with the preceding ones
pūrveśām	First, foremost
rāga	Desire, attachment, pleasure
rajas	One of the three qualities of nature, vibrancy
rājasic	Belonging to the quality of *rajas*
rakta	Blood, one of the seven constituents of the body
Rāmakṛṣṇa Paramahaṁsa	A great sage of the 19th century; a realized soul; guru of Svāmi Vivekānanda
Rāmaṇa Māharṣi	20th-century Saint of Aruṇācala
Rāmānūjācārya	Sri Vaiṣṇava teacher of the 12th century (exponent of *Viśiṣṭādvaita* or qualified monism)
rasa	Taste, flavour, chyle, one of the seven constituents of the body
rasātala	One of the seven regions under the earth
rasātmaka jñāna	Essence of true knowledge
ratna	Gem, precious thing
Ratnākara	Previous name of sage Vālmīki
ratna pūrita dhātu	The jewel of the blood
roga	Disease, malady, ailment
rogī	Diseased person
Ṛṣabha	Jaḍa Bhārata's father, king of Bhārata
ṛṣi	A patriarchal sage, a saint, seer
ṛtambharā	Full of truth, full of intellectual essence
ṛtambharā prajñā	Truth-bearing wisdom
rūdhaḥ	Having ascended, established
rūpa	Form, an outward appearance, beauty
ruta	Sound
sa	This

śabdha	Word, sound
śabdhādi	Sound and others
śabdha jñāna	Verbal knowledge
sabīja	With seed
Śachi	Wife of Indra, Lord of heaven
sadā	Always
sadājñātā	Ever alert and aware
Sadānandācārya	Pupil of Śrī Śaṅkarācārya who is also known as Padmapādācārya as he had the imprints of the lotus flower in his feet. He used to walk over water
sādhaka	Aspirant, a practitioner
sādhana	Practice
sādhana pāda	Second part of the *Yoga Sūtras*, on practice
sādhāraṇa	Common to all, universal
Sagara	King of Ayodhyā
saguṇa	Good qualities, virtuous qualities
saḥ	That
sahabhuvaḥ	Side by side, concurrent
sahaja	Natural
sahasrāra	*Cakra* or energy centre situated at the crown of the head, symbolized by thousand-petalled lotus
sahita	Deliberate
Sai Bābā	20th-century Saint of Śirḍi
śaithilya	Laxity
sākṣātkāraṇa	To see directly with one's eyes and mind
śakti	Power, capacity, faculty
sālambana	With support
samādhi	Putting together, profound meditation, eighth and final aspect of *aṣṭāṅga yoga*
samādhi pāda	First part of the *Yoga Sūtras* on total absorption
samādhi pariṇāma	Transformation towards tranquillity
samādhi saṁskāra	Imprints of tranquillity
samāhita citta	Cultured consciousness, stable consciousness
samāna	One of the *vāyus*, vital energy which aids digestion
samāpatti	Transformation, assuming the original form, contemplation
samāpti	The end
samaya	Condition, circumstance, time
saṁbandha	Relationship
saṁhananatva	Compactness, firmness
saṁhatya	Well-knitted, firmly united
saṁjñā	Resolution, understanding, knowledge

sāṁkhya	Minuteness, precision
Sāṁkhya	One of the divisions of philosophy enumerating the principles of nature and Soul
saṁpat	Wealth, perfection
saṁprajñāta	Distinguish, know actually
saṁprajñāta samāpatti	Untinged transformation of the consciousness
saṁprayoga	Communion
saṁskāra	Subliminal impressions
saṁskāra phala	Effect of subliminal impressions
saṁskāra śeṣaḥ	Balance of subliminal impressions
saṁvedana	Perception, consciousness, understanding, to be known, to be understood
saṁvega	Cheerful, quick
saṁyama	Holding together, integration
saṁyama yoga	Yoga of integration
sāmyatā	Equanimity
sāmye	Being equal
saṁyoga	Union
sānanda	Unalloyed bliss
sañcita karma	Merit or demerit accumulated from earlier lives
saṅgha	Association, coming together
saṅgṛhītatva	Held together
sañjīvanī	A plant that restores life
Śaṅkarācārya	8th-century teacher who expounded the philosophy of monism (*advaita*)
saṅkaraḥ	Commingle, intermixture, confusion
saṅkīrṇa	Strewn, pounded together
sannidhau	Vicinity
sannyāsāśrama	The fourth stage of religious order in which all worldly possessions and affections are relinquished
sannyāsī	One who casts off all worldly possessions and affections; an ascetic
śānta	Appeased, calmed, pacified
śānti	Quiet, peace, serenity, calm
saṇtoṣa	Contentment
saptadhā	Sevenfold
Saptaṛṣi	The seven *ṛṣis* or great sages: Agastya, Aṅgīrasa, Atri, Bhāradvāja, Jamadagni, Kaśyapa, Vasiṣṭha
Śāradā	A monastery built at Śṛṅgeri by Ādi Śaṅkarācārya in honour of Bhārati, the wife of Maṇḍana Miśra
śarīra	Body

śarīra jñāna	Knowledge of the body
śarīra prajñā	Awareness of the body
Śarmiṣṭha	Daughter of the king of demons and wife of Yayāti
sarpa	Snake, to go fast
sarpobhava	Become a snake
sārūpyam	Closeness, likeness, nearness
sarvabhaumāḥ	Universal
sarvajña	All-knowing, omniscient, all-wise
sarvam	Whole, all
sarvārthā	Wholly, in all ways, at all times
sarvārtham	All-pervading
sarvārthatā	All-pointedness, many-pointedness
sāsmitā	Sense of *sāttvic* individuality
śāstras	Treatises
sat	Being, pure
satcidānanda	(*sat* = purity; *cit* = consciousness; *ānanda* = unalloyed bliss) pure unalloyed bliss
sati	Being, being accomplished
sātkāra	Dedication, devotion
sattva	Luminosity, white, pure
sattva buddhi	Illuminative intelligence
sattvāpatti	Experiencing pure *sattva*
sattvaśuddhi	Purity in *sattva*
satya	Truthfulness, honest, faithful, one of the five *yamas*
satyaloka	One of the seven aerial regions
śauca	Cleanliness, purity
śavāsana	An *āsana*, used for practice of relaxation and meditation techniques
savicāra	Right reflection, deliberation, consideration
savitarkā	Right analysis
siddha	The perfect being
siddhi vidyā	Knowledge of attainments
siddhiḥ	Attainment, perfection
śīlam	Virtue
śīrṣāsana	Headstand
Śiva	Auspicious, prosperous, the third deity of the Hindu triad, the Destroyer
Śiva Saṁhitā	A classical text on *haṭha* yoga
smaya	Wonder
smṛti	Memory, recollection
sopakrama	Immediate effects of actions
sparṣa	Touch

śraddhā	Faith, reverence, confidence
śravaṇa	Faculty of hearing
Śrīmad Bhāgavatam	One of the sacred *purāṇas*
śṛṅgeri śaṅkarācārya maṭha	A hermitage for learning according to the teachings of Śañkara
Śṛṅgeri	A place of worship in South India
śrotra	Organ of hearing
staṁbha	Restraint, suspension
staṁbha vṛtti	Act of holding the breath
sthairya	Steadiness, immovability
sthāna	Position, rank
sthira	Firm
sthita	Constant, steady
sthita prajñā	A perfect yogī, a steadfast person
sthūla	Gross
styāna	Langour, sluggishness, lack of interest
śubhecchā	Right desire
śuci	Pure
śuddha buddhi	Pure intelligence
śuddhan	A pure person
śuddhi	Cleanliness, purity
śūdrā	Working class, one of the four *varṇas* or classes of Hinduism
Śuka	Son of Vyāsa
sukha	Happiness, delight
śukla	White
śukra	Semen, one of the seven constituents of the body
Śukrācārya	Preceptor of the demons and inventor of elixir of life
sūkṣma	Subtle, soft, fine, minute
sūkṣma śarīra	Subtle body
sūkṣmottama	Subtlest of the subtle
sūrya	Sun
sūrya sthāna	Energy centre for sympathetic nervous system
suṣumna	*Naḍī* which controls central nervous system
suṣupti	Sleep
suṣuptyāvasthā	State of sleep
sutala	One of the seven nether worlds
suvarloka	One of the seven aerial worlds
sva	One's own
svābhāsaṁ	Self-illuminative
svādhiṣṭāna cakra	Energy centre situated above the organ of generation

svādhyāya	Study of the Self, study of the spiritual scriptures
svāmi	Owner, master, lord, seer
svapnā	Dream
svapnāvasthā	Dream-filled state
svarasavāhī	Current of love of life
svarasavāhinī	Flow of the fragrance of consciousness
svārtha	One's own, self-interest
svarūpa	One's own state, of true form
svarūpamātrajyoti	Light of one's own form, one's visage, one's own sight
svarūpa śūnya	Devoid of one's nature
śvāsa	Inbreath, inhalation
śvāsa praśvāsa	Heavy or laboured or irregular respiration
svayaṁbhū	(*svayam* = of one's own account; *bhū* = existent) incarnation by one's own will
Swami Rāmdās	Saint of Mahārāṣṭra
syat	Would happen
tā	They
tad	Their, its, from that
tadā	Then, at that time
tadañjanatā	Taking the shape of the seer or the known
tadārthah	For that sake, for that purpose
tadeva	The same
tajjaḥ	Born from, sprung from
talātala	One of the seven worlds in the nether region
tamas	Inertia, darkness
tāmasic	One of the three *guṇas* of nature: inertia
tantraṁ	Dependent
tanu	Thin, attenuated
tanūkaraṇārthaḥ	Reducing for the purpose of thinning, weakening
tanumānasā	Disappearance of memory and mind
tāpa	Pain, sorrow, heat
tapas	Austerity, penance, spiritual practice, devoted discipline, religious fervour
tapoloka	One of the seven aerial worlds
tāra	Stars
tārakam	Shining, clear
tāsām	Those
tasmin	On this
tasya	In conjunction, its, that, him, his
tat	It, that, his, their
tataḥ	From that, then, thence, therefore

tathā	All the same
tatparaṁ	The highest, the purest, the supreme
tatprabhoḥ	Of its Lord
tatra	There, of these
tatstha	Becoming stable
tattva	Principle, real state, reality, truth, essence
tayoḥ	There, of the two
te	These, they
tejastattva	Element of fire
ṭha	In *Haṭhayoga Pradīpikā*, it represents consciousness or *citta* as 'moon' which waxes and wanes
Tirumangai Ālwār	A devotee from South India (8th century A.D.) who built the temple of Śrī Rañganātha at Śrīraṅgam by the bank of Kāveri near Trichy
tīvra	Vehement, intense, sharp, supreme
traya	Three
tridoṣa	Disorders of the three humours of the body, vitiation of the bile, blood and phlegm
Trimūrthi	The triad of Brahmā (creator), Viṣṇu (protector) and Śiva (destroyer)
trividham	Threefold
tu	And, but
Tukārām	A 17th-century saint of Mahārāṣṭra
tula	Cotton fibre
tūlya	Equal, exactly similar
tūryāvasthā	The fourth state of consciousness, *kaivalya*
tyāga	Abandonment, renunciation
ubhaya	Of both
udāna	One of the five principal *vāyus* (vital energies), situated in the throat region which controls the vocal cords and intake of air and food
udāraṇām	Highly active
udaya	The rise
udita	Ascended, manifested, generation
uditau	Raising
uktam	Described
upalabdhi	To find, perceive, recognize
upanimantraṇe	On invitation, on being invited
Upaniṣad	(*upa* = near; *ni* = down; *sat* = to sit) literally sitting down near the Guru to receive spiritual instructions

upaprāṇa	Five supporting *vāyus*
uparāga	Conditioning, colouring
uparaktam	Coloured, reflected
upasarga	Hindrances, obstacles
upasthānam	Approaching, coming up
upavāyu	Same as *upaprāṇa*
upāya	That by which one reaches one's aims, means, way, stratagem
upekṣā	Indifference or non-attachment towards pleasure and pain
upekṣitvāt	Expectations
Ūrvaśi	A famous mystical damsel, daughter of Nara Nārāyaṇa
utkrāntiḥ	Ascension, levitation
utpannā	Born, produced
utsāha	Cheerfulness
uttareṣām	That which follows, subsequent
vā	Or, an option, alternatively
vācā	Speech
vācakaḥ	Connoting, denoting, sign, signifying
Vācaspati Miśra	A great scholar of the sixth century who wrote a glossary on Vyāsa's commentary on the *Yoga Sūtras*
vāhī	Current
vāhinī (vāhita)	Flow
vaira	Hostility
vairāgi	A renunciate
vairāgya	Renunciation, detachment, dispassion
vairāgya mārga	Path of renunciation or detachment
vaiśāradye	Skilfulness, profound knowledge, undisturbed pure flow
vaiśya	Merchant class, one of the four *varṇas* or classes of Hinduism
vajra	Diamond, hard, firm
vāk	Power of speech
Vallabha	A 16th-century *ācārya* from South India who believed in pure monism
vāmadeva	A sage
vānaprastha	The third stage or order of life (*āśrama*); in which one begins to learn non-attachment while living in the family
varaṇam	Veil, obstacles

varṇa	A colour, a cover, an abode, a kind, a quality: four orders divided according to different stages of evolution in men known as *brāhmana*, *ksatriya*, *vaiśya* and *śūdra*
varṇa dharma	Duties of communities
vārthāha	Faculty of smell
vāsanā	Desires, impressions
vaśīkāra	Freeing oneself from cravings, bringing into subjugation
vaśīkāra prajñā	Knowing the ways to subjugate desires
vasiṣṭa	A *brahmarṣi* or sage
vaśitva	The power to subjugate anyone or anything, one of the supernatural powers
vastu	Thing, substance, object
vastuśūnyaḥ	Devoid of substances, devoid of things
vaśyatā	Air, one of the five elements of nature
Veda	Sacred scriptures of the Hindu religion
vedanā	Faculty of touch
vedanīyaḥ	To be known, to be experienced
vedānta	(*veda* = knowledge; *anta* = end – end of knowledge, one of the orthodox systems of Indian philosophy, considered as later (*uttara*) *mīmāṁsā*. The *Upaniṣads* are *Vedānta* (the final parts = ends of the vedas)
vibhaktaḥ	Separate, different, partition
vibhūti	Powers, properties of yoga
vibhūti pāda	Third part of the *Yoga Sūtras* which deals with the properties of yoga
vicāra	Reason, synthesis, discrimination
vicāraṇā	Right reflection
vicāra prajñā	Differentiating knowledge of refinement
viccedaḥ	Cessation, stoppage, interruptions
vicchinna	Interrupted
videha	Existing without body, incorporeal
vidhāraṇābhyām	Maintaining, holding, restraining
Vidura	Adviser to King Dhṛtarāṣṭra in the Mahābhārata
viduṣaḥ	A wise man, a scholar
vidyā	Discriminative knowledge
vigraha	Idol (*mūla-vigraha* = base idol and *utsava-vigraha* = replica of base idol)
vijñāna	Discerning knowledge
Vijñāna Bhikṣu	(1525–1580 A.D.) the great scholar, author of

	Yoga Vārttika, commentary on *Yoga Sūtras*
vijñāna jñāna	Stability in intelligence
vijñānamaya kośa	The intellectual or discriminative body
vikalpa	Imagination, fancy
vikaraṇābhāvah	Knowledge gained without the help of the senses, freedom from senses of perception
vikṣepa	Distraction
vikśipta	Agitated, scattered
viniyogaḥ	Application
vipāka	Ripe, mature, result, fruition
viparyaya	Perverse, contrary, unreal cognition
viprakṛṣṭa	Distant
virāma	Cessation, rest, repose, pause
virodhāt	Obstruction, on account of, opposite
vīrya	Vigour, energy, courage, potency, valour
viṣaya	An object of sense, an object, matter, region, sphere, reference, aim, realm
viṣayavatī	Attached to object, related to
viśeṣa	Peculiar, specially itself, particular, distinction
viśeṣa darśinaḥ	Distinction of seer
viśeṣa vidhi	Special injunctions
Viṣṇu	The second deity of the Hindu triad or Trimurthi, the sustainer or the protector of the Universe
viśoka	Sorrowless effulgent light
viśuddhi cakra	Energy centre situated behind the throat region
vitala	One of the nether worlds
vītarāga	(*vīta* = free from; *rāga* = desire) one who is free from desire; calm, tranquil
vitarka	Analytical thinking, being engrossed in analytical study
vitarka-bādhana	Dubious knowledge, obstructing to analytical thinking
vitarka prajñā	Intellectual analysis
vitṛṣṇa	Freedom from desire, contentment
viveka	Discrimination, discriminative understanding
vivekaja jñānam	Exalted knowledge, exalted intelligence, sacred spiritual knowledge
viveka-khyāti	Discriminative intelligence, crown of wisdom
vivekanimnam	Flow of exalted intelligence in consciousness
vivekī	One who distinguishes and separates the indivisible soul from the visible world

vivekinaḥ	The enlightened, man of discrimination
vṛtti	Waves, movements, changes, functions, operations, conditions of action or conduct in consciousness
vyādhi	Disease, physical disease
vyākhyātā	Related, narrated, explained, expounded, commented upon, described
vyakta	Manifest
vyāna	One of the vital energies pervading the entire body distributing the energy from the breath and food through the arteries, veins and nerves
Vyāsa	A sage, author of *Vyāsa Bhāsyā*, the oldest commentary on Patañjali's *Yoga Sūtras*
vyatireka	Keeping away from desire
vyavahita	Concealed
vyavahitānām	Separated
vyavasāyātmika buddhi	Experienced subjective knowledge
vyūha	Galaxy, orderly arrangement of a system, disposition
vyutthāna	Emergence of thoughts, rising thoughts, outgoing mind
yama	The first of the eight limbs of *aṣṭāṅga yoga*; five ethical disciplines of yoga: non-violence, truthfulness, non-misappropriation, celibacy and non-greediness
Yama	God of death
yathābhimata	A pleasing thing, a selected thing
yatamāna	Disengaging the senses from action
yatnaḥ	Effort, continuous effort
Yayāti	Son of King Nahūṣa
yoga	Yoking, uniting, joining, contacting, union, association, connection, deep meditation, concentration, contemplation on the supreme union of body, mind and soul, union with God
yoga-bhraṣṭa	One who has fallen from the position of yoga, deprived of virtue, fallen from the grace of yoga
Yoga cuḍāmaṇi upaniṣad	One of the *Yoga Upaniṣads*
yoga darśana	(*yoga* = union; *darśana* = mirror, insight) like a mirror, yoga reflects one's soul through one's thoughts and actions

yogāgni	The fire of yoga
yogānuśāsanam	The yogic code of conduct
yogāsana	A yogic posture
yogaśāstra	Science of yoga
yoga sūtras	Yoga aphorisms of Patañjali
yoga-svarūpa	Natural constitution of yoga, natural states of yoga
Yoga Vāsiṣṭa	Treatise on yoga, spoken by Vāsiṣṭa to Lord Rāma, the king of Ayodhyā, seventh incarnation of Lord Viṣṇu
yogeśvara	Lord Kṛṣṇa, Lord of Yoga
yogī	Adept of yoga
yoginaḥ	Of a yogi
yoginī	Female adept of yoga
yogirāja	King among yogis
yogyatā manasaḥ	(*yogyatā* = fitness, ability, capability; *manasaḥ* = of the mind) a ripe mind
yogyatvāni	Fitness to see
Yudhiṣṭira	Son of Pāndu of Mahābhārata

Index

Absorption (*samādhi*), profound meditation and spiritual integration, 4–6, 8, 26, 30, 34, 35, 39, 45–103, 175, 180–1, 182, 192, 194, 219, 242, 246
compared with ultimate emancipation (*kaivalya*), 8
hindrances to, 37
and integration (*saṁyama*), 182, 183–4, 185–6, 188, 190, 201–2
and pure state (*samāpatti*), 93–4, 98–9
stages of awareness, with seed (*saṁprajñāta samādhi*, or *sabīja samādhi*), 5, 18, 68–70, 71, 72, 98–9, 100, 103
first stage: intellectual analysis (*vitarka*), 18, 68, 69, 70, 72, 100; with deliberation (*savitarkā*), 68, 69, 98, 100, 111n; with non-deliberation (*nirvitarka*), 68, 69, 95–6, 98, 100, 111n
second stage: differentiating knowledge (*vicāra*), 18, 68, 69, 70, 72, 100; with reasoning (*savicāra*), 68, 69, 96–7, 98, 100, 111n; with non-reasoning (*nirvicāra*), 68, 69, 96–7, 98, 99, 100, 111n
third stage: bliss (*ānanda*), 18, 68–9, 70, 72, 97, 98, 100, 111n
fourth stage: state of 'I' (*asmitā* or *asmitā rūpa saṁprajñāta samādhi*), 68, 69, 70, 72, 97, 98, 100, 111n
passive and transitory stage of quietness (*virāma pratyaya*, *asaṁprajñāta samādhi* or *manolaya*), 18–20, 22, 56, 69, 70–2, 99, 100, 127
final seedless stage of yoga (*nirbīja samādhi*) or rain-cloud of virtue (*dharma meghasamādhi*), 5, 6, 9, 18, 22, 69, 71, 72, 74, 99, 100, 103, 182, 278–9, 281–2
Actions and reactions, 24, 40
four types of (*karma*), 40, 243, 253–5
see also cause and effect (*karma*)
Ādiśeṣa, Lord of serpents, 1–2, 162–3
Afflictions (*kleśas*), 6–7, 23–4, 31, 78–9, 109, 111–13, 117–19, 291
attachment (*rāga*), 17, 23, 111, 112, 115, 132
aversion (*dveṣa*), 23, 111, 112, 116, 132
clinging to life (*abhiniveśa*), 23, 111, 112, 116–17, 132
egoism (*asmitā*), 11–12, 23, 42, 111, 112, 114–15, 132
ignorance (*avidyā*), 6–7, 17, 23–4, 28, 41, 42, 111, 112, 113–14, 132, 134
Ahalyā, 8

Aims of life (*puruṣārtha*): science of duty (*dharma*), livelihood (*artha*), enjoyments of life (*kāma*)
and liberation from worldly life (*mokṣa*), 3–4, 283–7
see also emancipation (*kaivalya*)
Attachment (*rāga*), 17, 23, 111, 112, 115, 132
Āuṁ *see* sacred syllable Āuṁ
Aversion (*dveṣa*), 23, 111, 112, 116, 132
Awareness (*prajñā*), seven states of, 29, 77, 132, 137–8

Bhagavad Gīta, 3, 71–2, 110, 189, 224–5, 254, 268, 273, 277, 279, 284, 286–7
Bhakti Sūtras, 225
Bhāratī, Śrīmatī, 220–1
Body (*śarīra*), 32, 162–3, 195
see also sheaths (*kośa*)
Brahma, 81, 162
Brahma Sūtra, 49
Brain, 13, 69, 96, 98–9, 100, 111n,
Breath (*prāṇa*), 33, 81, 87, 89, 92, 160–6, 199
Breath control (*prāṇāyāma*), 3, 7, 29, 30, 32–4, 69–70, 92, 140, 142, 160–7, 180, 185, 189, 198, 199, 262, 263
in concentration (*dhāraṇā*) and meditation (*dhyāna*), 167, 178, 180

Cause and effect (*karma*), law of, 24, 39, 40, 42, 43, 243, 256
Celestial beings, 233
Cellular body, 57, 235
Cleanliness (*śauca*), 30, 144, 153–4
Compassion (*karuṇā*), 86
Concentration (*dhāraṇā*), 7, 30, 34, 35, 51–2, 140, 142, 167, 175, 178–9, 182, 185
and breath control (*prāṇāyāma*), 167, 178, 180
and integration (*saṁyama*), 182, 185, 186, 188
and meditation (*dhyāna*), 180
Conscience (*antaḥkaraṇa*), 14, 50, 51, 92, 128
Consciousness (*citta*), 4, 14–17, 22, 35–6, 38–9, 42–3, 49–51, 53–4, 55, 58, 62, 65, 67, 88, 89, 92, 96, 97, 132, 137–8, 182, 190–202, 251–3, 262–77, 291
cosmic, universal (*mahat*), 12, 14, 25, 50, 87, 97, 100, 132, 160, 165, 169, 264
distractions (*citta vikṣepa*), 83, 86
divine (*divya citta*), 14, 29, 252, 270
evolution of, 127

five fluctuations, 56–61
correct knowledge (*pramāṇa*), 56, 57–8, 61, 132
fanciful knowledge (*vikalpa*), 15, 56, 59, 61, 132
illusory perceptions (*viparyaya*), 15, 56, 58–9, 61, 132
memory (*smṛti*), 15, 56, 61,132
sleep (*nidrā*), 15, 56, 59–60, 61, 90, 132
five qualities of intelligence: ignorance (*mūḍa*), distracted (*kṣiptā*), agitated (*vikśipta*), attentive (*ekāgra*) and controlled (*niruddha*), 56, 61, 186,
fluctuations (*vṛtti*) and movement in, 4, 7, 14, 49–50, 51–2, 53–5, 56–7, 60, 63, 64, 132, 265, 268, 291; as visible state (*dṛṣṭa*), invisible state (*adṛṣṭa*), painful (*kliṣṭā*) and non-painful (*akliṣṭā*), 55, 62
four planes of: unconscious (*nidrā*), subconscious (*svapnā*), conscious (*jāgrata*) and superconscious (*tūryā* or *samādhi*), 90, 197–8
and *nirbīja samādhi*, 103
order of transformations (*pariṇāma*), 190–4
restraining (*nirodha pariṇāma*), 188, 190, 191, 192, 194, 200, 252, 258
to *samādhi* (*samādhi pariṇāma*), 188, 189, 190, 192, 194, 200
to no-pointed (*ekāgratā pariṇāma*), 188, 190, 193–4, 195, 199, 200
restraint of (*citta vṛtti nirodha*), 11, 14, 49–52, 61–2, 103, 187–91
seven states of awareness, 29, 77, 132, 137–8
three facets: mind (*manas*), intelligence (*buddhi*), ego (*ahaṁkāra*), 47
universal and individual (*cit, citta*), the 'seer' and the 'seen' , 14, 42–3, 131–2, 262–73, 274–7
Contemplation *see* absorption (*samādhi*)
Contentment (*santoṣa*), 30, 144, 155
Continence, chastity (*brahmacarya*), 30, 142–3, 151–2

Death, fear of (*abhiniveśa*), 23, 111, 112, 116–7, 132
Desires, impressions (*vāsanā*), 15, 41, 255, 273–4
freedom from, 8, 55, 61–2, 64–5, 89, 241
Detachment (*vairāgya*), 16, 17–19, 24, 61–70, 134
five states (*yatamāna, vyatireka, ekendriya, vaśīkāra, paravairāgya*), 65, 66, 67
path of renunciation (*vairāgya mārga* or *virakti mārga*), 241
and renunciation, 17–18, 19, 61–2, 232
and sense-withdrawal (*pratyāhāra*), 168–71
supreme (*paravairāgya*), 65, 66
Dhammapada, 75
Dhruva, Prince, 4, 211–12, 247
Direct perception (*pratyakṣa*), 15, 56, 57

Disciplined code of conduct (*anuśāsanam*), 16, 48–9
Discrimination (*viveka*), 27, 61
Discriminative intelligence (*viveka-khyāti*), 278
Disease, physical (*vyādhi*), 83
(*rogas*), three types: self-inflicted, genetic, caused by imbalance of elements, 7, 84, 149
Divine cosmic energy (*kuṇḍalini*), 184
Dream-state (*svapnā*), 89–90
Drugs and herbs, 246
Duty (*dharma*), 4, 283, 284–5

Effort (*yatnaḥ*), 63
Ego (*ahaṁkāra*), 8, 11–12, 26, 34, 35, 47, 49, 50, 67, 92, 98, 128, 132
Egoism, sense of self (*asmitā*), 11–12, 23, 42, 97–8, 111, 112, 114–15, 132, 229, 250–1
pure state (*sāsmitā*), 70, 100, 250
Eightfold path of yoga (*aṣṭāṅga yoga*), 4, 6, 24, 29–30, 140–2, 178–9, 184
Elements (*mahābhuta*) of nature (*prakṛti*), 226–7
and corresponding *kośas*, 12, 51, 100
earth, water, fire, air, ether, 25, 51, 100, 195, 227
subtle (*tanmatra*), 26, 100
Emancipation *see* liberation (*kaivalya*)
Energy centres (*cakras*)
anus (*mūlādhāra*), 210
sacral (*svādhiṣṭāna*), 210
navel (*nābhi* or *maṇipūraka*), 210, 212–13
heart (*anāhata*), 210, 216
throat (*viśuddhi*), 210, 213
brow (*ājñā*), 198, 210
crown (*sahasrāra*), 210, 215
Energy of nature (*prakṛti shakti* or *kuṇḍalini*), 184
Ethical disciplines (*yama*), 6, 29, 30, 31, 38, 62, 86, 92, 140–2, 171, 176
effects of, 30
and freedom from avarice (*aparigraha*), 30
non-violence (*ahiṁsā*), truthfulness (*satya*), non-stealing (*asteya*), continence (*brahmacarya*), 30, 142–3, 149, 150, 151–2
Evolution and involution, 25–6, 62, 67, 199, 132–3
stages of (*avasthā*), 19, 194–6, 197

Faith (*śraddhā*), 73, 75
Flawless jewel (*abhijāta maṇi*), 94
Friendliness (maitrī), 21, 86, 208

Gāndhi, Mahātma, 156, 184
God (*Īśvara*), 13, 20, 78–81
  surrender to (*Īśvara praṇidhāna*), 6, 23, 30, 78, 85, 108, 157
Goṇikā, yoginī, 2
Greed, abstention from (*aparigraha*), 30, 142–3, 152–3

Hanumān, Lord, 4, 225
Happiness (*sukha*), 86, 114, 115, 155, 157

Ignorance (*avidyā*), 6–7, 17, 23–4, 28, 41, 42, 111, 112, 113–14, 132, 134
  seven states of, 28
Illuminative (*sattvic*) quality of nature, 11
Imagination and fancy (*vikalpa*), 15, 56, 59, 61, 132
Impressions, subliminal (*saṁskāra*), 5, 8, 15, 40, 71, 102, 191
Indifference to pleasures and pains (*upekṣā*), 86
Indra, Lord, 162
Inertia, darkness (*tamas*), 5, 127, 128
Inference (*anumāna*), 57, 101–2
Integration (*saṁyama*) of concentration, meditation and absorption, 34–5, 175, 182–5, 201, 216–17, 234–6, 242
  compared with *nirbīja samādhi*, 186
  and supernatural powers, 202, 207, 208, 209–18, 220–30
Intelligence (*buddhi*), 11, 34, 35–6, 47, 49, 50–1, 57–8, 98, 100, 128
  pure, 58

Jaḍa Bharata, 74–5, 85
Jñāneśvar, Saint, 224
Joy (*muditā*), 86

Kālimātā, Goddess, 74–5
Kapilā, 224
Karma see cause and effect
Knowledge, wisdom (*jñāna*), 90, 101–2
  highest (*vidyā*), 114
  illusory (*mīthyā jñāna*) or wrong, 58–9
  true (*vivekaja jñānam*), 38, 58, 234–8
  verbal (*śabdha jñāna*), 59
  see also awareness (*prajñā*); ignorance (*avidyā*)
Kṛṣṇa, Lord, 124
  see also Bhagavad Gītā
Kuṇḍalini see energy of nature

Liberation, emancipation and freedom (*kaivalya*), 3, 4, 8–9, 26, 38, 39, 43, 67, 127, 135–6, 232, 237–8, 239–87
Life, clinging to (*abhiniveśa*), 23, 111, 112, 116–17, 132
Life force (*prāṇa*) *see* breath
Light, sorrowless (*viśoka jyotiṣmati*), 88
  of awareness (*prajñā ālokah*), 183
Luminosity (*sattva*), 5, 39, 99

Mahābhārata, 123–4, 24
Mahābhāsya, 2
Māṇḍavya, Sage, 246–7
Matsya, yogi, 8
Matter, primary (*pradhāna*), 97
Meditation (*dhyāna*), 3, 7, 30, 34, 35, 51–2, 90–1, 92, 118, 140–2, 175, 179–81
  and absorption (*samādhi*), 181
  and breath control (*prāṇāyāma*), 167, 178, 180
  and integration (*saṁyama*), 182, 185, 186, 188
Memory (*smṛti*), 15, 40, 56, 61, 95–6, 132, 256
Mind (*manas*), 11, 12–13, 14–15, 25, 41–2, 47, 49, 81, 92, 12
  ripeness of (*yogyata manasāḥ*), 167
  see also consciousness
Misconception (*viparyaya*), 15, 56, 58–9, 61, 132
Miśra, Maṇḍana, 220–1
Moment (*kṣaṇa*), 187–90, 234–6, 281–2
  experience of 'now', 235–6
Moment and movement, 38, 259–60
Muṇḍakopaniṣad, 270

Nahūṣa, King, 7–8, 120, 247
Nandi, 8, 119–20
Nature (*prakṛti*), 11, 24, 25–6, 27–8, 43, 66, 88, 97–8, 125–6, 128, 160
  cosmology, 25–6
    cosmic intelligence (*mahat*), 12, 14, 25, 50, 67, 87, 97, 100, 128, 132, 160, 165, 169
    non-specific (*aviśeṣa*) and manifest (*viśeṣa*) stages, 25, 26, 66, 67, 126, 132–3
    noumenal (*aliṅga*) and phenomenal (*liṅga*) stages, 25, 26, 66, 67, 133
    root of nature (*mūla prakṛti*), 25, 26, 98, 100, 132
  elements (*mahābhuta*) of (earth, water, fire, air, ether), 25, 51, 100, 195, 227

energy of (*prakṛti shakti* or *kuṇḍalini*), 184
evolution and involution of, 25, 26, 132–3
and stages of, 66
freedom from (*guṇātītan, guṇavaitṛṣṇyam*), 39, 66
merging in (*prakṛtilaya*), 72–3
and order of transformations (*dharma*, *lakṣaṇa* and *avasthā pariṇāma*), 190, 194–6, 200, 201
principles (*tattvas*) of, 25, 128
qualities of (*guṇas*), 3, 25, 26, 39, 40, 41–2, 67, 125–6, 127, 128
Nerves (*nāḍi*)
sympathetic, parasympathetic and central nervous systems, 147, 212, 214–15
Non-attachment *see* detachment (*vairāgya*)
Non-existence (*abhāva*), 59–60
Non-physical state of existence (*videha*), 72–3, 225–6
Non-stealing (*asteya*), 30, 142–3, 150
Non-violence (*ahiṁsā*), 30, 149
Now (*atha*), 44, 48, 49

Obstacles (*antarāyā*), 21, 83–4

Painful states (*kliṣṭā*), 54–5
Painless states (*akliṣṭā*), 54–5
Passive and transient state of quietness (*manolaya*), 18–20, 22, 56, 69, 70–2, 99, 100, 127
Peace (*śānti*), 193, 196–9
Personal disciplines (*niyama*), 6, 29, 30–1, 38, 62, 92, 144–5, 147, 158, 176
Personality, split, 59
Postures (*āsana*), 3, 7, 12, 29, 30, 31–2, 57, 69–70, 89, 91, 92, 95–6, 140–2, 146–7, 157–9, 171, 180, 199, 235, 292
effects of, 31–2
Powers and properties of Yoga (*vibhūti*), 3, 7–8, 36–9, 173–238
and integration (*saṁyama*), 202, 207, 208, 209–18, 220–30, 234–6
as obstacles to progress, 37–8, 175, 176–7, 219, 232
supernatural powers (*siddhis*), 36–7, 175–7, 201–16, 218, 219–31,
Practice (*sādhanā*), 3, 5, 6–7, 19, 21, 22, 26, 34, 37, 38, 55, 62, 65, 75, 105–71, 177, 242
Practice (*abhyāsa*), repetitive, mechanical, 5–6, 16–20, 21–2, 61–5, 67, 85, 140
and detachment (*vairāgya*), 5–6, 61–2, 65, 67
levels of, 19
religious, devotional (*anuṣṭhāna*), 62, 140

Practitioner (*sādhaka*)
four levels of, 18, 19
Principles of nature (*tattva*), 25, 128

Religious fervour (*tapas*), 6, 8, 23, 30, 39
Renunciation *see* detachment
Restraint of consciousness (*citta vṛtti nirodha*), 11, 14, 49–52, 61–2, 103, 187–91
see also detachment (vairāgya)

Sacred syllable Āuṁ (*praṇava*), 20, 80–2
Samkhya philosophy, 25, 33
Śaṅkara, Sage, 220–1
Self-Realization, 3, 21, 23, 27, 34, 65, 82, 98
Self-study (*svādhyāya*), 6, 23, 30, 144, 156
Sense-withdrawal (*pratyāhāra*), 7, 29–30, 34, 92, 168–70
Senses of perception, freedom from (*vikaraṇābhāvah*), 230–1
Sensual enjoyment (*bhoga*), 121, 125, 126, 245
Sheaths (*kośa*), 12, 47, 100
and corresponding elements, 51
mental and intellectual, 47
Śiva, Lord, 1–2, 81, 120, 162, 163
Sleep (*nidrā*), 15, 56, 59–60, 61, 73, 89–90, 132
three types, 60
Sorrow (*duḥkha*), 84, 86, 116, 122, 148
Soul, spirit, 13–14
(*ātmā*, *ātman*), 11, 12, 25,
great (*mahātmā*), 81
individual in human body (*jīvātmā*), 13
merging with nature (*prakṛti*), 25, 26, 51
(*puruṣa*), 13, 25–6
special entity (*puruṣa viśeṣaḥ*), 97
supreme (*paramātmā*), 4, 13, 90
universal self (*antarātmā*), 243
vision of (*ātmadarśana*), 47
Speech (*vācā*), 81
Spiritual lustre, radiance (*dīpti*), 140
Spiritual science (*mokṣa śāstra*), 48
Śrīmad Bhāgavatam, 162
Stages of life (*āśrama*), 3
Sun (*Sūrya*), 209

Time (*kāla*), 41, 201–2, 234–6, 259–61
Tirumangai Ālwār, Saint, 222–3
Transformation (*pariṇāma*) *see* consciousness
Truth-bearing wisdom (*ṛtambharā prajñā*), 9, 101
Truthfulness (*satya*), 30, 142–3, 150

Universal cosmic consciousness (*mahat*), 12, 14, 25, 50, 67, 87, 97, 100, 128, 132, 160, 165, 169, 264
Ūrvaṣi, 8
Uttānapāda, King, 211, 247

Vedanta philosophy, 49
Vibrancy, energy (*rajas*), 5, 125–6, 127
Vice (*apuṇya*), 86
Vigour (*vīrya*), 73, 75, 151
Violence *see* non-violence (*ahiṁsā*)
Virtue (*puṇya*), 86
Viṣṇu, Lord, 1–2, 81, 162, 163, 212
Viṣṇu Purāṇa, 9
Vyāsa, Sage, 7, 9, 72, 74, 138, 179, 184

Wakeful state (*jāgratāvasthā*), 89–90, 197
Wisdom, 7, 9, 22, 64, 69, 72, 100
  Illuminating, 102
  (*prajñā*), seven states of, 28
  see also knowledge (*jñāna*)
Word (*śabdha*), 94, 202–3

Yayāti, King, 246, 247
Yoga of action (*kriyāyoga*), 6, 22, 108–9, 110
Yogis, 43–4, 233
  characteristics of perfect, 244–5
  five types of, 39, 246
  King among (*Yogirāja*), 43